MRI in Practice

Other MRI books from Blackwell Publishing

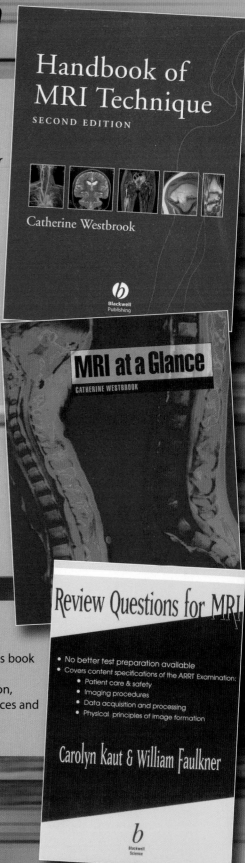

Handbook of MRI Technique

Second Edition

Catherine Westbrook

"Essential for many MRI courses in the UK and USA and is a very popular source of information to radiographers, radiologists and all interested MRI practitioners...This publication should have a mandatory place in the department library of all imaging centres with access to MRI." RAD MAGAZINE

Handbook of MRI Technique has proved hugely successful in guiding the uninitiated through scanning techniques and helping more experienced technologists to improve image quality. This edition continues to build on the strengths of the first edition and considers new technologies and developments essential to good practice. Technologists and radiographers from the US and Australia have contributed large sections to the book to ensure that information on techniques and image optimization is comprehensive.

464 pages| Paperback | 978-0-632-05264-6 | 1999

MRI at a Glance

Catherine Westbrook

Students of radiology and radiography at both undergraduate and postgraduate level often experience difficulty in MRI techniques. This book provides concise, easily accessible information on MRI physics which can be used as a ready reference revision tool.

128 pages |Paperback | 978-0-632-05619-4 | 2002

Review Questions for MRI

Carolyn Kaut Roth & William Faulkner

The authors, experts in the field of MRI education, have compiled this book to help students prepare for the registry examination. The book is extremely comprehensive, covering all the aspects of the examination, including patient care and safety, imaging procedures, pulse sequences and data acquisition, along with imaging artifacts and options.

144 pages | Paperback | 978-0-632-03905-0 | 1995

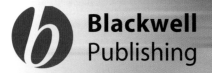

Blackwell
Publishing

MRI in Practice

Third edition

Catherine Westbrook MSc, DCRR, CTC
Senior Lecturer
Anglia Polytechnic University
Cambridge
UK

and

Carolyn Kaut Roth RT (R)(MR)(CT)(M)(CV)
Fellow SMRT (Section for Magnetic Resonance Technologists)
Director Technologist Continuing Education and MRI Internship
Programs for Technologists
University of Pennsylvania Heal Systems, Philadelphia, Pennsylvania,
USA

with

John Talbot MSc, DCRR
Senior Lecturer
Anglia Polytechnic University
Cambridge
UK

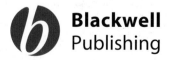

Blackwell
Publishing

© 1993, 1998 by Blackwell Science Ltd, 2005 by Blackwell Publishing Ltd

Editorial offices:
Blackwell Publishing Ltd, 9600 Garsington Road, Oxford OX4 2DQ, UK
 Tel: +44 (0)1865 776868
Blackwell Publishing Inc., 350 Main Street, Malden, MA 02148-5020, USA
 Tel: +1 781 388 8250
Blackwell Publishing Asia Pty Ltd, 550 Swanston Street, Carlton, Victoria 3053, Australia
 Tel: +61 (0)3 8359 1011

First published 1993
Reprinted 1994 (four times), 1995
Second edition published 1998
Reprinted 1999 (twice), 2000, 2001, 2002, 2003 (twice)
Third edition published 2005
7   2011

ISBN: 978-1-4051-2787-5

Library of Congress Cataloging-in-Publication Data
Westbrook, Catherine.
    MRI in practice / Catherine Westbrook, Caroline Roth, and John Talbot.
 – 3rd ed.
      p.   cm.
    Includes index.

    ISBN-13: 978-1-4051-2787-5 (pbk. : alk. paper)
 1. Magnetic resonance imaging.   I. Kaut-Roth, Carolyn.
 II. Talbot, John, Msc.   III. Title.
    RC78.7.N83W48 2005
    616.07′548–dc22   2004026945

A catalogue record for this title is available from the British Library

Set in 10/12pt Sabon
by Graphicraft Limited, Hong Kong
Printed and bound in USA
by Sheridan Books, Inc., Chelsea, MI, USA

For further information on Blackwell Publishing, visit our website:
www.blackwellpublishing.com

Contents

Foreword

Magnetic resonance imaging has seen many changes over the many years of its evolution, into a highly sophisticated tool and, perhaps arguably, the cornerstone of medical imaging. The improvements in technology and scientific discoveries have made it possible to acquire, in a matter of seconds, what used to take upwards of a quarter of an hour or longer. As an MR technologist, after the initial challenge of beginning to learn the basic and advanced concepts and then how to apply them, the next challenge is to keep up with the advancements in our profession.

Of all the changes in MRI I have witnessed over the years, one of the constants I could count on has always been *MRI in Practice*. In this third edition, Catherine Westbrook and Carolyn (Candi) Roth continue their tradition of providing both the new and experienced MRI technologist with the most comprehensive MRI textbook for technologists available. Topics include the basic concepts, current pulse sequences, cardiac and blood flow imaging, as well as functional techniques such as diffusion and spectroscopy.

I have known Cathy and Candi for many years and feel fortunate to have them as colleagues and friends. I can state without reservation that the third edition of *MRI in Practice* is a must-have for every MRI department or facility as a reference for their MR technologists. Congratulations to Cathy and Candi on an excellent job and thanks from all the MRI technologists out there for continuing the tradition 'MRI in Practice'.

William Faulkner, BS, RT(R)(MR)(CT), FSMRT
William Faulkner & Associates, L.L.C.
Director of Education
Chattanooga Imaging

Preface to the third edition

Magnetic Resonance Imaging (MRI) is an exciting imaging modality that has changed clinicians' ability to visualise anatomy, pathology and physiology. Despite being used in clinical practice for nearly 20 years, MRI is still evolving at a rapid pace. As technologists, we have been privileged, not only to have been involved in this field for nearly all of those 20 years, but also to teach countless generations of technologists, radiographers, radiologists, nurses and medical students in the science of MRI.

Over 10 years have elapsed since *MRI in Practice* was first published. Although we knew that there was a need for a book that breached the middle ground between simple and complicated texts, little did we know how popular this book would be. Its success is down to many things, not least the tremendous support we have received from colleagues in the field of MRI who have used and recommended this book to others.

However, we were aware that the format of the book was becoming rather out-dated, hence the radical changes that are seen in the third edition. Not only is it now gloriously technicolored, but we have also included ideas that we have used successfully in our teaching courses. First of all, we have increased the use of analogies – which are highlighted to the reader by icons in the margin. Analogies are a great way of explaining topics that are difficult to visualize or conceptualize by grounding them in something more real to the reader. An example of this is using the analogy of a chest of drawers to explain K space! Secondly, we have increased the use of learning points to emphasize areas of special importance. These, along with summaries, bullet points and tables are now color-coded to assist the reader. Thirdly, all of the diagrams have been beautifully re-drawn by our gifted illustrator, MR technologist and teacher John Talbot, and complement the text in a new and exciting way.

We have also taken the opportunity to update the book to include recent developments: parallel imaging, functional imaging techniques, new sequences such as balanced gradient echo, and updates in equipment and coils. The result is a completely fresh look that keeps the simple, logical approach of previous editions but also incorporates new explanations and concepts.

We hope that the third edition will appeal to those who have read the book in the past as well as clinicians new to MRI.

Catherine Westbrook

Acknowledgments

We continue to be extremely grateful to colleagues and family members who have supported us both professionally and personally, and who continue to encourage us. Again, without you, none of this would have been possible. We are also eternally grateful to the staff at Blackwell Publishing, who have continued to support us in this edition. In particular to Caroline Connelly, for paving the way toward color reproduction. In addition, many of the images and photographs were supplied with the kind permission of Philips Medical Systems. General Electric Medical Systems and Seimens Medical have also been very generous in this respect.

A special thank you goes to: my children Adam, Ben and Madeleine Westbrook. I am constantly amazed that I managed to produce such wonderful kids; to my parents Joe and Maggie Barbieri; my family, the Bellavista's of Florida, the Barbieri's of Texas and the Haworth's of Lancashire; my friends Chris Kendel, John Talbot, Rachael Blundell, Peter Sharpe and Peter Cox; to Nicky, Kate, Mandy, Micky, Rhona, Fizz, Shandy, Liz, Jill and all the other girls; and Toni, who makes me coffee every morning.

CW

1

Basic principles

Introduction

The basic principles of magnetic resonance imaging (MRI) form the foundation for further understanding of this complex subject. It is important that these ideas are fully grasped before continuing on to areas that are more complicated. There are essentially two ways of explaining the fundamentals of MRI; classically and via quantum physics. Any discussion requires both, so we have attempted to integrate the two versions. Within this chapter, the properties of atoms and their interactions with magnetic fields, excitation and relaxation are discussed.

Atomic structure

All things are made of **atoms**, including the human body. Atoms are very small. Half a million lined up together are narrower than a human hair. Atoms are organized in **molecules**, which are two or more atoms arranged together. The most abundant atom in the body is **hydrogen**. This is most commonly found in molecules of water (where two hydrogen atoms are arranged with one oxygen atom, H_2O) and fat (where hydrogen atoms are

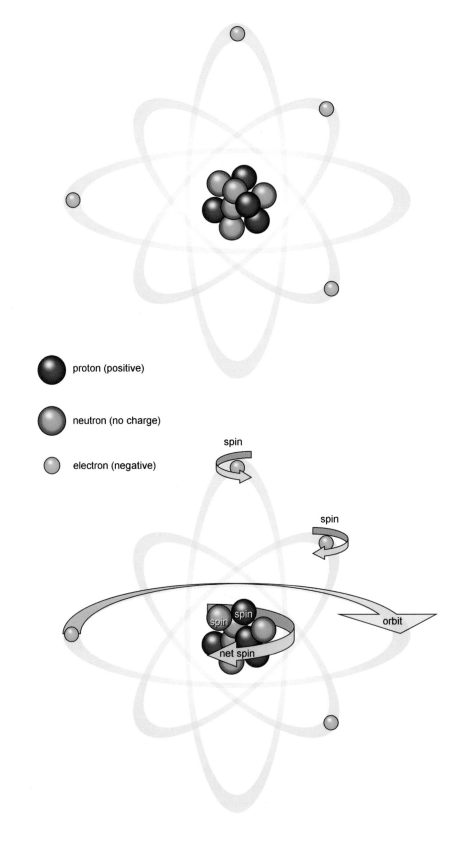

Figure 1.1 The atom.

1

arranged with carbon and oxygen atoms; the number of each depends on the type of fat).

The atom consists of a central nucleus and orbiting **electrons** (Figure 1.1). The nucleus is very small, one millionth of a billionth of the total volume of an atom, but it contains all the atom's mass. This mass comes mainly from particles called **nucleons**, which are subdivided into **protons** and **neutrons**. Atoms are characterized in two ways. The **atomic number** is the sum of the protons in the nucleus. This number gives an atom its chemical identity. The **mass number** is the sum of the protons and neutrons in the nucleus. The number of neutrons and protons in a nucleus are usually balanced so that the mass number is an even number. In some atoms, however, there are slightly more or fewer neutrons than protons. These atoms are called **isotopes** and result in an odd mass number. It is these atoms that are important in MRI (*see* later).

Electrons are particles that spin around the nucleus. Traditionally this is thought of as being analogous to planets orbiting around the Sun. In reality, electrons exist around the nucleus in a cloud; the outermost dimension of the cloud is the edge of the atom. The position of an electron in the cloud is not predictable as it depends on the energy of an individual electron at any moment in time (physicists call this Heisenberg's Uncertainty Principle). The number of electrons, however, is usually the same as the number of protons in the nucleus.

Protons have a positive electrical charge, neutrons have no net charge, and electrons are negatively charged. So atoms are electrically stable if the number of negatively charged electrons equals the number of positively charged protons. This balance is sometimes altered by applying external energy to knock out electrons from the atom. This causes a deficit in the number of electrons compared with protons and causes electrical instability that leads to an emission of energy called **radioactivity**. Atoms in which this has occurred are called **ions**.

Motion in the atom

Three types of motion are present within the atom (Figure 1.1). These are:

- electrons spinning on their own axis
- electrons orbiting the nucleus
- the nucleus itself spinning about its own axis.

The principles of MRI rely on the spinning motion of specific nuclei present in biological tissues. This spin derives from the individual spins of protons and neutrons within the nucleus. Pairs of subatomic particles automatically spin in opposite directions but at the same rate as their partners. In nuclei that have an even mass number, i.e. the number of protons equals the number of neutrons, half spin in one direction and half in the other. The nucleus itself has no net spin. However, in nuclei with odd mass

1

numbers, i.e. where the number of neutrons is slightly more or less than the number of protons, spin directions are not equal and opposite, so the nucleus itself has a net spin or **angular momentum**. These are known as **MR active nuclei**.

MR active nuclei

MR active nuclei are characterized by their tendency to align their axis of rotation to an applied magnetic field. This occurs because they have angular momentum or spin and, as they contain positively charged protons, they possess electrical charge. The laws of electromagnetic induction refer to three individual forces – motion, magnetism and charge – and state that if two of these are present, then the third is automatically induced. MR active nuclei that have a net charge and are spinning (motion), automatically acquire a **magnetic moment** and can align with an external magnetic field.

Important examples of MR active nuclei, together with their mass numbers are listed below:

hydrogen	1
carbon	13
nitrogen	15
oxygen	17
fluorine	19
sodium	23
phosphorus	31

Although neutrons have no net charge, their subatomic particles are not evenly arranged over the surface of the neutron and this imbalance enables the nucleus in which the neutron is situated to be MR active as long as the mass number is odd. Alignment is measured as the total sum of the nuclear magnetic moments and is expressed as a vector quantity. The strength of the total magnetic moment is specific to every nucleus and determines the sensitivity to magnetic resonance.

The hydrogen nucleus

The hydrogen nucleus is the MR active nucleus used in clinical MRI. The hydrogen nucleus contains a single proton (atomic and mass number 1). It is used because it is very abundant in the human body, and because its solitary proton gives it a relatively large magnetic moment. Both of these characteristics enable utilization of the maximum amount of available magnetization in the body.

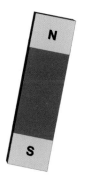

magnetic moment

The hydrogen nucleus as a magnet

The laws of electromagnetism state that a magnetic field is created when a charged particle moves. The hydrogen nucleus contains one positively charged proton that spins, i.e. it moves. Therefore the hydrogen nucleus has a magnetic field induced around it, and acts as a small magnet. The magnet of each hydrogen nucleus has a north and a south pole of equal strength. The north/south axis of each nucleus is represented by a **magnetic moment** and is used in the classical theory of the principles of MRI. The magnetic moment of each nucleus has vector properties, i.e. it has size and direction and is denoted by an arrow. The direction of the vector designates the direction of the magnetic moment, and the length of the vector designates the size of the magnetic moment as in Figure 1.2.

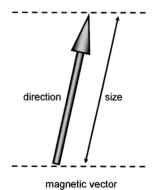

bar magnet

Alignment

In the absence of an applied magnetic field, the magnetic moments of the hydrogen nuclei are randomly orientated. When placed in a strong static external magnetic field, however, (shown as a white arrow on Figure 1.3 and termed B_0), the magnetic moments of the hydrogen nuclei align with this magnetic field. Some of the hydrogen nuclei align parallel with the magnetic field (in the same direction), while a smaller number of the nuclei align anti-parallel to the magnetic field (in the opposite direction) as in Figure 1.3.

Quantum theory (first described by Max Planck in 1900) describes the properties of electromagnetic radiation in terms of discrete quantities of energy called quanta. Applying quantum theory to MRI, hydrogen nuclei possess energy in two discrete quantities or populations termed low and high (Figure 1.4). Low-energy nuclei align their magnetic moments

Figure 1.2 The magnetic moment of the hydrogen nucleus.

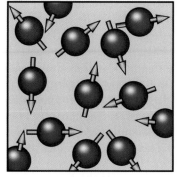

random alignment
no external field

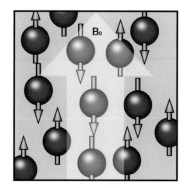

alignment
external magnetic field

Figure 1.3 Alignment – classical theory.

low energy spin-up nucleus

low energy spin-up population

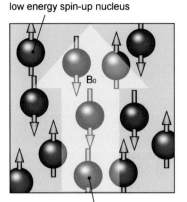

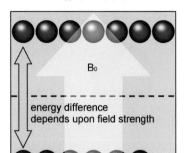

energy difference
depends upon field strength

Figure 1.4 Alignment –
quantum theory.

high energy spin-down nucleus

high energy spin-down population

parallel to the external field (shown as a white arrow on Figure 1.4) and are termed **spin-up** nuclei (drawn in blue in Figure 1.4). High-energy nuclei align their magnetic moments in the anti-parallel direction and are termed **spin-down** nuclei (drawn in red in Figure 1.4).

Learning point: magnetic moments

It is the *magnetic moments* of the hydrogen nuclei that align with B_0 not the hydrogen nuclei themselves. In addition they are only capable of aligning in one of two directions: parallel or anti-parallel to B_0. This is because they represent the only two possible energy states of hydrogen. The hydrogen nucleus itself does not change direction but merely spins on its axis.

The factors affecting which hydrogen nuclei align parallel and which align anti-parallel are determined by the strength of the external magnetic field and the thermal energy level of the nuclei. Low thermal energy nuclei do not possess enough energy to oppose the magnetic field in the anti-parallel direction. High thermal energy nuclei, however, do possess enough energy to oppose this field, and as the strength of the magnetic field increases, fewer nuclei have enough energy to do so. The thermal energy of a nucleus is mainly determined by the temperature of the patient. In clinical applications this cannot be significantly altered and is not important. This is called **thermal equilibrium**. Under these circumstances it is the strength of the external field that determines the relative quantities of spin-up to spin-down nuclei.

In thermal equilibrium there are always fewer high-energy nuclei than low-energy nuclei, therefore the magnetic moments of the nuclei aligned

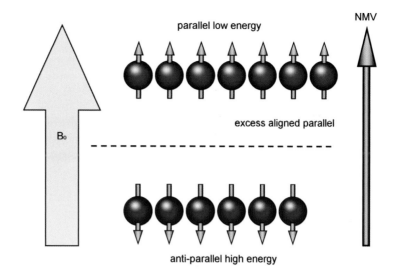

parallel low energy

NMV

B_0

excess aligned parallel

anti-parallel high energy

Figure 1.5 The net magnetization vector.

parallel to the magnetic field cancel out the smaller number of magnetic moments aligned anti-parallel. As there is a larger number aligned parallel, there is always a small excess in this direction that produces a net magnetic moment (Figure 1.5). Other MR active nuclei also align with the magnetic field and produce their own small net magnetic moments.

These magnetic moments are not used in clinical MRI because they do not exist in enough abundance in the body to be imaged adequately as their net magnetic moments are very small. However, with RF (**radio frequency**) coils tuned to the appropriate frequency and with adequate B_0 homogeneity it is possible to image other MR active nuclei. The net magnetic moment of hydrogen, however, produces a significant magnetic vector that is used in clinical MRI. This is called the **net magnetization vector** (**NMV**) and reflects the relative balance between spin-up and spin-down nuclei.

Learning point: NMV vs field strength

When a patient is placed in the bore of the magnet, the magnetic moments of hydrogen nuclei within the patient align parallel and anti-parallel to B_0. A small excess line up parallel to B_0 and constitute the NMV of the patient (Figure 1.5). The energy difference between the two populations increases as B_0 increases. At high field strengths fewer nuclei have enough energy to join the high-energy population and align their magnetic moments in opposition to the stronger B_0 field. This means that the magnitude of the NMV is larger at high field strengths than low field strengths, resulting in improved signal. This is discussed further in Chapter 4.

Summary

- The net magnetic moment of hydrogen is called the net magnetization vector (NMV)
- The static external magnetic field is called B_0
- The interaction of the NMV with B_0 is the basis of MRI
- The unit of B_0 is tesla or gauss. 1 tesla (T) is the equivalent of 10 000 gauss (G)

Precession

Each hydrogen nucleus is spinning on its axis as in Figure 1.6. The influence of B_0 produces an additional spin, or wobble of the magnetic moments of hydrogen around B_0. This secondary spin is called **precession** and causes the magnetic moments to follow a circular path around B_0. This path is called the **precessional path** and the speed at which they wobble around B_0 is called the **precessional frequency**. The unit of precessional frequency is megahertz (MHz) whereby 1 Hz is 1 cycle per second and 1 MHz is 1 million cycles per second.

Combining Figure 1.6 with what we now know about quantum physics, it is possible to appreciate that there are two populations of hydrogen

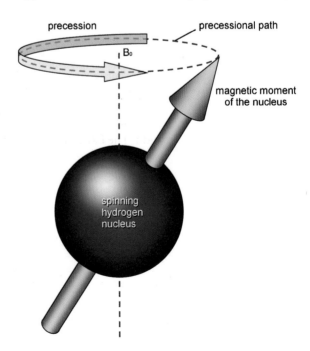

Figure 1.6   Precession.

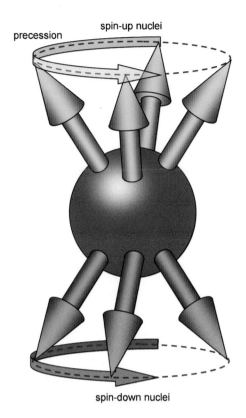

precession spin-up nuclei

spin-down nuclei

Figure 1.7 Precession of the spin-up and spin-down populations.

nuclei: some high-energy, spin-down nuclei and a greater number of low-energy, spin-up hydrogen nuclei. The magnetic moments of all these nuclei precess around B_0 on a circular precessional path (Figure 1.7).

The Larmor equation

The value of the precessional frequency is governed by the Larmor equation. The Larmor equation states that:

$$\omega_0 = B_0 \times \lambda$$

where:

ω_0 is the precessional frequency
B_0 is the magnetic field strength of the magnet
λ is the gyro-magnetic ratio.

The **gyro-magnetic ratio** expresses the relationship between the angular momentum and the magnetic moment of each MR active nucleus. It is constant and is expressed as the precessional frequency of a specific MR active nucleus at 1 T. The unit of the gyro-magnetic ratio is therefore MHz/T.

The gyro-magnetic ratio of hydrogen is 42.57 MHz/T. Other MR active nuclei have different gyro-magnetic ratios, so have different precessional frequencies at the same field strength. In addition, hydrogen has a different precessional frequency at different field strengths. For example:

At *1.5 T* the precessional frequency of hydrogen is *63.86 MHz* (42.57 MHz × 1.5 T)
At *1.0 T* the precessional frequency of hydrogen is *42.57 MHz* (42.57 MHz × 1.0 T)
At *0.5 T* the precessional frequency of hydrogen is *21.28 MHz* (42.57 MHz × 0.5 T).

The precessional frequency is often called the **Larmor frequency**, because it is determined by the Larmor equation.

Learning point: the Larmor equation

The Larmor equation tells us two important facts:

1   All MR active nuclei have their own gyro-magnetic constant so that when they are exposed to the same field strength, they precess at different frequencies, i.e. hydrogen precesses at a different frequency to either fluorine or carbon. This allows us to specifically image hydrogen and ignore the other MR active nuclei in the body. The way in which this is done is discussed later.

2   As the gyro-magnetic ratio is a constant of proportionality, B_0 is proportional to the Larmor frequency. Therefore if B_0 increases, the Larmor frequency increases and vice versa.

Resonance

Resonance is a phenomenon that occurs when an object is exposed to an oscillating perturbation that has a frequency close to its own natural frequency of oscillation. When a nucleus is exposed to an external perturbation that has an oscillation similar to its own natural frequency, the nucleus gains energy from the external force. The nucleus gains energy and resonates if the energy is delivered at exactly the same precessional frequency. If energy is delivered at a different frequency to that of the Larmor frequency of the nucleus, resonance does not occur.

Energy at the precessional frequency of hydrogen at all field strengths in clinical MRI corresponds to the **radio frequency (RF)** band of the

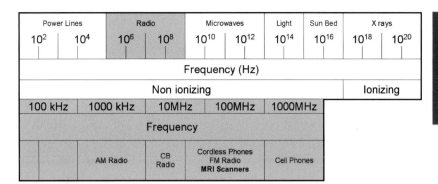

Power Lines		Radio		Microwaves		Light	Sun Bed	X rays	
10^2	10^4	10^6	10^8	10^{10}	10^{12}	10^{14}	10^{16}	10^{18}	10^{20}

Frequency (Hz)

Non ionizing	Ionizing

100 kHz	1000 kHz	10MHz	100MHz	1000MHz

Frequency

		AM Radio	CB Radio	Cordless Phones FM Radio **MRI Scanners**	Cell Phones

Figure 1.8 The electromagnetic spectrum.

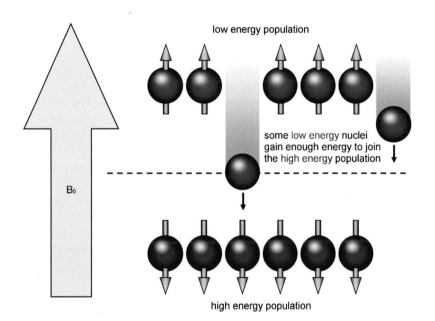

low energy population

some low energy nuclei gain enough energy to join the high energy population

B_0

high energy population

Figure 1.9 Energy transfer during excitation.

electromagnetic spectrum (Figure 1.8). For resonance of hydrogen to occur, an **RF pulse** of energy at exactly the Larmor frequency of hydrogen must be applied. Other MR active nuclei that have aligned with B_0 do not resonate, because their precessional frequencies are different to that of hydrogen.

The application of an RF pulse that causes resonance to occur is termed **excitation**. This absorption of energy causes an increase in the number of spin-down hydrogen nuclei as some of the spin-up (drawn in blue in Figure 1.9) nuclei gain energy via resonance and become high-energy nuclei (drawn in red in Figure 1.9). The energy difference between the two populations corresponds to the energy required to produce resonance via excitation. As the field strength increases, the energy difference between the two populations also increases so that more energy (higher frequencies) are required to produce resonance.

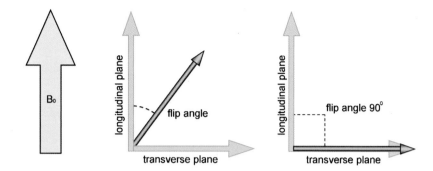

Figure 1.10   The flip angle.

The results of resonance

One of the results of resonance is that the NMV moves out of alignment away from B_0. This occurs because some of the low-energy nuclei are given enough energy via resonance to join the high-energy population. As the NMV reflects the balance between the low and high-energy populations, resonance causes the NMV to no longer lie parallel to B_0 but at an angle to it. The angle to which the NMV moves out of alignment is called the **flip angle** (Figure 1.10). The magnitude of the flip angle depends upon the amplitude and duration of the RF pulse. Usually the flip angle is 90°, i.e. the NMV is given enough energy by the RF pulse to move through 90° relative to B_0. However, as the NMV is a vector even if flip angles other than 90° are used, there is always a component of magnetization in a plane perpendicular to B_0. *See* learning point on p. 18.

- B_0 is now termed the longitudinal axis/plane
- the plane at 90° to B_0 is termed the **transverse plane**.

With a flip angle of 90° the nuclei are given sufficient energy so that the longitudinal NMV is completely transferred into a transverse NMV. This transverse NMV rotates in the transverse plane at the Larmor frequency. When flip angles less than 90° are used, only a portion of the NMV is transferred to the transverse plane. This reflects a smaller number of low-energy spins becoming high-energy spins as a result of excitation. If flip angles greater than 90° are used this reflects a larger number of high-energy spins than low-energy spins. The NMV merely represents the balance between the spin-up to spin-down populations.

The other result of resonance is that the magnetic moments of hydrogen nuclei move into phase with each other. Phase is the position of each magnetic moment on the precessional path around B_0. Magnetic moments that are **in phase** (or **coherent**) are in the same place on the precessional path around B_0 at any given time. Magnetic moments that are **out of phase** (or **incoherent**) are not in the same place on the precessional path. When resonance occurs, all the magnetic moments move to the same position on the precessional path and are then in phase (Figure 1.11).

1

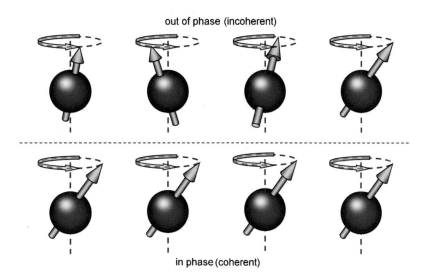

out of phase (incoherent)

in phase (coherent)

Figure 1.11 In phase (coherent) and out of phase (incoherent).

Learning point: the watch analogy

The terms frequency and phase are used many times in this book and it is important to understand the difference between them and how they relate to each other. The easiest analogy is the little hand on an analogue watch. **Frequency** is the time it takes the little hand to make one revolution of the watch face, i.e. 12 hours. The unit of frequency is hertz (Hz), where 1 Hz is 1 cycle or revolution per second. Using the watch analogy, the frequency of the little hand is 1/43 200 s = 0.0000231 Hz as it moves around the watch face once every 12 hours. The **phase** of the little hand, measured in degrees or radians, is the time on the watch, e.g. 1 o'clock, 2 o'clock, which corresponds to its position around the watch face when you look to see what time it is (Figure 1.12).

The phase of the little hand depends on its frequency. If the frequency is correct then the little hand always tells the correct time. If the watch goes fast or slow, i.e. the frequency either increases or decreases, then the watch tells an incorrect time. There are 360° in a circle, so 360 possible phase positions. However, there are an infinite number of frequencies.

Imagine a room full of people with watches that tell perfect time who are asked to synchronize their watches at 12 noon. One hour later, all their watches will say 1 o'clock because they have kept perfect time. They are in phase or coherent because they all tell the same time and their little hands are all at the same place on the watch face at the same time. If however, after synchronization, the watches on the left-hand side of the room go fast for one hour and the watches on the right-hand side of the room go slow for one hour, then at 1 o'clock they will be telling different times. The watches on the left-hand side of the room will be telling a time greater than 1 o'clock, e.g. 1.15 pm, and those on the right-hand side of the room will be telling a time less than 1 o'clock, e.g. 12.45 pm. Therefore the watches are out of phase or incoherent because they tell different times and their little hands are not at the same place on the watch face at the same time. How much they are out of phase depends on their relative frequencies between 12 noon and 1 o'clock.

If the difference in frequencies is large then the difference in phase is greater than if the frequency difference is small. Phase and frequency are therefore connected. In this context the frequency of the little hand is related to its change of phase over time. In other contexts used later in this book, frequency is a change of phase over distance. We refer to the watch analogy many times in this book. Look out for the watch symbol in the margin.

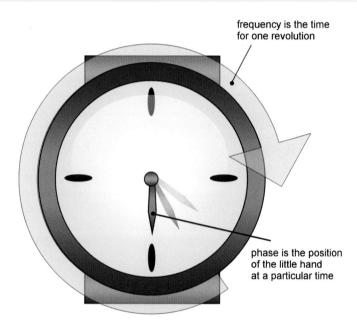

frequency is the time for one revolution

phase is the position of the little hand at a particular time

Figure 1.12   Phase and frequency.

Summary

- For resonance of hydrogen to occur, RF at exactly the Larmor frequency of hydrogen must be applied
- The result of resonance is magnetization in the transverse plane that is in phase
- This in phase transverse magnetization precesses at the Larmor frequency

The MR signal

As a result of resonance, in phase magnetization precesses at the Larmor frequency in the transverse plane. Faraday's laws of induction state that if a receiver coil or any conductive loop is placed in the area of a moving magnetic field, i.e. the magnetization precessing in the transverse plane, a voltage is induced in this receiver coil. The **MR signal** is produced when coherent (in phase) magnetization cuts across the coil. Therefore the coherent moving transverse magnetization produces magnetic field fluctuations inside the coil that induce an electrical voltage in the coil. This voltage constitutes the MR signal. The frequency of the signal is the same as the Larmor frequency – the magnitude of the signal depends on the amount of magnetization present in the transverse plane. Why would you expect the MR signal in Figure 1.13 to be alternating?

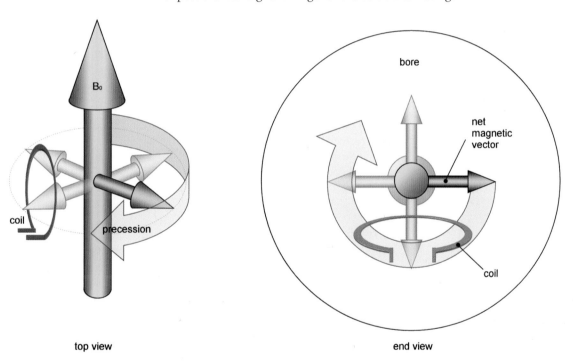

top view   end view

Figure 1.13 Generation of the signal.

The free induction decay (FID) signal

When the RF pulse is switched off, the NMV is again influenced by B_0 and it tries to realign with it. To do so, the hydrogen nuclei must lose the energy given to them by the RF pulse. The process by which hydrogen loses this energy is called **relaxation**. As relaxation occurs, the NMV returns to realign with B_0 because some of the high-energy nuclei return to the low-energy population and align their magnetic moments in the spin-up direction.

- The amount of magnetization in the **longitudinal plane** gradually increases – this is called **recovery**.
- At the same time, but independently, the amount of magnetization in the transverse plane gradually decreases – this is called **decay**.

As the magnitude of transverse magnetization decreases, so does the magnitude of the voltage induced in the receiver coil. The induction of reduced signal is called the **free induction decay (FID)** signal.

Relaxation

During relaxation hydrogen nuclei give up absorbed RF energy and the NMV returns to B_0. At the same time but independently the magnetic moments of hydrogen lose coherency due to dephasing. Relaxation results in recovery of magnetization in the longitudinal plane and decay of magnetization in the transverse plane.

- The recovery of longitudinal magnetization is caused by a process termed **T1 recovery**.
- The decay of transverse magnetization is caused by a process termed T2 decay.

T1 recovery

T1 recovery is caused by the nuclei giving up their energy to the surrounding environment or lattice, and it is termed **spin lattice relaxation**. Energy released to the surrounding lattice causes the magnetic moments of nuclei to recover their longitudinal magnetization (magnetization in the longitudinal plane). The rate of recovery is an exponential process, with a recovery time constant called the **T1 relaxation time**. This is the time it takes 63% of the longitudinal magnetization to recover in the tissue (Figure 1.14).

T2 decay

T2 decay is caused by nuclei exchanging energy with neighboring nuclei. The energy exchange is caused by the magnetic fields of each nucleus

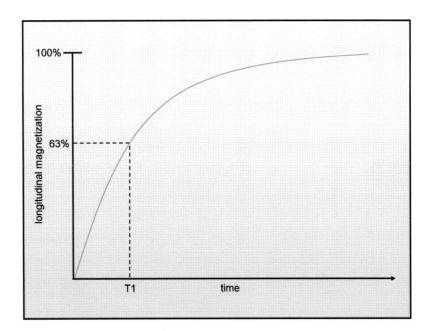

Figure 1.14 The T1 recovery curve.

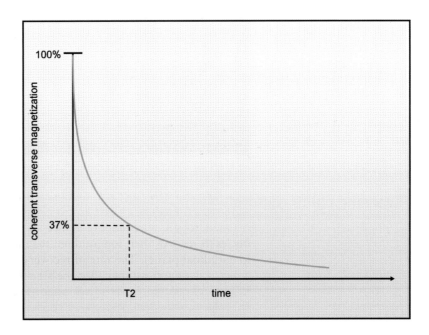

Figure 1.15 The T2 decay curve.

interacting with its neighbor. It is termed **spin-spin relaxation** and results in decay or loss of coherent transverse magnetization (magnetization in the transverse plane). The rate of decay is also an exponential process, so that the **T2 relaxation time** of a tissue is its time constant of decay. It is the time it takes 63% of the transverse magnetization to be lost (Figure 1.15).

1

Summary

- T1 relaxation results in the recovery of longitudinal magnetization due to energy dissipation to the surrounding lattice
- T2 relaxation results in the loss of coherent transverse magnetization due to interactions between the magnetic fields of adjacent nuclei
- A signal or voltage is only induced in the receiver coil if there is coherent magnetization in the transverse plane, that is, in phase (Figure 1.16)

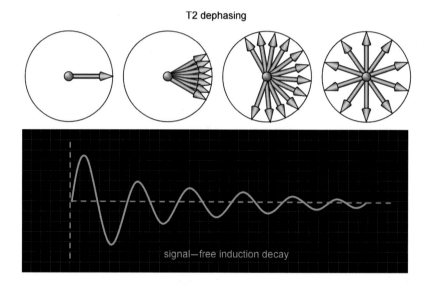

Figure 1.16   Dephasing and the FID.

Learning point: vectors

The NMV is a vector quantity. It is created by two components at 90° to each other. These two components are magnetization in the longitudinal plane and magnetization in the transverse plane (Figure 1.17). Before resonance, there is full longitudinal magnetization parallel to B_0. After the application of the RF pulse, and assuming a flip angle of 90°, the NMV is flipped fully into the transverse plane. There is now full transverse magnetization and zero longitudinal magnetization.

Once the RF pulse is removed, the NMV recovers. As this occurs, the longitudinal component of magnetization grows again, while the transverse component decreases (shown later in Figure 2.1). As the received signal amplitude is related to the magnitude of the coherent transverse component, the signal in the coil decays as relaxation takes place.

1

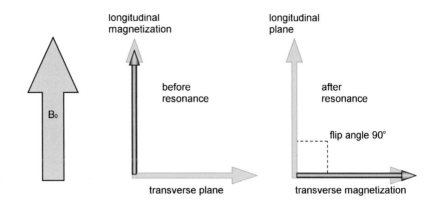

Figure 1.17 Longitudinal and transverse magnetization.

The magnitude and timing of the RF pulses form part of the **pulse sequences,** which are the basis of contrast generation in MRI.

Pulse timing parameters

A very simplified pulse sequence is a combination of RF pulses, signals and intervening periods of recovery (Figure 1.18). It is important to note that a pulse sequence as shown diagrammatically in Figure 1.18 merely shows in simple terms the separate timing parameters used in more complicated sequences, i.e. TR and TE.

A pulse sequence consists of several components: the main ones are outlined below.

- The **repetition time (TR)** is the time from the application of one RF pulse to the application of the next RF pulse for each slice and is

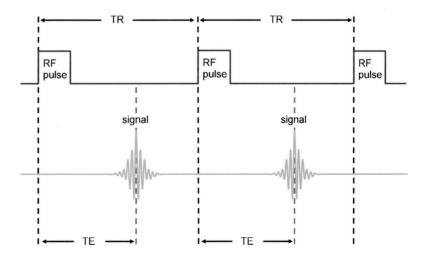

Figure 1.18 A basic pulse sequence.

measured in milliseconds (ms). The TR determines the amount of relaxation that is allowed to occur between the end of one RF pulse and the application of the next. The TR thus determines the amount of T1 relaxation that has occurred when the signal is read.

- The **echo time (TE)** is the time from the application of the RF pulse to the peak of the signal induced in the coil and is also measured in ms. The TE determines how much decay of transverse magnetization is allowed to occur. The TE thus controls the amount of T2 relaxation that has occurred when the signal is read.

The basic principles of signal creation have now been described. The application of RF pulses at certain repetition times and the receiving of signals at predefined echo times produce contrast in MRI images. This concept is discussed fully in the next chapter.

Questions

1   What are the two theories used to describe the basic principles of MRI?

2   Can you define the following?
atoms
molecules
nucleons
protons
neutrons
electrons
isotopes
ions.

3   What is the mass number and why is it important in MRI?

4   What conditions are necessary for resonance?

5   What is the difference between phase and frequency?

2 Image weighting and contrast

2

Introduction

All clinical diagnostic images must demonstrate contrast between normal anatomical features and between anatomy and any pathology. If there is no contrast difference, it is impossible to detect abnormalities within the body. One of the main advantages of MRI compared with other imaging modalities is the excellent soft tissue discrimination of the images. The contrast characteristics of each image depend on many variables, and it is important that the mechanisms that affect image contrast in MRI are understood.

Image contrast

The factors that affect image contrast in diagnostic imaging are usually divided into two categories.

- **Intrinsic contrast parameters** are those that cannot be changed because they are inherent to the body's tissues.
- **Extrinsic contrast parameters** are those that can be changed.

For example, in X-ray imaging, intrinsic contrast parameters include the density of structures the X-ray beam passes through and is attenuated by, while extrinsic contrast parameters are the exposure factors set by the

X-ray technician. Both of these determine X-ray image contrast. In MRI there are several parameters in each group.

Intrinsic contrast parameters are:

- T1 recovery time
- T2 decay time
- proton density
- flow
- apparent diffusion coefficient (ADC)

All these are inherent to the body's tissues and cannot be changed. T1 recovery time and T2 decay time and proton density are discussed in this chapter. Flow and ADC are discussed later.

Extrinsic contrast parameters are:

- TR
- TE
- flip angle
- TI
- turbo factor/echo train length
- b value

These are all selected at the operator console. The parameters selected depend on the pulse sequence used. TR and TE were discussed in Chapter 1. The others are described in Chapters 5 and 12.

Contrast mechanisms

An MR image has contrast if there are areas of high signal (white on the image), and areas of low signal (dark on the image). Some areas have an intermediate signal (shades of gray in between white and black). The NMV can be separated into the individual vectors of the tissues present in the patient, such as fat, cerebrospinal fluid (CSF) and muscle.

A tissue has a high signal if it has a large transverse component of coherent magnetization at time TE. If there is a large component of coherent transverse magnetization the amplitude of the signal received by the coil is large, resulting in a bright area on the image. A tissue returns a low signal if it has a small transverse component of coherent magnetization at time TE. If there is a small component of transverse coherent magnetization, the amplitude of the signal received by the coil is small, resulting in a dark area on the image.

Images obtain contrast mainly through the mechanisms of T1 recovery, T2 decay and proton or spin density. T1 recovery and T2 decay were discussed in Chapter 1. The **proton density** of a tissue is the number of protons per unit volume of that tissue. The higher the proton density of a tissue, the more signal available from that tissue. T1 and T2 relaxation depend on three factors:

- *The inherent energy of the tissue.* If the inherent energy is low, then the molecular lattice is more able to absorb energy from hydrogen nuclei. Tissues with a low inherent energy are like sponges that can easily absorb energy from hydrogen nuclei during relaxation. The reverse is true in tissues with a high inherent energy that cannot easily absorb energy from hydrogen nuclei. These tissues are like kitchen paper, which is less able to absorb energy via relaxation. This is especially important in T1 relaxation processes.
- *How closely packed the molecules are.* In tissues where molecules are closely spaced, there is more efficient energy exchange between hydrogen nuclei. The reverse is true when molecules are spaced apart. This is especially important in T2 decay processes, where energy is exchanged from one hydrogen nucleus to another (spin-spin energy transfer or 'pass the parcel').
- *How well the molecular tumbling rate matches the Larmor frequency of hydrogen.* If there is a good match between the two, energy exchange between hydrogen nuclei and the molecular lattice is efficient. (This is similar to resonance where energy exchange occurs when energy is applied at the same frequency as the Larmor frequency of hydrogen.) When there is a bad match, energy exchange is not as efficient. This is important in both T1 and T2 relaxation processes.

Relaxation in different tissues

As discussed in Chapter 1, T1 relaxation and T2 decay are exponential processes with a time constant T1 and T2 that represent the time it takes for 63% of the total energy to be regained in the longitudinal plane via spin lattice energy transfer (T1), or lost in the transverse plane via spin-spin energy transfer (T2). This section relates the exponential curves to energy transfer within tissues.

Generally, the two extremes of contrast in MRI are fat and water (Figure 2.1). In this book fat vectors are drawn in yellow and water vectors in blue.

Fat and water

Fat molecules contain atoms of hydrogen arranged with carbon and oxygen. They consist of large molecules called lipids that are closely packed together and whose molecular tumbling rate is relatively slow. Water molecules contain two hydrogen atoms arranged with one oxygen atom (H_2O). Its molecules are spaced apart and their molecular tumbling rate is relatively fast. The oxygen in water tends to steal the electrons away from around the hydrogen nucleus. This renders it more available to the effects of the main magnetic field.

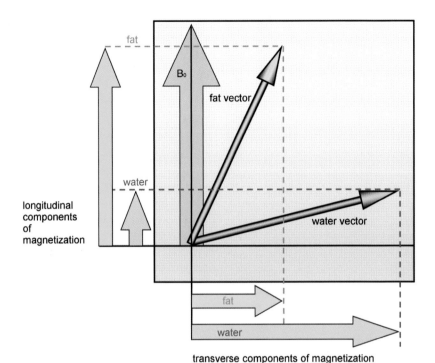

Figure 2.1   The magnitude of transverse magnetization versus amplitude of signal.

In fat, the carbon does not take the electrons from around the hydrogen nucleus. They remain in an electron cloud, protecting the nucleus from the effects of the main field. The Larmor frequency of hydrogen in water is higher than that of hydrogen in fat. Hydrogen in fat recovers more rapidly along the longitudinal axis than water and loses transverse magnetization faster than in water. Subsequently, fat and water appear differently in MR images.

T1 recovery in fat

T1 recovery occurs due to nuclei giving up their energy to the surrounding environment. Fat has a low inherent energy and can easily absorb energy into its lattice from hydrogen nuclei. The slow molecular tumbling in fat allows the recovery process to be relatively rapid, because the molecular tumbling rate matches the Larmor frequency and allows efficient energy exchange from hydrogen nuclei to the surrounding molecular lattice. This means that the magnetic moments of fat nuclei are able to relax and regain their longitudinal magnetization quickly. The NMV of fat realigns rapidly with B_0 so the T1 time of fat is short (Figure 2.2).

T1 recovery in water

T1 recovery occurs due to nuclei giving up the energy acquired from the RF excitation pulse to the surrounding lattice. Water has a high inherent energy and cannot easily absorb energy into its lattice from hydrogen

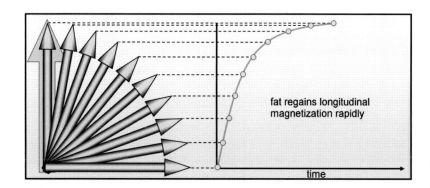

Figure 2.2   T1 recovery in fat.

fat regains longitudinal
magnetization rapidly

time

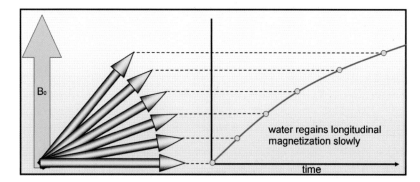

Figure 2.3   T1 recovery in
water.

B₀

water regains longitudinal
magnetization slowly

time

nuclei. In water, molecular mobility is high, resulting in less efficient T1 recovery because the molecular tumbling rate does not match the Larmor frequency and does not allow efficient energy exchange from hydrogen nuclei to the surrounding molecular lattice. The magnetic moments of water take longer to relax and regain their longitudinal magnetization. The NMV of water takes longer to realign with B_0 and so the T1 time of water is long (Figure 2.3).

T2 decay in fat

T2 decay occurs as a result of the magnetic fields of the nuclei interacting with each other, thereby exchanging their energy to their neighbors. Energy exchange is efficient in hydrogen in fat as the molecular tumbling rate of fat is similar to the Larmor frequency and the molecules are packed closely together. As a result spins dephase quickly and the loss of transverse magnetization is rapid. The T2 time of fat is therefore short (Figure 2.4).

T2 decay in water

Energy exchange in water is less efficient than in fat as the molecular tumbling rate of fat is different to the Larmor frequency and the molecules are spaced apart. As a result, spins dephase slowly and the loss of transverse magnetization is gradual. The T2 time of water is therefore long (Figure 2.5).

2

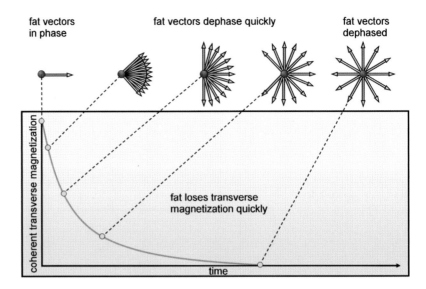

Figure 2.4   T2 decay in fat.

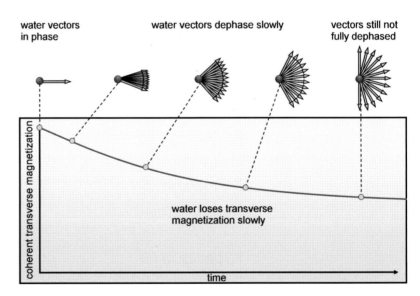

Figure 2.5   T2 decay in water.

T1 contrast

As the T1 time of fat is shorter than that of water, the fat vector realigns with B_0 faster than the water vector. The longitudinal component of magnetization of fat is therefore larger than that of water. After a certain TR that is shorter than the total relaxation times of the tissues, the next RF excitation pulse is applied. The RF excitation pulse flips the longitudinal components of magnetization of both fat and water into the transverse plane (assuming a 90° pulse is applied) as in Figure 2.6. As there is more

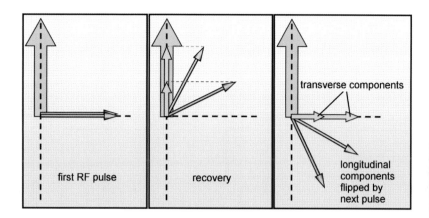

transverse components

longitudinal components flipped by next pulse

first RF pulse

recovery

Figure 2.6 T1 contrast generation.

longitudinal magnetization in fat before the RF pulse, there is more transverse magnetization in fat after the RF pulse. Fat therefore has a high signal and appears bright on a T1 contrast image. As there is less longitudinal magnetization in water before the RF pulse, there is less transverse magnetization in water after the RF pulse. Water therefore has a low signal and appears dark on a T1 contrast image. Such images are called **T1 weighted images**. (*See* Figures 2.23 and 2.26.)

T2 contrast

The T2 time of fat is shorter than that of water, so the transverse component of magnetization of fat decays faster. The magnitude of transverse magnetization in water is large. Water has a high signal and appears bright on a T2 contrast image. However, the magnitude of transverse magnetization in fat is small. Fat therefore has a low signal, and appears dark on a T2 contrast image (Figure 2.7). Such images are called **T2 weighted images** (Figure 2.25).

Proton density contrast

Proton density contrast refers to differences in signal intensity between tissues that are a consequence of their relative number of protons per unit volume. To produce contrast due to the differences in the proton densities between the tissues, the transverse component of magnetization must reflect these differences. Tissues with a high proton density (e.g. brain tissue) have a large transverse component of magnetization (and therefore a high signal), and are bright on a proton density contrast image. Tissues with a low proton density (e.g. cortical bone) have a small transverse component

2

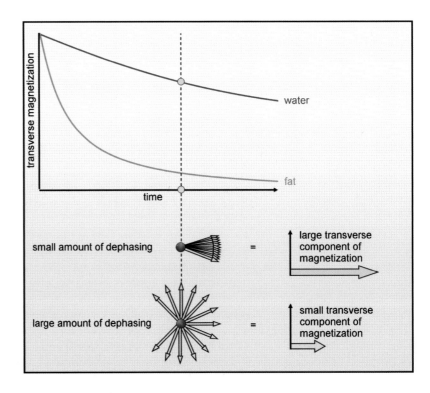

Figure 2.7 T2 contrast generation.

of magnetization (and therefore a low signal), and are dark on a proton density contrast image (Figure 2.24). Proton density contrast is always present and depends on the patient and the area being examined. It is the basic MRI contrast and is called **proton density weighting.**

Summary

- Fat has short T1 and T2 times
- Water has long T1 and T2 times
- To produce high signal, there must be a large component of coherent magnetization in the transverse plane to induce a large signal in the coil
- To produce a low signal, there must be a small component of coherent magnetization in the transverse plane to induce a small signal in the coil
- T1 weighted images are characterized by bright fat and dark water
- T2 weighted images are characterized by bright water and dark fat
- Proton density weighted images are characterized by:
  - areas with high proton density (bright)
  - areas with low proton density (dark)

Table 2.1   T1 and T2 relaxation times of brain tissue at 1 T.

Tissue	T1 time (ms)	T2 time (ms)
Water	2500	2500
Fat	200	100
Cerebrospinal fluid	2000	300
White matter	500	100

The T1 and T2 relaxation times of a tissue, although inherent to that tissue, are dependent on the field strength of the magnet. As field strength increases, tissues take longer to relax. Table 2.1 shows the T1 and T2 relaxation times of brain tissue at 1 T.

Weighting

All the intrinsic contrast parameters listed at the beginning of this chapter simultaneously affect image contrast and would therefore produce images of mixed contrast. This means that, when reading an image, it would be very difficult to determine the relative contribution of each parameter to the contrast observed. This makes image interpretation very challenging. So we need to *weight* image contrast towards one of the parameters and away from the others. This is done by using our understanding of how extrinsic contrast parameters control the relative contribution of each intrinsic contrast parameter. Flow and ADC are discussed in later chapters and are controlled in a specialized way. The other types of weighting mechanisms (T1, T2 and proton density) are discussed here.

To demonstrate either T1, proton density or T2 contrast, specific values of TR and TE are selected for a given pulse sequence. The selection of appropriate TR and TE weights an image so that one contrast mechanism *predominates* over the other two.

T1 weighting

A T1 weighted image is one where the contrast depends predominantly on the differences in the T1 times between fat and water (and all the tissues with intermediate signal). Because the TR controls how far each vector recovers before it is excited by the next RF pulse, to achieve T1 weighting the TR must be short enough so that neither fat nor water has sufficient time to fully return to B_0. If the TR is too long, both fat and water return to B_0 and recover their longitudinal magnetization fully. When this occurs, T1 relaxation is complete in both tissues and the differences in their T1 times are not demonstrated on the image (Figure 2.8).

2

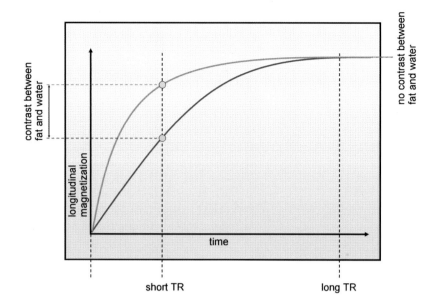

Figure 2.8 The T1 differences between fat and water.

- *TR controls the amount of T1 weighting*
- *for T1 weighting the TR must be short.*

T2 weighting

A T2 weighted image is one where the contrast predominantly depends on the differences in the T2 times between fat and water (and all the tissues with intermediate signal). The TE controls the amount of T2 decay that is allowed to occur before the signal is received. To achieve T2 weighting, the TE must be long enough to give both fat and water time to decay. If the TE is too short, neither fat nor water has had time to decay, and therefore the differences in their T2 times are not demonstrated in the image (Figure 2.9).

- *TE controls the amount of T2 weighting.*
- *For T2 weighting the TE must be long.*

Proton density weighting

A proton density image is one where the difference in the numbers of protons per unit volume in the patient is the main determining factor in forming image contrast. Proton density weighting is always present to some extent. To achieve proton density weighting, the effects of T1 and T2 contrast must be diminished, so that proton density weighting can dominate. A long TR allows both fat and water to fully recover their longitudinal magnetization, and so diminishes T1 weighting. A short TE does not give fat or water time to decay and so diminishes T2 weighting.

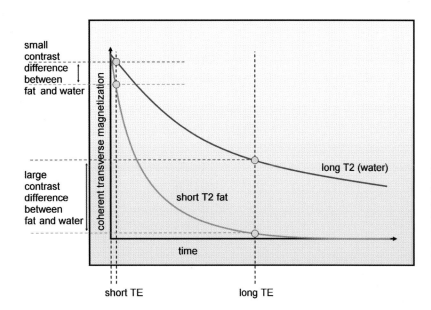

Figure 2.9 The T2 differences between fat and water.

In any image, the contrast due to the inherent proton density together with T1 and T2 mechanisms occur simultaneously and contribute to image contrast. To weight an image so that one process is dominant, the other processes must be diminished.

Learning point: the heat analogy

The mechanisms of weighting are well described using an analogy of a gas oven that has two knobs labeled TR and TE. The TR knob controls the amount of T1 contrast; the TE knob controls the amount of T2 contrast. The TR knob turns the heat up or down on T1 contrast. The TE knob turns the heat up or down on T2 contrast.

Turning the *TR knob down*, turns the *heat up on T1 contrast*, i.e. T1 contrast is increased. Turning the *TE knob up*, turns the *heat up on T2 contrast*, i.e. T2 contrast is increased. To weight an image in a particular direction we need to turn the heat up on one intrinsic contrast parameter and the heat down on the others. For example:

For *T1 weighting* turn the heat up on T1 and the heat down on T2 so the image is weighted towards T1 contrast and away from T2 contrast (proton density depends on the relative number of protons and cannot be changed for a given area).

- To turn the heat up on T1 contrast the TR is short (TR knob down).

- To turn the heat down on T2 the TE is short (TE knob down) (Figure 2.10).

For *T2 weighting* turn the heat up on T2 and the heat down on T1. In this way the image is weighted towards T2 contrast and away from T1 contrast (proton density depends on the relative number of protons and cannot be changed for a given area).

- To turn the heat up on T2 contrast the TE is long (TE knob up).
- To turn the heat down on T1 contrast the TR is long (TR knob up) (Figure 2.11).

For *PD weighting* turn the heat down on T1 and the heat down on T2. In this way proton density contrast predominates.

- To turn the heat down on T1 contrast the TR is long (TR knob up).
- To turn the heat down on T2 the TE is short (TE knob down) (Figure 2.12).

The heat analogy is used elsewhere in this book. Look out for the heat symbol in the margin.

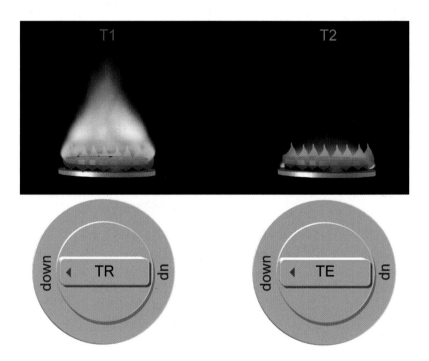

Figure 2.10   T1 weighting and the heat analogy.

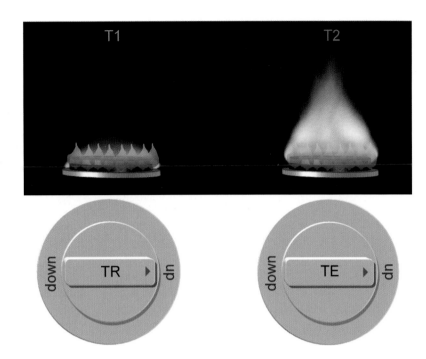

Figure 2.11 T2 weighting and the heat analogy.

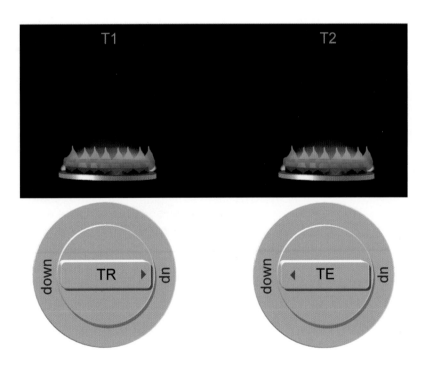

Figure 2.12 Proton density weighting and the heat analogy.

Learning point: saturation

Whenever the NMV is pushed beyond 90° it is said to be **partially saturated**. When the NMV is pushed to a full 180° it is said to be **fully saturated**. If partial saturation of the fat and water vectors occurs, T1 weighting results. If, however, saturation of the fat and water vectors does not occur, proton density weighting results. To understand this, the processes of T1 recovery should be reviewed.

Look at Figure 2.13. Before the application of the first RF pulse, the fat and water vectors are aligned with B_0. When the first 90° RF pulse is applied, the fat and water vectors are flipped into the transverse plane. The RF pulse is then removed, and the vectors begin to relax and return to B_0. Fat has a shorter T1 than water, and so returns to B_0 faster than water. If the TR is shorter than the T1 of the tissues, the next (and all succeeding) RF pulses flip the vectors beyond 90° and into partial saturation because their recovery was incomplete. The fat and water vectors are saturated to different degrees because they were at different points of recovery before the 90° flip. The transverse component of magnetization for each vector is therefore different.

The transverse component of fat is greater than that of water because its longitudinal component grows to a greater degree before the next RF pulse is applied, and so more longitudinal magnetization is available to be flipped into the transverse plane. The fat vector therefore generates a higher signal than water – fat is bright and water is dark. A T1 weighted image results.

Now look at Figure 2.14. If the TR is longer than the T1 times of the tissues, both fat and water fully recover before the next (and all succeeding) RF pulses are applied. Both vectors are flipped directly into the transverse plane and are never saturated. The magnitude of the transverse component of magnetization for fat and water depends only on their individual proton densities, rather than the rate of recovery of their longitudinal components. Tissues with a high proton density are bright, while tissues with a low proton density are dark. A proton density weighted image results. Clearly the flip angle (how far the RF excitation pulse moves the vectors via resonance) and the TR (how long we allow the vectors to recover in between excitation pulses) have a significant impact on saturation effects. This is discussed in more detail later.

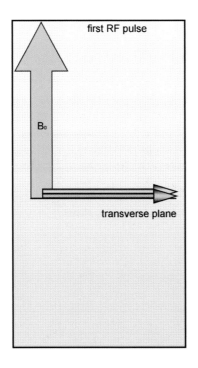

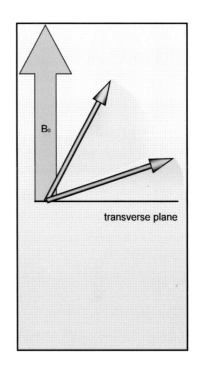

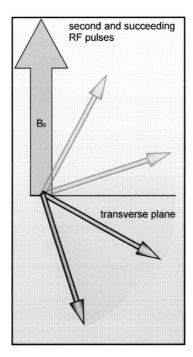

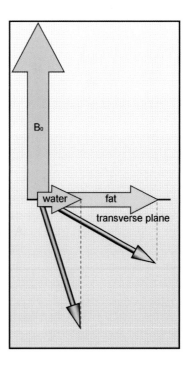

Figure 2.13 Saturation with a short TR.

2

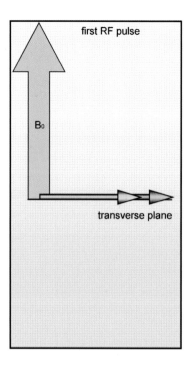

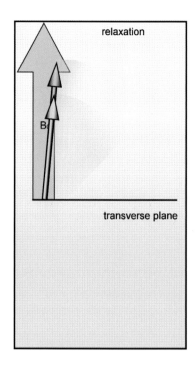

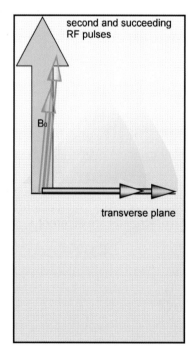

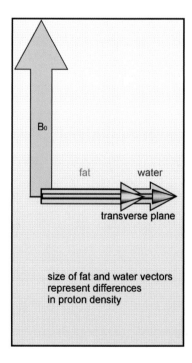

Figure 2.14 No saturation with a long TR.

T2* decay

When the RF excitation pulse is removed, the relaxation and decay processes occur immediately. T2* decay is the decay of the FID following the RF excitation pulse. This decay is faster than T2 decay since it is a combination of two effects:

- T2 decay itself
- dephasing due to magnetic field **inhomogeneities**.

Inhomogeneities are areas within the magnetic field that do not exactly match the external magnetic field strength. Some areas have a magnetic field strength slightly less than the main magnetic field (shown in blue in Figure 2.15), while other areas have a magnetic field strength slightly more than the main magnetic field (shown in red in Figure 2.15).

As the Larmor equation states, the Larmor frequency of a nucleus is proportional to the magnetic field strength it experiences. If a nucleus lies in an area of inhomogeneity with a higher field strength, the precessional frequency of the nucleus increases, i.e. it speeds up. However, if a nucleus lies in an area of inhomogeneity with a lower field strength, the precessional frequency of the nucleus decreases, i.e. it slows down. This is shown in Figure 2.15. This relative acceleration and deceleration, as a result of magnetic field inhomogeneities and differences in the precessional frequency in certain tissues, causes immediate dephasing of the NMV and produces an FID as shown in Figure 2.15. This dephasing is predominantly responsible for T2* decay. The rate of dephasing due to inhomogeneities is an exponential process.

Learning point: inhomogeneities

Do you remember the watch analogy in Chapter 1? The change of phase of magnetic moments due to inhomogeneities in the field is the same as several watches telling different times because the frequencies of their little hands are different.

Pulse sequences

Dephasing caused by inhomogeneities produces a rapid loss of coherent transverse magnetization and therefore signal, so that it reaches zero before most tissues have had time to attain their T1 or T2 relaxation times. To measure relaxation times and produce an image with good contrast, we need to compensate for T2* dephasing so that the signal can

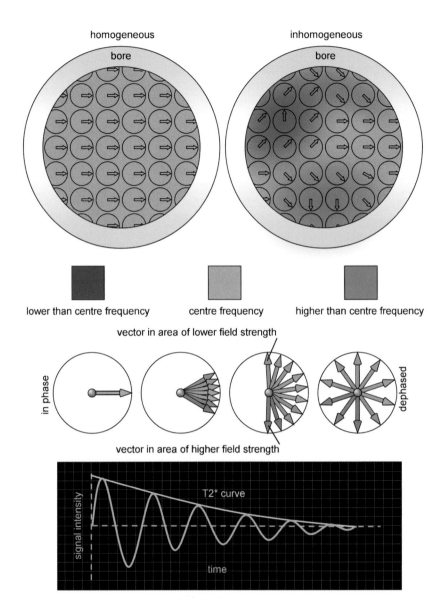

Figure 2.15 T2* decay and field inhomogeneities.

be regenerated and T1 and T2 properly measured. There are two ways of doing this – by using an additional 180° RF pulse or by using gradients. Sequences that use a 180° pulse to regenerate signal are called **spin echo sequences**; those that use a gradient are called **gradient echo sequences**. These are now discussed in more detail.

The spin echo pulse sequence

The **spin echo pulse sequence** uses a 90° excitation pulse to flip the NMV into the transverse plane. The NMV precesses in the transverse plane

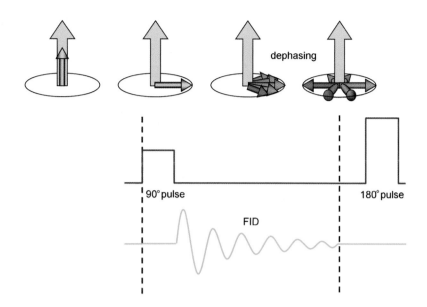

Figure 2.16 T2* dephasing.

inducing a voltage in the receiver coil. The precessional paths of the magnetic moments of the nuclei within the NMV are translated into the transverse plane. When the 90° RF pulse is removed a free induction decay signal (FID) is produced. T2* dephasing occurs immediately, and the signal decays. A 180° RF pulse is then used to compensate for this dephasing (Figure 2.16).

The 180° RF pulse is an RF pulse that has sufficient energy to move the NMV through 180°. The T2* dephasing causes the magnetic moments to dephase or 'fan out' in the transverse plane. The magnetic moments are now out of phase with each other, i.e. they are at different positions on the precessional path at any given time. The magnetic moments that slow down form the trailing edge of the fan (shown in blue in Figure 2.17). The magnetic moments that speed up form the leading edge of the fan (shown

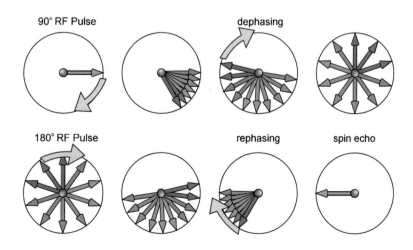

Figure 2.17 180° rephasing.

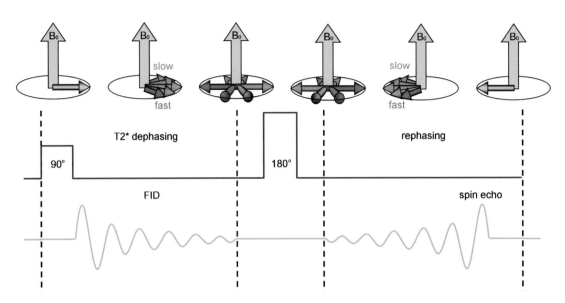

Figure 2.18 A basic rephasing sequence.

in red in Figure 2.17). The 180° RF pulse flips these individual magnetic moments through 180°. They are still in the transverse plane, but now the magnetic moments that formed the trailing edge before the 180° pulse form the leading edge. Conversely, the magnetic moments that formed the leading edge before the 180° pulse, now form the trailing edge (as shown in the bottom half of Figure 2.17). The red spin that formed the leading edge before the 180° pulse now forms the trailing edge. The blue spin that formed the trailing edge before the 180° pulse now forms the leading edge.

The direction of precession remains the same, and so the trailing edge begins to catch up with the leading edge. At a specific time later, the two edges are superimposed. The magnetic moments are now momentarily in phase because they are momentarily at the same place on the precessional path. At this instant, there is transverse magnetization in phase, and so a maximum signal is induced in the coil. This signal is called a **spin echo**. The spin echo now contains T1 and T2 information as T2* dephasing has been reduced and more time has been allowed for tissues to reach their T1 and T2 relaxation times (Figure 2.18).

Learning point: the Larmor Grand Prix

An easy way to understand 180° rephasing is to imagine three cars on a circular racetrack. The cars relate to three magnetic moments and the circular racetrack to the precessional path of the magnetic moments. The cars have varying speeds; one is a racing car, one a family saloon, and one a tractor (*see* Figure 2.19).

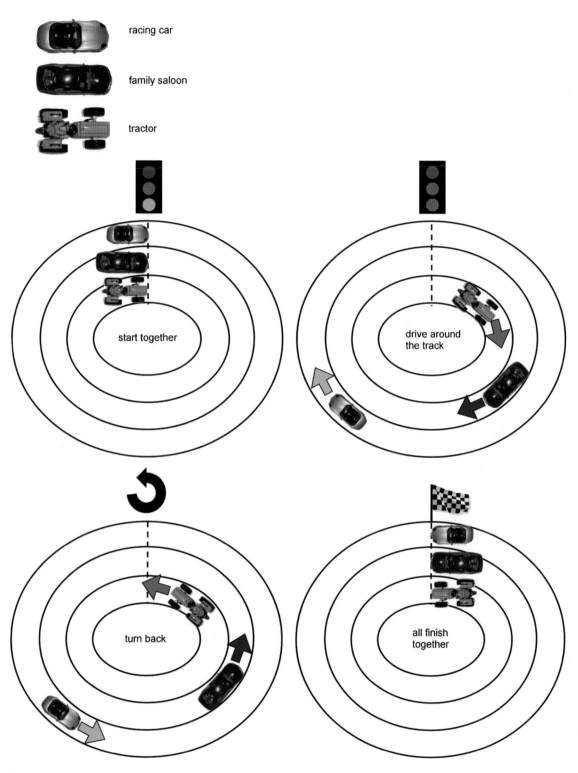

Figure 2.19 The Larmor Grand Prix.

At the sound of the start gun the cars set off around the track. Very shortly, the racing car pulls ahead of the family car, which in turn sprints ahead of the tractor. They are now out of phase with each other, as they are in a different place on the track to each other at a given time. The longer the race is allowed to run, the more dephasing between the vehicles occurs.

The starting gun is fired again. The starting gun now refers to the 180° RF pulse. On hearing the gun, the cars turn around and head back towards the start line. The racing car is now at the back, because it traveled furthest at the beginning of the race. The tractor is at the front because it traveled slower at the beginning of the race. The family saloon is somewhere in between. Assuming the cars travel back to the start line at exactly the same speed as they traveled out at the beginning of the race, the racing car and family saloon catch up with the tractor, and are at exactly the same place at the same time when they get back to the start line. So they are back in phase, and if they were magnetic moments they would generate a spin echo at this point. The time taken for the cars to complete the whole race (from the starting line to the point where they turn around and back to the starting line again) corresponds to the TE.

Timing parameters in spin echo

TR is the time between each 90° excitation pulse for each slice. TE is the time between the 90° excitation pulse and the peak of the spin echo (Figure 2.20). The time taken to rephase after the application of the 180° RF pulse equals the time the NMV took to dephase when the 90° RF pulse was withdrawn. This time is called the **TAU** time. The TE is therefore twice the TAU. Look at Figure 2.20 and note the symmetry of the spin echo. As spins gradually come into phase, the signal gradually builds reaching a peak at the TE when all the spins are in phase. However, the fast spins soon overtake the slow ones and dephasing occurs again. This results

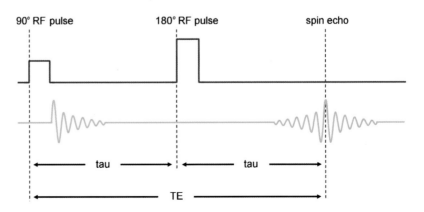

Figure 2.20 TAU.

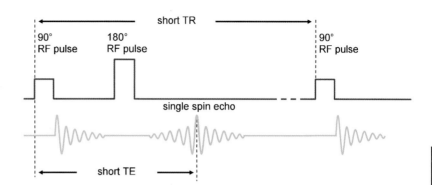

Figure 2.21 Spin echo with one echo.

2

in a gradual loss of signal, which mirrors the gradual growth before the peak of the echo. This accounts for its symmetry.

In most spin echo pulse sequences, more than one 180° RF pulse can be applied after the 90° excitation pulse. Each 180° pulse generates a separate spin echo that can be received by the coil and used to create an image. Although any number of echoes can be created, spin echo sequences are typically used generating either 1 or 2 echoes.

Spin echo using one echo

This pulse sequence can be used to produce T1 weighted images if a short TR and TE are used (Figure 2.21). One 180° RF pulse is applied after the 90° excitation pulse. The single 180° RF pulse generates a single spin echo. The timing parameters used are selected to produce a T1 weighted image. A short TE ensures that the 180° RF pulse and subsequent echo occur early, so that only a little T2 decay has occurred. The differences in the T2 times of the tissues do not dominate the echo and its contrast. A short TR ensures that the fat and water vectors have not fully recovered, and so the differences in their T1 times dominate the echo and its contrast (Figure 2.23).

Spin echo using two echoes

This can be used to produce both a proton density and a T2 weighted image in the TR time (Figure 2.22). The first spin echo is generated early by

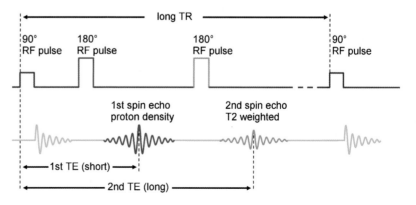

Figure 2.22 Spin echo with two echoes.

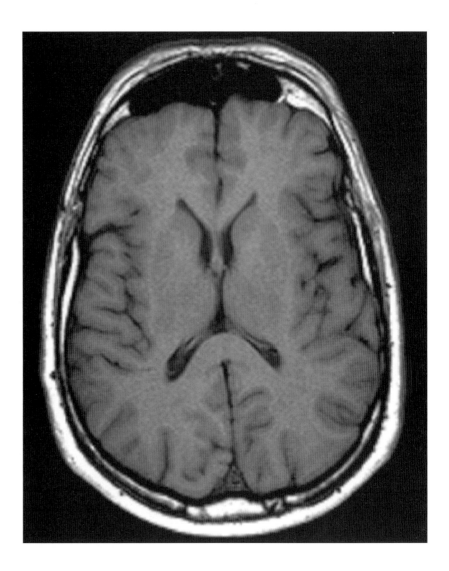

Figure 2.23 Axial T1 weighted spin echo image through the brain.

selecting a short TE. Only a little T2 decay has occurred and so T2 differences between the tissues are minimized in this echo. The second spin echo is generated much later by selecting a long TE. A significant amount of T2 decay has now occurred, and so the differences in the T2 times of the tissues are maximized in this echo. The TR selected is long, so that T1 differences between the tissues are minimized. The first spin echo therefore has a short TE and a long TR and is proton density weighted. The second spin echo has a long TE and a long TR and is T2 weighted. Figure 2.23 shows a T1 weighted image; Figure 2.24 shows a proton density weighted image; and Figure 2.25 shows a T2 weighted image.

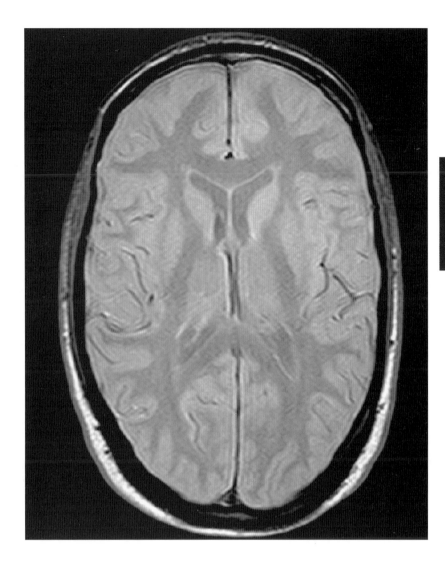

Figure 2.24 Axial PD weighted spin echo image through the brain.

Summary

- Spin echo pulse sequences produce either T1, T2 or proton density weighting
- TR controls the T1 weighting (see the heat analogy)
- Short TR maximizes T1 weighting
- Long TR maximizes proton density weighting
- TE controls the T2 weighting
- Short TE minimizes T2 weighting
- Long TE maximizes T2 weighting

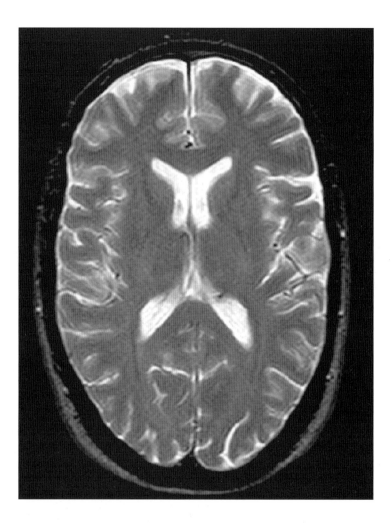

Figure 2.25   Axial T2 weighted spin echo image through the brain.

Typical values of TR and TE

Long TR	2000 ms
Short TR	300–700 ms
Long TE	60 ms+
Short TE	10–25 ms

Learning point: understanding weighting

Understanding image weighting is a fundamental skill in MRI. One of the basic rules is to look for the water content in the image and if it has a high signal, the image must be T2 weighted and have been acquired with a long TE. Generally speaking, if water has a low signal it is likely to be T1 weighted and have been acquired with a short TR, but depending on the area of the body, some proton density images have dark water. Fat is an unreliable marker as it can be bright on many types of weighting depending on the pulse sequence used.

To demonstrate the variables in image contrast, look at Figure 2.26. It was acquired using a standard spin echo sequence and is a T1 weighted image so the contrast is predominantly due to differences in the T1 recovery times of the tissues. It has contrast we would expect from an image acquired with a short TR and TE, e.g. fat in the scalp and bony marrow of the clivus is bright and water in the CSF is dark. However, looking more closely it is clear that not all areas of high signal are fat and not all areas of low signal are water. For example, the area labeled A, which has a high signal, is not fat but slow-flowing blood in the superior sagittal sinus. The area labeled B, which has a low signal, is not water but air in the sphenoid sinus. Although this image is predominantly T1 weighted, there are also flow and proton density effects contributing to image contrast. Now look at Figures 2.24 and 2.25 and see if you can identify areas that demonstrate contrast not typical of the weighting shown.

2

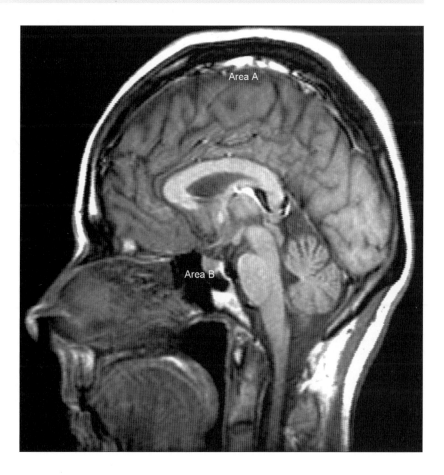

Figure 2.26 Midline sagittal T1 weighted spin echo image through the brain.

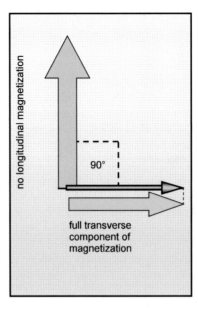

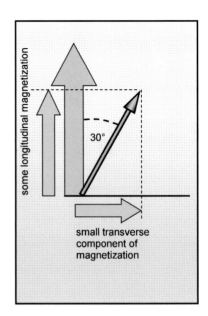

Figure 2.27   How the flip angle controls the amplitude of the signal.

The gradient echo pulse sequence

A gradient echo pulse sequence uses an RF excitation pulse that is variable, and therefore flips the NMV through any angle (not just 90°). A transverse component of magnetization is created, the magnitude of which is less than in spin echo, where all the longitudinal magnetization is converted to the transverse plane. When a flip angle other than 90° is used, only part of the longitudinal magnetization is converted to transverse magnetization, which precesses in the transverse plane and induces a signal in the receiver coil (Figure 2.27).

After the RF pulse is withdrawn, the FID signal is immediately produced due to inhomogeneities in the magnetic field and T2* dephasing therefore occurs. The magnetic moments within the transverse component of magnetization dephase, and are then rephased by a gradient. A gradient causes a change in the magnetic field strength within the magnet and is discussed in more detail later. The gradient rephases the magnetic moments so that a signal is received by the coil, which contains T1 and T2 information. This signal is called a **gradient echo**.

Gradients

Gradients perform many tasks, which are explored fully in Chapter 3. **Magnetic field gradients** are generated by coils of wire situated within the bore of the magnet. The laws of electromagnetic induction state that when charge moves through a gradient coil, a magnetic field (or gradient field as it is now known) is induced around it. This gradient field interacts with

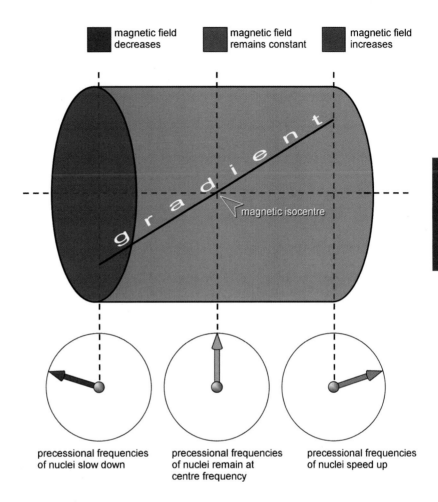

| magnetic field decreases | magnetic field remains constant | magnetic field increases |

magnetic isocentre

precessional frequencies of nuclei slow down

precessional frequencies of nuclei remain at centre frequency

precessional frequencies of nuclei speed up

Figure 2.28   The gradients.

the main static magnetic field, so that the magnetic field strength along the axis of the gradient coil is altered in a linear way. The middle of the axis of the gradients remains at the field strength of the main magnetic field. This is called **magnetic isocentre**.

The magnetic field strength increases relative to the isocentre in one direction of the gradient axis because the magnetic field produced by the gradient adds to the main magnetic field (shown in red on Figure 2.28). It decreases relative to the isocentre in the other direction of the gradient axis because the magnetic field produced by the gradient subtracts from the main magnetic field (shown in blue in Figure 2.28). Whether a gradient field adds or subtracts from the main magnetic field depends on the direction of the current passing through the gradient coils. This is called the **polarity** of the gradient.

When a gradient is switched on, the magnetic field strength along its axis is sloped or graded. The Larmor equation states that the precessional frequency of the magnetic moments increases or decreases, depending on the magnetic field strength they experience at different points along the gradient (Figure 2.28).

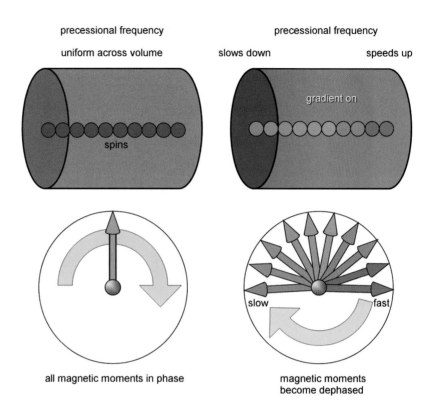

precessional frequency

uniform across volume

precessional frequency

slows down   speeds up

gradient on

spins

all magnetic moments in phase

slow   fast

magnetic moments
become dephased

Figure 2.29 How gradients dephase.

The precessional frequency increases when the magnetic field increases, and decreases when the magnetic field decreases. Magnetic moments experiencing an increased field strength due to the gradient speed up, i.e. their precessional frequency increases. Magnetic moments experiencing a decreased magnetic field strength slow down, i.e. their precessional frequency decreases. As gradients cause nuclei to speed up or slow down, they can be used either to dephase or rephase their magnetic moments.

How gradients dephase. Look at Figure 2.29. With no gradient applied, all spins precess at the same frequency as they experience the same field strength (in reality they do not because of inhomogeneities in the field but these changes are relatively small compared with those imposed by a gradient). A gradient is applied to coherent (in phase) magnetization (all the magnetic moments are in the same place at the same time). The gradient alters the magnetic field strength experienced by the coherent magnetization. Depending on their position along the gradient axis some of the magnetic moments speed up and some slow down. Thus the magnetic moments fan out or dephase because their frequencies have been changed by the gradient (*see* the watch analogy in Chapter 1).

The trailing edge of the fan (shown in blue) consists of nuclei that have slowed down, as they are situated on the gradient axis that has a lower magnetic field strength relative to the isocentre. The leading edge of the fan (shown in red) consists of nuclei that have sped up as they are situated on

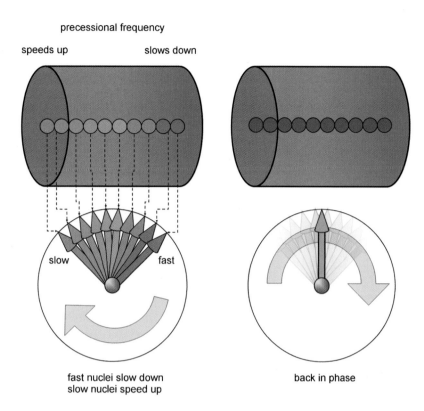

precessional frequency

speeds up   slows down

slow   fast

fast nuclei slow down
slow nuclei speed up

back in phase

Figure 2.30 How gradients rephase.

the gradient axis that has a higher magnetic field strength relative to the isocentre. The magnetic moments of the nuclei are therefore no longer in the same place at the same time and so the magnetization has been dephased by the gradient. Gradients that dephase are called **spoilers**.

How gradients rephase. Look at Figure 2.30. A gradient is applied to incoherent (out of phase) magnetization. The magnetic moments have fanned out due to T2* dephasing and the fan has a trailing edge consisting of slow nuclei (shown in blue), and a leading edge consisting of faster nuclei (shown in red). A gradient is then applied, so that the magnetic field strength is altered in a linear fashion along the axis of the gradient. The direction of this altered field strength is such that the slow nuclei in the trailing edge of the fan experience an increased magnetic field strength and speed up.

In Figure 2.30 the blue spins are experiencing the red 'high end' of the gradient. The faster nuclei in the leading edge of the fan experience a decreased magnetic field strength and slow down. In Figure 2.30 the red spins are experiencing the blue 'low end' of the gradient. After a short period of time, the slow nuclei have sped up sufficiently to meet the faster nuclei that are slowing down. When the two meet, all the magnetic moments are in the same place at the same time and have been rephased by the gradient. A maximum signal is therefore induced in the receiver coil and this signal is called a *gradient echo*. Gradients that rephase are called **rewinders**.

2

The advantages of gradient echo pulse sequences

Since gradients rephase faster than 180° RF pulses, the minimum TE is much shorter than in spin echo pulse sequences, and so the TR can also be reduced. The TR can also be reduced because flip angles other than 90° are used. With low flip angles, full recovery of the longitudinal magnetization occurs sooner than with large flip angles. The TR can therefore be shortened without producing saturation. The TR plays an important part in the time of the scan (*see* Chapter 3), so as the TR is reduced, the scan time is also reduced. Gradient echo pulse sequences are therefore usually associated with much shorter scan times than spin echo pulse sequences.

The disadvantages of gradient echo pulse sequences

The most important disadvantage is that there is no compensation for magnetic field inhomogeneities. Gradient echo pulse sequences are therefore very susceptible to magnetic field inhomogeneities. Gradient echo pulse sequences contain a magnetic susceptibility artefact (*see* Chapter 7). As the T2* effects are not eliminated, in gradient echo imaging T2 weighting is termed T2* weighting and T2 decay is termed T2* decay.

Timing parameters in gradient echo

As in spin echo, the TR is the time between each RF excitation pulse, while the TE is the time from the excitation pulse to the peak of the gradient echo. Although not a timing parameter, in gradient echo sequences the flip angle is an extrinsic contrast parameter that is changed to affect image contrast. Its value, combined with the TR, determines whether T1 effects are maximized or minimized.

Weighting and contrast in gradient echo

The TR, TE and flip angle affect image weighting and contrast and the TR can be much shorter than in spin echo pulse sequences. As the TR controls that amount of T1 recovery that has been allowed to occur before the application of the next RF pulse, a short TR produces T1 weighting and never permits a T2 or proton density weighted image to be obtained. To give gradient echo imaging more flexibility, the flip angle is reduced to less than 90°. If the flip angle is less than 90°, it does not take the NMV as long to recover full longitudinal magnetization, and so the TR can be shortened to reduce the scan time without producing saturation.

In gradient echo pulse sequences, the TR and the flip angle control the amount of T1 relaxation that has occurred before the next RF pulse is applied. The TE controls the amount of T2* decay that has occurred

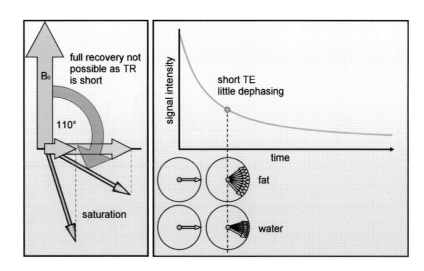

Figure 2.31 T1 weighting in gradient echo.

before the gradient echo is received by the coil. Apart from the added variable of the flip angle, the rules of weighting in gradient echo are exactly the same as in spin echo (*see* the heat analogy in Chapter 1).

T1 weighting in gradient echo. To obtain a T1 weighted image, the differences in the T1 times of the tissues are maximized, and the differences in the T2 times of the tissues are minimized. To maximize T1 differences, neither the fat nor the water vectors must have had time to recover full longitudinal magnetization before the next RF pulse is applied. To avoid full recovery, the flip angle is large and the TR short, so that the fat and water vectors are still in the process of relaxing when the next RF is applied. To minimize T2* differences, the TE is short so that neither fat nor water has had time to decay (Figure 2.31).

T2* weighting in gradient echo. To obtain a T2* weighted image, the differences in the T2* times of the tissues are maximized, and the differences in the T1 times are minimized. To maximize T2* decay, the TE is long so that the fat and water vectors have had time to decay sufficiently to show their decay differences. To minimize T1 recovery, the flip angle is small and the TR long enough to permit full recovery of the fat and water vectors. In this way, T1 differences are not demonstrated. In practice, small flip angles produce such little transverse magnetization that the TR can be kept relatively short and full recovery still has time to occur (Figure 2.32).

Proton density weighting in gradient echo. To obtain a proton density weighted image both T1 and T2* processes are minimized so that the differences in proton density of the tissues can be demonstrated. To minimize T2* decay, the TE is short so that neither the fat nor the water vectors have had time to decay. To minimize T1 recovery, the flip angle is small and the TR long enough to permit full recovery of longitudinal magnetization.

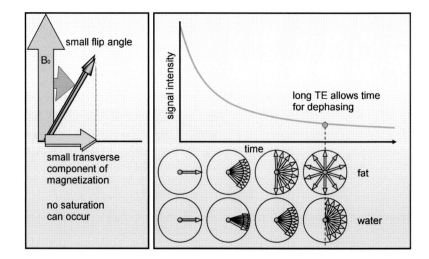

Figure 2.32 T2* weighting in gradient echo.

Learning point: weighting and gradient echo using the heat analogy

For *T1 weighting* turn the heat up on T1 and the heat down on T2*. Flip angle and TR control T1 contrast, TE controls T2* contrast (proton density depends on the relative number of protons and cannot be changed for a given area).

- To turn the heat up on T1 contrast the TR is short (TR knob down)and the flip angle is high.
- To turn the heat down on T2* the TE is short (TE knob down) (Figure 2.33).

For *T2* weighting* turn the heat up on T2* and the heat down on T1. Flip angle and TR control T1 contrast, TE controls T2* contrast (proton density depends on the relative number of protons and cannot be changed for a given area).

- To turn the heat up on T2* contrast the TE is long (TE knob up).
- To turn the heat down on T1 contrast the TR is long (TR knob up) and the flip angle is low (Figure 2.34).

For *PD weighting* turn the heat down on T1 and the heat down on T2*. In this way proton density contrast predominates.

- To turn the heat down on T1 contrast the TR is long (TR knob up) and the flip angle low.
- To turn the heat down on T2* the TE is short (TE knob down) (Figure 2.35).

Look at Figures 2.36 and 2.37. Both were acquired using a gradient echo sequence and the same TR. To change the weighting one other parameter has been altered. Is it the flip angle or TE?

To answer this question, first determine their weighting. Figure 2.36 is clearly T2* weighted as the CSF has a high signal. Figure 2.37 is more difficult to interpret. Although the CSF is darker than on Figure 2.36 and could be thought to be T1 weighted, the hydrated intervertebral discs have a high signal, which we would not expect on a T1 weighted image. In fact this image is proton density weighted. As neither image is T1 weighted, neither was acquired with a high flip angle. Both have a low flip angle and – as the TR is the same – the parameter we have changed is the TE.

On Figure 2.37, low flip angles have minimized saturation and therefore T1 contrast and a short TE has minimized T2* contrast, resulting in a proton density weighted image. Figure 2.36 has also been acquired with a low flip angle minimizing T1 contrast but has a long TE maximizing T2* contrast resulting in a T2* weighted image. The parameter that has been changed is therefore the TE.

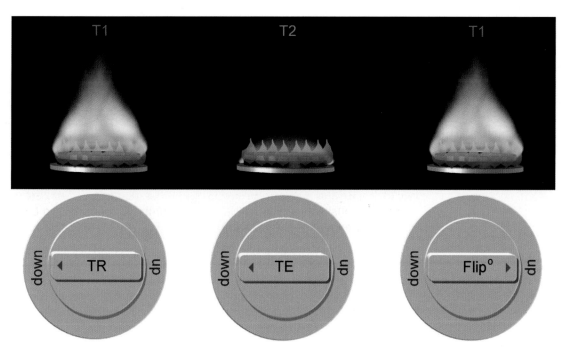

Figure 2.33 T1 contrast in gradient echo and the heat analogy.

2

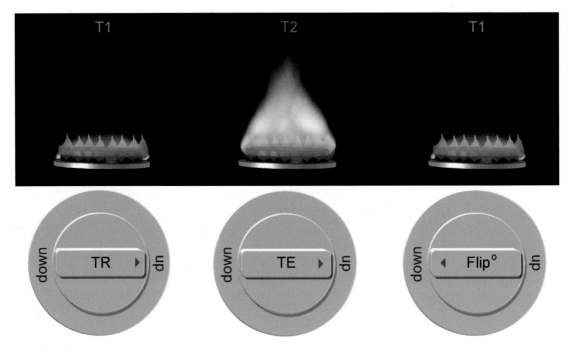

Figure 2.34 T2* contrast in gradient echo and the heat analogy.

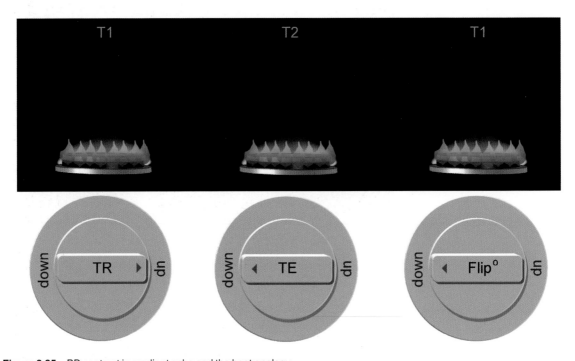

Figure 2.35 PD contrast in gradient echo and the heat analogy.

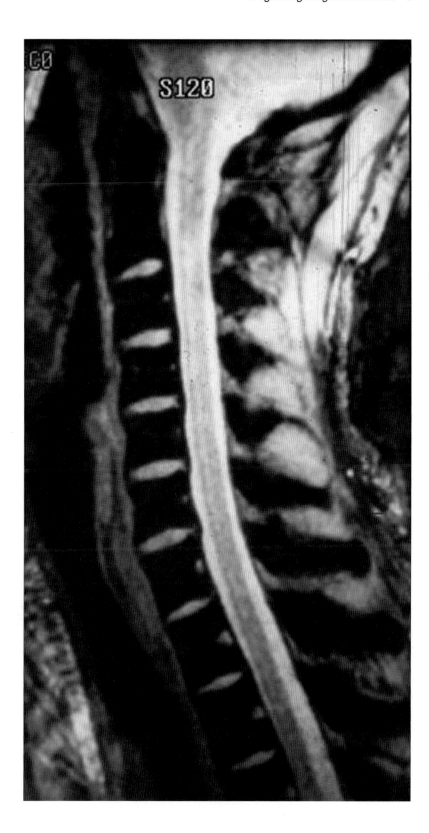

2

Figure 2.36   Midline sagittal
T2* weighted gradient echo
through the cervical spine.

2

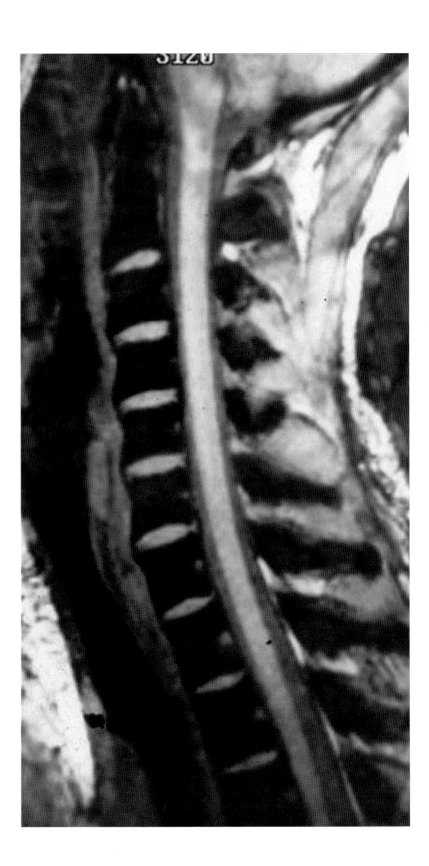

Figure 2.37 Midline sagittal PD weighted gradient echo through the cervical spine.

Summary

- Gradient echo pulse sequences use a gradient to rephase the magnetic moments
- Variable flip angles are used
- The TE can be much shorter than in spin echo imaging
- Gradients do not eliminate effects from magnetic field inhomogeneities

2

Typical values in gradient echo imaging

Long TR	100 ms+
Short TR	less than 50 ms
Short TE	5–10 ms
Long TE	15–25 ms
Small flip angles	5°–20°
Large flip angles	70°–110°

Table 2.2 summarizes the differences between spin echo and gradient echo. Table 2.3 gives the parameters used in gradient echo. Signal creation and how it can be manipulated to produce image contrast has now been discussed. In the next chapter, the process of image formation is described.

Table 2.2 Summary of the differences between spin echo and gradient echo.

Sequence	TR	TE	Flip angle
Spin echo	long 2000 ms+	long 60 ms+	90°
	short 250–700 ms+	short 10–25 ms+	90°
Gradient echo	long 100 ms+	long 15–25 ms	small 5°–20°
	short less than 50 ms	short less than 10 ms	medium 30°–45°
			large 70°–110°

Table 2.3 Parameters used in gradient echo.

Weighting	TR	TE	Flip angle
T1	short	short	large
T2	long	long	small
Proton density	long	short	small

Questions

1   What factors determine the T1 and T2 relaxation times of a tissue?

2   Why does fat have short T1 and T2 relaxation times?

3   Define the term weighting.

4   What values of TR and TE are needed for PD weighting in a spin echo sequence and why?

5   List the main factors that make gradient echo sequences different from spin echo.

6   What parameter controls T2 decay and why?

7   What types of contrast will the following produce?
    (a)   TR 50 ms, TE 5 ms, flip 120°.
    (b)   TR 400 ms, TE 15 ms, flip 35°.

3

Encoding and image formation

3

ENCODING

Introduction

As previously described, for resonance to occur, a RF must be applied at 90° to B_0 at the precessional frequency of hydrogen. The RF pulse gives hydrogen nuclei energy so that transverse magnetization is created. The RF pulse also puts the individual magnetic moments of hydrogen into phase. The resultant coherent transverse magnetization precesses at the Larmor frequency of hydrogen in the transverse plane. A voltage or signal is therefore induced in the receiver coil that is positioned in the transverse plane. This signal has a frequency equal to the Larmor frequency of hydrogen, regardless of the origin of signal in the patient.

The system must be able to locate signal spatially in three dimensions, so that it can position each signal at the correct point on the image. To do this, it first locates a slice. Once a slice is selected, the signal is located or **encoded** along both axes of the image. These tasks are performed by gradients.

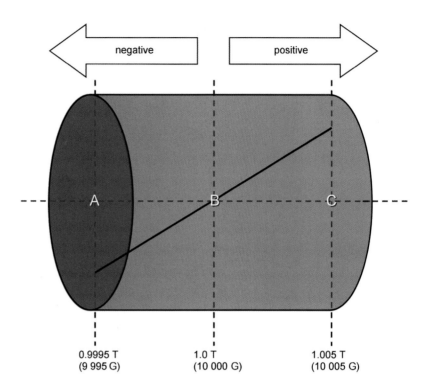

negative

positive

A   B   C

0.9995 T   1.0 T   1.005 T
(9 995 G)   (10 000 G)   (10 005 G)

Figure 3.1 Gradients and changing field strength.

Gradients

The mechanisms of gradients were introduced in Chapter 2 and are further discussed in Chapter 9. To recap, gradients are alterations to the main magnetic field and are generated by coils of wire located within the bore of the magnet through which current is passed. The passage of current through a gradient coil induces a gradient (magnetic) field around it, which either subtracts from, or adds to, the main static magnetic field B_0. The magnitude of B_0 is altered in a linear fashion by the gradient coils, so that the magnetic field strength and therefore the precessional frequency experienced by nuclei situated along the axis of the gradient can be predicted (Figure 3.1). This is called **spatial encoding**.

Look at Figure 3.1. A gradient has been applied that increases the magnetic field strength towards the right-hand side of the magnet (shown in red) and decreases it towards the left-hand side (purple). The change in magnetic field strength is linear and with this particular amplitude at point A, a nucleus experiences a field of 0.9995 T, a nucleus at point B (the isocentre) experiences exactly 1 T, and at point C, a nucleus experiences a field of 1.005 T. In all gradient diagrams in this book, magnetic fields higher than the isocentre are shown in red or pink and those lower, blue or purple.

Nuclei that experience an increased magnetic field strength due to the gradient speed up, i.e. their precessional frequency increases; while nuclei

Table 3.1 Frequency changes along a linear gradient.

Position along gradient	Field strength	Larmor frequency
At isocentre	10 000 G	42.5700 MHz
1 cm negative to isocentre	9 999 G	42.5657 MHz
2 cm negative to isocentre	9 998 G	42.5614 MHz
1 cm positive to isocentre	10 001 G	42.5742 MHz
2 cm positive to isocentre	10 002 G	42.5785 MHz
10 cm negative to isocentre	9 990 G	42.5274 MHz

that experience a lower magnetic field strength due to the gradient slow down, i.e. their precessional frequency decreases. Therefore the position of a nucleus along a gradient can be identified according to its precessional frequency.

Table 3.1 gives the frequency changes along a linear gradient that alters the magnetic field strength by 1G/cm.

There are three gradient coils situated within the bore of the magnet, and these are named according to the axis along which they act when they are switched on. Figure 3.2 shows these directions in a superconducting magnet.

- The *Z gradient* alters the magnetic field strength along the Z- (*long*) axis of the magnet
- The *Y gradient* alters the magnetic field strength along the Y- (*vertical*) axis of the magnet
- The *X gradient* alters the magnetic field strength along the X- (*horizontal*) axis of the magnet
- The magnetic isocentre is the center point of the axis of all three gradients, and the bore of the magnet. The magnetic field strength and therefore the precessional frequency remain unaltered here even when the gradients are applied.

Permanent magnets (*see* Chapter 9) have different axes. The Z-axis is vertical, not horizontal, as shown in Figure 3.2. The magnetic field strength at the isocentre is always the same as B$_0$ (e.g. 1.5 T, 1.0 T, 0.5 T),

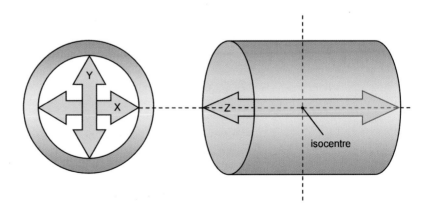

Figure 3.2 Gradient axes.

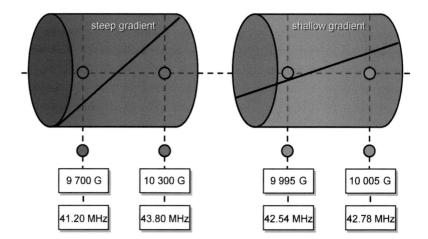

Figure 3.3 Steep and shallow slopes.

even when the gradients are switched on. When a gradient coil is switched on, the magnetic field strength is either subtracted from or added to B_0 relative to the isocentre. The slope of the resulting magnetic field is the amplitude of the magnetic field gradient and it determines the rate of change of the magnetic field strength along the gradient axis. Steep gradient slopes alter the magnetic field strength between two points more than shallow gradient slopes. Steep gradient slopes therefore alter the precessional frequency of nuclei between two points more than shallow gradient slopes (Figure 3.3).

It is convenient (for easy mathematics) to now use the unit gauss to describe magnetic field strength rather than tesla where 1.0 T is equal to 10 000 G. Gauss is the unit used to show the relative change in field strength between two points in Figure 3.3.

Gradients perform many important tasks during a pulse sequence as previously described in Chapter 2. Can you remember what these are? Gradients can be used to either dephase or rephase the magnetic moments of nuclei. Gradients also perform the following three main tasks in encoding:

- **Slice selection** – locating a slice within the scan plane selected
- Spatially locating (encoding) signal along the long axis of the anatomy – this is called **frequency encoding**
- Spatially locating (encoding) signal along the short axis of the anatomy – this is called **phase encoding**.

Slice selection

When a gradient coil is switched on, the magnetic field strength, and therefore the precessional frequency of nuclei located along its axis, is altered in a linear fashion. Therefore a specific point along the axis of the gradient has a specific precessional frequency (*see* Figure 3.3). Therefore nuclei situated within a slice have a particular precessional frequency. A slice can therefore be selectively excited, by transmitting RF with a band of frequencies coinciding with the Larmor frequencies of spins in a particular slice as defined by the slice select gradient. Resonance of nuclei within the slice occurs because RF appropriate to that position is transmitted. However, nuclei situated in other slices along the gradient do not resonate, because their precessional frequency is different due to the presence of the gradient (Figure 3.4).

Learning point: slice selection and the tuning fork analogy

Look at Figure 3.4 in which tuning forks are used to illustrate how slice selection is performed. In the top diagram a gradient has been applied to change the magnetic field strength from low (blue) to high (red). Imagine we are trying to select Slice A. With this particular amplitude of gradient the spins in this slice have a precessional frequency of 41.20 MHz when the gradient is switched on. Spins on either side of this slice have a different frequency because the gradient has changed the field strength across the bore of the magnet. Without the gradient all spins would precess at the same frequency and therefore we would not be able to differentiate them. As the gradient has been applied, however, the precessional frequency of spins has changed across the bore, so that along the Z-axis spins in different slices precess at different frequencies.

This is analogous to having tuning forks tuned to different frequencies located across the Z axis of the magnet. To produce resonance and excite spins in Slice A, an RF excitation pulse that matches the precessional frequency of spins in Slice A, i.e. 41.20 MHz, must be applied. Doing so causes resonance just in spins in Slice A; spins in other slices do not resonate because they are precessing at different frequencies. To produce the same affect in Slice B (bottom diagram) an RF excitation pulse with a frequency of 43.80 MHz must be applied to produce resonance in spins in Slice B. In this example, axial slices are being excited (assuming the patient is lying either supine or prone on the scan table) by applying the slice select gradient during the application of the excitation pulse.

3

The scan plane selected determines which of the three gradients performs slice selection during the excitation pulse (Figure 3.5).

- The *Z gradient* alters the field strength and precessional frequency along the Z-axis of the magnet and therefore selects *axial* slices.
- The *X gradient* alters the field strength and the precessional frequency along the X-axis of the magnet and therefore selects *sagittal* slices.
- The *Y gradient* alters the field strength and the precessional frequency along the Y-axis of the magnet and therefore selects *coronal* slices.
- Oblique slices are selected using two gradients in combination.

3

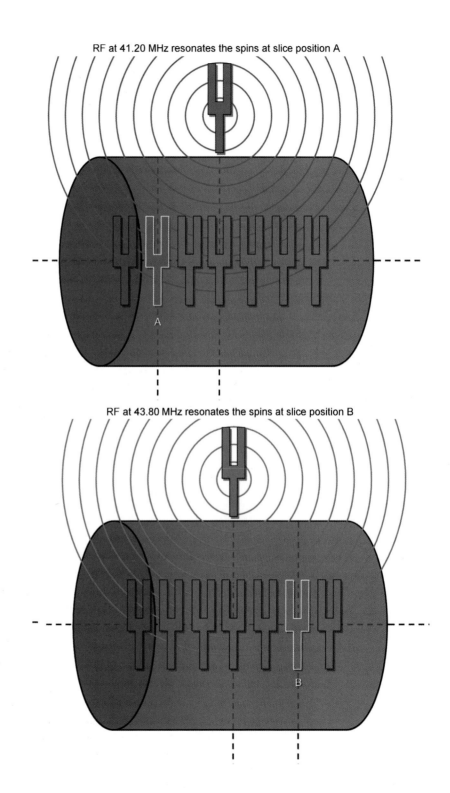

RF at 41.20 MHz resonates the spins at slice position A

RF at 43.80 MHz resonates the spins at slice position B

Figure 3.4 Slice selection.

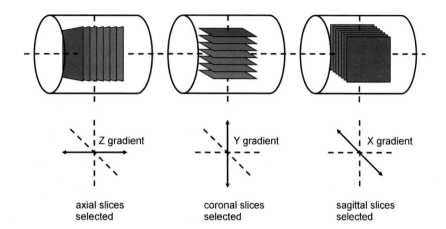

Figure 3.5 X, Y, Z as slice selectors.

axial slices selected

coronal slices selected

sagittal slices selected

Slice thickness

To give each slice a thickness, a 'band' of nuclei must be excited by the excitation pulse. The slope of the slice select gradient determines the difference in precessional frequency between two points on the gradient. Steep gradient slopes result in a large difference in precessional frequency between two points on the gradient, while shallow gradient slopes result in a small difference in precessional frequency between the same two points. Once a certain gradient slope is applied, the RF pulse transmitted to excite the slice must contain a range of frequencies to match the difference in precessional frequency between two points. This frequency range is called the **bandwidth**, and as the RF is being transmitted at this point it is specifically called the **transmit bandwidth** (Figure 3.6).

- To achieve *thin slices*, a *steep slice* select slope and/or *narrow transmit bandwidth* is applied.
- To achieve *thick slices, a shallow slice* select slope and/or *broad transmit bandwidth* is applied.

In practice, the system automatically applies the appropriate gradient slope and transmit bandwidth according to the thickness of slice required. The slice is excited by transmitting RF at the center frequency corresponding to the precessional frequency of nuclei in the middle of the slice, and the bandwidth and gradient slope determine the range of nuclei that resonate on either side of the center.

The gap between the slices is determined by the gradient slope and by the thickness of the slice. The size of the gap is important in reducing image artefact (*see* Chapter 7). In spin echo pulse sequences, the slice select gradient is switched on during the application of the 90° excitation pulse and during the 180° rephasing pulse, to excite and rephase each slice selectively (Figure 3.7). In gradient echo pulse sequences, the slice select gradient is switched on during the excitation pulse only. The significance of this is explored in Chapter 6.

3

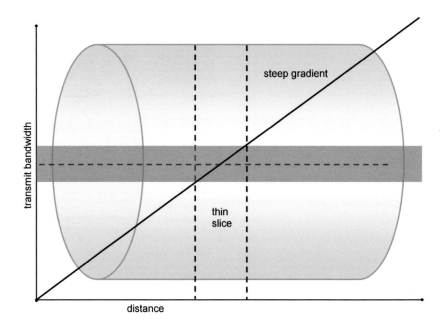

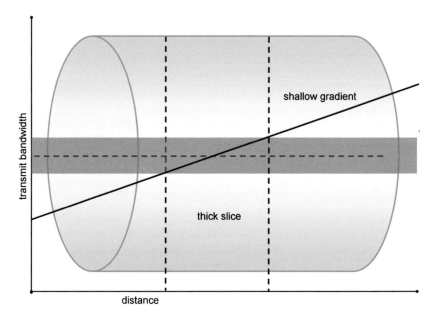

Figure 3.6 Transmit bandwidth, gradient slope and slice thickness.

Frequency encoding

Once a slice has been selected, the signal coming from it must be located along both axes of the image. The signal is usually located along the long axis of the anatomy by a process known as frequency encoding. When the frequency encoding gradient is switched on, the magnetic field strength

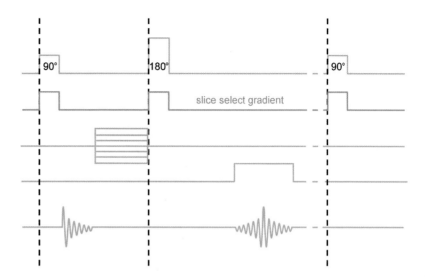

Figure 3.7 Timing of slice selection in a pulse sequence.

and therefore the precessional frequency of signal along the axis of the gradient is altered in a linear fashion. The gradient therefore produces a frequency difference or shift of signal along its axis. The signal can now be located along the axis of the gradient according to its frequency (Figure 3.8).

Learning point: the keyboard analogy

Within the echo many different frequencies are present. This is because initially spins with a range of frequencies are excited and rephased within each slice. This is what gives a slice its thickness. In addition, the phase encoding gradient produces a change of phase across the slice that remains when the gradient is switched off. Finally, the application of the frequency encoding gradient produces a change of frequency across the remaining axis of the slice. This frequency change depends on the spatial location of frequencies along the frequency encoding gradient.

In some ways the result is similar to a piano keyboard. Each key is tuned to produce a certain note when pressed. Different notes are characterized by the fact that they resonate a piano wire at different frequencies so that, for example, note A has a different frequency to note B. Each note has a different position or spatial location on the keyboard. Experienced pianists, on hearing a particular note, will know which key has been pressed and where on the keyboard it is located. In other words, they have spatially located that key by its frequency. This is the basis of spatial encoding.

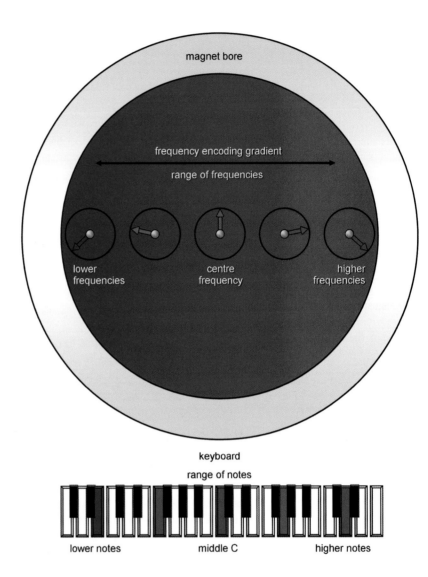

Figure 3.8 Frequency encoding.

The operator can select the direction of frequency encoding so that it encodes the signal along the long axis of the anatomy. It may help to refer back to the images in Chapter 2 to work out which gradient was used for each spatial encoding function. Always remember that the patient is usually lying supine along the Z-axis while lying on the table (in a superconducting system). Using this standard, it is easy to work out the long and short axis of the anatomy.

- In *coronal* and *sagittal* images, the long axis of the anatomy lies along the Z-axis of the magnet and therefore, the *Z gradient* performs frequency encoding.

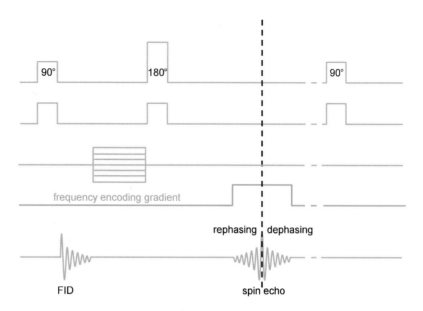

Figure 3.9 Timing of frequency encoding in a pulse sequence.

3

- In *axial* images, the long axis of the anatomy usually lies along the horizontal axis of the magnet and, therefore, the X *gradient* performs frequency encoding. However, in imaging of the head, the long axis of the anatomy usually lies along the anterior posterior axis of the magnet, so in this case, the Y gradient performs frequency encoding.

The frequency encoding gradient is switched on when the signal is received and is often called the **readout gradient**. The echo is usually centered in the middle of the frequency encoding gradient, so that the gradient is switched on during the rephasing and dephasing part of the echo and the peak (Figure 3.9). Typically, the frequency encoding gradient is switched on for 8 ms, during 4 ms of rephasing and 4 ms of dephasing of the echo. The steepness of the slope of the frequency encoding gradient determines the size of the anatomy covered along the frequency encoding axis during the scan. This is called the **field of view (FOV)**.

Phase encoding

The signal must now be located along the remaining short axis of the image and this localization of signal is called phase encoding. When the phase encoding gradient is switched on, the magnetic field strength and therefore the precessional frequency of nuclei along the axis of the gradient is altered. As the speed of precession of the nuclei changes, so does the accumulated phase of the magnetic moments along their precessional path. Nuclei that have sped up due to the presence of the gradient move further around their precessional path than if the gradients had not been applied. Nuclei that have slowed down due to the presence of the gradient move further back around their precessional path than if the gradient had not been applied.

Learning point: phase encoding and the watch analogy

The watch analogy referred in Chapter 1 is a very easy way of under-standing how phase encoding works. Imagine a watch telling the time of 12 o'clock and that this is equivalent to the phase of a magnetic moment of a nucleus experiencing B_0. When the phase encoding gradient is switched on, the magnetic field strength, precessional frequency, and phase of the magnetic moments of nuclei change according to their position along the gradient. Magnetic moments of nuclei experiencing a higher field strength gain phase, i.e. move fur-ther around the watch to say 4 o'clock, because they travel faster while the gradient is switched on. Magnetic moments of nuclei experien-cing a lower field strength lose phase, i.e. move back around the watch to say 8 o'clock, because they travel slower while the gradient is switched on. Magnetic moments of nuclei at isocentre do not experi-ence a changed field strength and their phase remains unchanged, i.e. 12 o'clock (Figure 3.10).

There is now a phase difference or shift between magnetic moments of nuclei positioned along the axis of the gradient. When the phase encoding gradient is switched off, the magnetic field strength experienced by the nuclei returns to the main field strength B_0 and therefore the precessional frequency of all the nuclei returns to the Larmor frequency. However, the phase difference between the nuclei remains. The nuclei travel at the same speed around their preces-sional paths, but their phases or positions on the watch are different because a gradient was previously switched on. This difference in phase between the nuclei is used to determine their position along the phase encoding gradient.

The phase encoding gradient is usually switched on just before the application of the 180° rephasing pulse (Figure 3.11). The steepness of the slope of the phase encoding gradient determines the degree of phase shift between two points along the gradient (Figure 3.12).

A steep phase encoding gradient causes a large phase shift between two points along the gradient, for example 8 o'clock and 4 o'clock, while a shallow phase encoding gradient causes a smaller phase shift between the

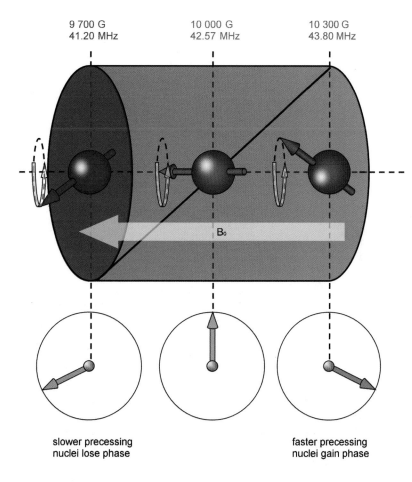

9 700 G
41.20 MHz

10 000 G
42.57 MHz

10 300 G
43.80 MHz

B_0

slower precessing
nuclei lose phase

faster precessing
nuclei gain phase

Figure 3.10 Phase encoding.

3

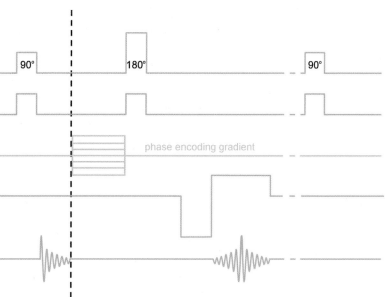

90°

180°

90°

phase encoding gradient

Figure 3.11 Timing of phase
encoding in a pulse sequence.

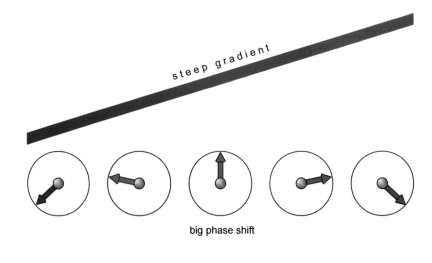

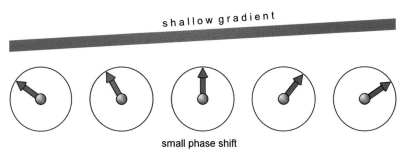

Figure 3.12 Steep and shallow phase gradients.

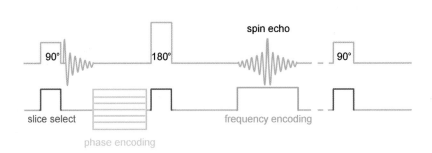

Figure 3.13 Gradient timing in a spin echo pulse sequence.

same two points along the gradient, for example 10 o'clock and 2 o'clock as shown in Figure 3.12.

Figure 3.13, Table 3.2 and the following list summarize the essential concepts of spatial encoding.

- The *phase encoding gradient* alters the phase along the remaining axis of the image, which is usually the short axis of the anatomy.

Table 3.2 Gradient axes in orthogonal imaging.

Plane	Slice selection	Frequency encoding	Phase encoding
Sagittal	X	Y	Z
Axial (body)	Z	Y	X
Axial (head)	Z	X	Y
Coronal	Y	X	Z

- In *coronal images* the short axis of the anatomy usually lies along the horizontal axis of the magnet and, therefore, the X *gradient* performs phase encoding.
- In *sagittal images* the short axis of the anatomy usually lies along the vertical axis of the magnet and, therefore, the Y *gradient* performs phase encoding.
- In *axial images*, the short axis of the anatomy usually lies along the vertical axis of the magnet and, therefore, the Y *gradient* performs phase encoding. However, when imaging the head, the short axis of the anatomy lies along the horizontal axis of the magnet and therefore the X gradient performs phase encoding.

3

Summary

- The slice select gradient is switched on during the 90° and 180° pulses in spin echo pulse sequences, and during the excitation pulse only in gradient echo pulse sequences
- The slope of the slice select gradient determines the slice thickness and slice gap (along with the transmit bandwidth)
- The phase encoding gradient is switched on just before the 180° pulse in spin echo, and between excitation and the signal collection in gradient echo
- The slope of the phase encoding gradient determines the degree of phase shift along the phase encoding axis. This determines the phase matrix (*see* later)
- The frequency encoding gradient is switched on during the collection of the signal
- The amplitude of the frequency encoding gradient determines the two dimensions of the FOV
- The timing of all these gradient functions during a pulse sequence is shown in Figure 3.13

Learning point: Using the watch analogy to understand spatial encoding

The watch analogy is a nice way of remembering how all gradients encode. Imagine two people wearing watches that are synchronized and tell perfect time. They walk into the MRI scan room for 15 minutes. The magnetic field of the scanner affects the timekeeping of the watches because it magnetizes the hands of the watches. The person standing nearest to the magnet is affected the most because the magnetic field here is strongest. The person standing furthest away is affected to a lesser degree because the magnetic field here is less strong.

If they then walk out of the room so they are no longer affected by the magnetic field, a stranger looking at their watches will be able to tell which person was standing nearer to the magnet and which was standing further away simply by looking at their watches. This is because the hands of the watch of the person standing closer to the magnet will be more out of phase from the synchronized time than the watch of the person standing further away. In other words, the stranger has used the frequency and phase shift of the hands of the watch, produced as a result of applying a magnetic field to the watches, to spatially encode the relative positions of each person while they were in the room.

Sampling

The frequency encoding gradient is switched on while the system reads frequencies present in the signal and samples or digitizes them. It is therefore sometimes called the readout gradient. The duration of the readout gradient is called the **sampling time** or **acquisition window**. During the sampling time, the system samples or digitizes frequencies up to 1024 different times (using current technology). The **sampling rate** *or* **sampling frequency** is the rate at which frequencies are sampled or digitized during readout. It determines how many samples are taken during readout.

Each sample is stored as a **data point**. Each data point contains information about the phase and frequency of signal at a particular point in time during readout. In MRI several data points are collected during the readout process. The number of these data points corresponds to the frequency matrix, i.e. if a frequency matrix of 256 is required, 256 data points must be collected for each slice every TR during readout. If the sampling time is 8 ms, and 256 data points are collected during this time, then frequencies in the signal are sampled once every 0.00003125 s or at sampling frequency of 32 000 Hz.

Learning point: sampling using the photograph analogy

This difficult concept is perhaps best understood by using the analogy of taking photographs. Imagine you have been asked to take several photographs of a runner completing a 100 m sprint race. Each photograph is a data point showing the position of the runner's arms and legs at particular points of the race. The time you have available to take the photographs is the length of the race, e.g. 10 s. This is equivalent to a sampling time of 10 s. The number of photographs taken during the race is equivalent to the number of data points. How fast you take the photographs is equivalent to the sampling rate and will determine how many you take during the race. For example, if you need to take 10 photographs during the race you must take one photograph per second for the whole 10 s of the race.

The sampling rate is stated by the **Nyquist theorem**, which tells us how fast to sample when several frequencies are to be digitized. This is relevant in MRI because an echo contains many different frequencies, some of which represent signal frequencies and some that represent noise (*see* Chapter 4). The Nyquist theorem states that when digitizing a signal with a range of analogue frequencies or bandwidth, the highest frequency must be sampled at least twice per cycle to accurately digitize or represent it. In other words, the sampling frequency must be at least twice the highest frequency in the signal.

Look at Figure 3.14. Sampling once per cycle or at the same frequency as the frequency we are trying to digitize results in a representation of a straight line or an absent frequency in the data (middle diagram). Sampling at less than once per cycle represents a completely incorrect frequency that leads to an artefact called **aliasing** (*see* Chapter 7). Sampling twice per cycle or at twice the frequency, we are trying to digitize results in correct representation of that frequency in the data (top diagram). As long as the highest frequency in the bandwidth is sampled twice it will be represented correctly in the data. Lower frequencies are sampled more often at the same sampling frequency and are also represented accurately in the data.

In addition, enough frequencies must occur during readout to achieve sufficient data points. This is determined by the **receive bandwidth**. The receive bandwidth is the range of frequencies we wish to sample or digitize during readout. The bandwidth is determined by applying a filter on the frequency encoding gradient. This is achieved by selecting the center frequency and defining the upper and lower limits of frequencies to be digitized on each side of the center frequency of the echo. The receive bandwidth therefore determines the number of frequencies available to be digitized during readout and it is proportional to the sampling rate or frequency.

By increasing the receive bandwidth, the difference between the highest and lowest frequencies we wish to sample is increased. To sample them

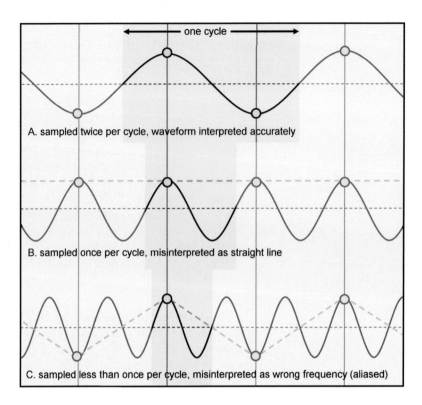

A. sampled twice per cycle, waveform interpreted accurately

B. sampled once per cycle, misinterpreted as straight line

C. sampled less than once per cycle, misinterpreted as wrong frequency (aliased)

Figure 3.14 The Nyquist theorem.

correctly, the sampling frequency must also be increased. If this does not occur, the lowest and highest frequencies are not represented in the image and an artefact called aliasing occurs (*see* Chapter 7). In addition, the sampling time is inversely proportional to the sampling frequency and to the receive bandwidth. Therefore if the receive bandwidth is reduced, the sampling time increases. This concept is explored in the following learning point.

Learning point: sampling and receive bandwidth

The receive bandwidth, frequency matrix and minimum TE we are permitted to select in a sequence are related to one another and have a significant impact on data acquisition. To understand this more clearly let us recap:

- The receive bandwidth determines the range or number frequencies we wish to digitize during readout,
- The frequency matrix determines the number of data points we must collect during readout,
- The minimum TE is affected by the sampling time because the echo is usually centered in the middle of the readout window, i.e. the peak of the echo corresponds the middle of the application

of the frequency encoding gradient. If the frequency encoding gradient is switched on for 8 ms (i.e. sampling time is 8 ms) then the peak of the echo occurs after 4 ms. If the sampling time is increased, the frequency encoding gradient is switched on for longer. Hence the peak of the echo occurs later, increasing the time from the peak of the echo to the RF excitation pulse that created it (i.e. TE increased). The opposite is true if the sampling time is decreased.

Suppose we wish to take 10 photographs of our runner in the 100 m race but with a camera that only takes a photograph every 2 s instead of every 1 s. We still require 10 photographs of the sprinter to work out exactly how he was running during the race. One option would be to take more photographs per second but in the context of MR, to do this would mean sampling more noise frequencies and would therefore be undesirable. The only ways to achieve this are either to make the race twice as long, i.e. a 200 m race that takes 20 s, or to ask the runner to run more slowly. The former is equivalent to doubling the sampling time; the latter is equivalent to reducing the receive bandwidth. The same would be true if we needed 20 photographs instead of 10. Assuming we are taking 1 photograph per second, to achieve this we either have to double the length of the race or ask the runner to run more slowly as before.

Using our previous example of a sampling time of 8 ms and a frequency matrix of 256, we need to sample at a frequency of 32 000 Hz (once every 0.00003125 s) to acquire 256 data points during the sampling time. According to the Nyquist theorem, this is twice the highest frequency in the receive bandwidth, so corresponds to a bandwidth of 16 000 Hz. If the receive bandwidth is halved to 8000 Hz, the sampling frequency also halves to 16 000 Hz. This means that in 8 ms, only 128 data points can be collected instead of the required 256. To collect the necessary data points at that bandwidth, the sampling time must be doubled to 16 ms and results in an 8 ms increase in the minimum permissible TE. For example, if the minimum TE was 10 ms using a bandwidth of 16 000 Hz and a frequency matrix of 256, by halving the receive bandwidth to 8000 Hz the minimum TE increases to 18 ms (Figure 3.15). There are occasions when changing the receive bandwidth is desirable and when the resultant change in TE becomes significant. These considerations are discussed later.

In addition, increasing the frequency matrix has the same effect. Again, using the example above, if the frequency matrix is increased to 512, then 512 data points are required and frequencies must be sampled 512 times during readout. If the receive bandwidth is maintained at 16 000 Hz then the sampling time and therefore the minimum TE must be increased to attain the required number of data points. Table 3.3 outlines this more clearly. The default is shown in the top line where a sampling time of 8 ms is used with a 32 KHz bandwidth when acquiring a frequency matrix of 256. If the bandwidth is halved, not enough data points are acquired (128 instead of the required 256). To solve this, the sampling time is doubled to 16 ms, which increases the TE by 8 ms (as the peak of the echo is situated in the middle of the acquisition window as shown in Figure 3.15). The same occurs if a frequency matrix of 512 is required. The sampling time must be doubled to acquire 512 data points. This also increases the TE.

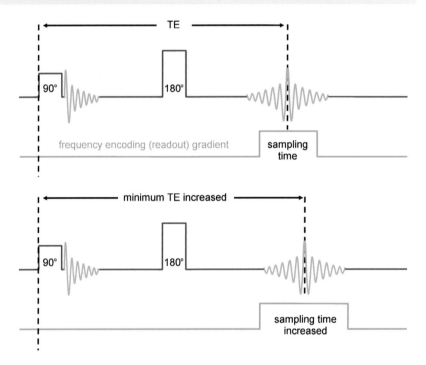

Figure 3.15 Sampling time and the TE.

Table 3.3 Receive bandwidth, sampling time and frequency matrix.

Frequency matrix	Receive bandwidth	Sampling time
256	32 KHz	8 ms
128	16 KHz	8 ms
256	16 KHz	16 ms
512	32 KHz	16 ms

Summary

- Sampling frequency is proportional to the receive bandwidth
- Sampling time is inversely proportional to the sampling frequency and the receive bandwidth

DATA COLLECTION AND IMAGE FORMATION

Introduction

The application of all the gradients selects an individual slice and produces a frequency shift along one axis of the slice, and a phase shift along the other. The system can now locate an individual signal within the image by measuring the number of times the magnetic moments cross the receiver coil (frequency) and their position around their precessional path (phase). This information now has to be translated on to the image. When data of each signal position are collected, the information is stored as data points in the array processor of the system computer. The data points are stored in **K space**.

K space description

Figure 3.16 illustrates K space for one slice. K space is rectangular in shape and has two axes perpendicular to each other. The frequency axis of K space is horizontal and is centered in the middle of several horizontal lines. The phase axis of K space is vertical and is centered in the middle of

3

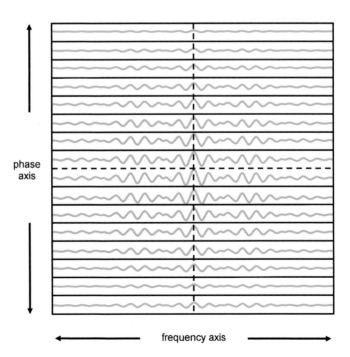

phase axis

frequency axis

Figure 3.16   K space – axes.

K space perpendicular to the frequency axis. K space is a spatial frequency domain, i.e. where information about the frequency of a signal and where it comes from in the patient is stored. In other words, it is where information of frequencies in space or distance is stored. Frequency is defined as phase change over distance (or over time in other contexts) and is measured in radians (a unit of degrees in a circle). The unit of K space is therefore radians per cm.

Learning point: the chest of drawers

K space is analogous to a chest of drawers. Look at Figure 3.17 in which K space with its lines parallel to the phase axis are illustrated. These lines look like drawers in a chest of drawers, which, like K space, is a storage device. The number of drawers corresponds to the number of lines of K space that must be filled with data points to complete the scan. The number of lines or drawers to be filled equals the phase matrix selected, i.e. if a phase matrix of 256 is selected then 256 lines or drawers must be filled with data points to complete the scan. As we will see shortly, the number of data points in each line or drawer corresponds to the frequency matrix selected. The chest of drawers analogy is referred to many times in this book. Look out for the chest of drawers symbol in the margin.

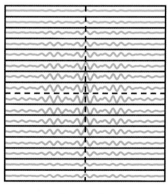
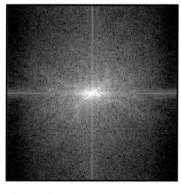
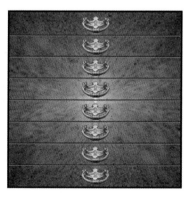

diagramatic   data   the chest of drawers

Figure 3.17 K space – the chest of drawers.
Note: this is K space for **one** slice. If 10 slices are selected, there are **10** areas of K space, or 10 chests of drawers.

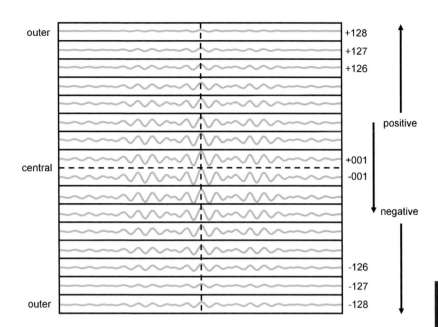

Figure 3.18 K space characteristics.

3

K space filling

Lines of K space are usually numbered with the lowest number near to the central axis (e.g. lines +/– 1,2,3) and the highest numbers towards the outer edges (e.g. +/– 128,127,126) (Figure 3.18). The lines in the top half of K space are called positive lines, those in the bottom half are called negative lines. This is because the line to be filled with data in a given TR is determined by the polarity and slope of the phase gradient. As previously discussed, the phase gradient is altered every TR. This is necessary to fill different lines of K space with data. If the phase encoding gradient is not changed, then the same line is filled every TR. As the number of lines filled determines the phase matrix, not changing the phase encoding gradient results in an image with only one pixel in the phase direction of the image. Therefore we need to alter both the polarity and the slope of the phase gradient every TR to give the image resolution in the phase direction.

The phase gradient therefore picks which line of K space or which drawer is filled with data in a particular TR period. Positive polarity phase gradients pick lines in the top half of K space; negative polarity gradients pick lines in the bottom half. In addition, the slope of the phase gradient determines which line is selected. Steep gradients, both positive and negative, select the most **outer lines** while shallow gradients select the **central lines**. As the slope of the phase gradient decreases from its steepest amplitude, so the lines through K space are stepped down from the most outer lines to the more central lines (Figure 3.19). Usually K space is filled in a linear fashion from top to bottom or bottom to top, although as we will

3

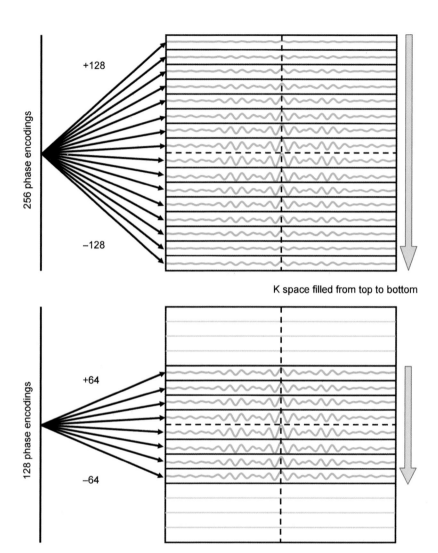

Figure 3.19 K space – phase matrix and the number of drawers.

see later, there are many different permutations. Using the linear filling model and the chest of drawers analogy, let us look more closely at exactly what happens during a pulse sequence.

Look at Figure 3.20 showing a typical spin echo sequence. The top half of the diagram shows when gradients are applied to each slice during the pulse sequence. The bottom half shows the equivalent areas of K space, drawn as a chests of drawers.

The slice select gradient is applied during the excitation and rephasing pulses to selectively excite and rephase a slice. The slope of the slice select gradient determines which slice is excited, or which chest of drawers is to be selected. Each slice has its own area of K space, or chest of drawers. Although 3 chests of drawers are shown in Figure 3.20, they do not represent K space for 3 separate slices in this diagram. In Figure 3.20, each chest of drawers represents the *same* slice at 3 different times in the sequence when each of the 3 gradients are switched on.

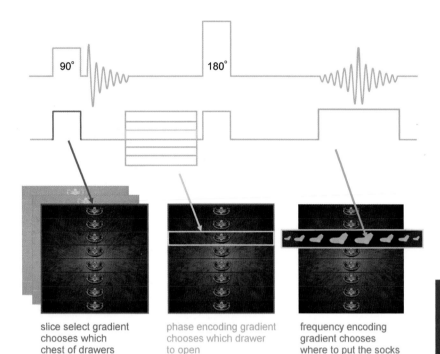

Figure 3.20 K space filling in a spin echo sequence.

slice select gradient chooses which chest of drawers

phase encoding gradient chooses which drawer to open

frequency encoding gradient chooses where to put the socks

3

The phase encoding gradient is then applied. This determines which line, or drawer, to fill with data. Normally, K space is filled linearly, with line +128 filled first (assuming a 256 phase matrix has been selected), followed by line +127, and so on. In Figure 3.20, lines + 128 and + 127 have already been filled, so the next line to be filled is line + 126. To open this drawer, the phase encoding gradient must be applied positively and steeply, corresponding to line + 126. Application of this gradient selects line +126 in K space.

The frequency encoding gradient is now switched on. The amplitude of this determines the FOV. During application of the frequency encoding gradient, frequencies in the echo are digitized to acquire data points which fill the line of K space selected by the phase encoding gradient. These data points are laid out in a line of K space (or in a drawer in the chest of drawers) during the sampling time, usually from left to right. In Figure 3.20, data points are represented as socks being put away in each drawer. The number of data points collected determines the frequency matrix of the image, e.g. 256. When sampling is completed, the frequency encoding gradient switches off and the slice select is applied again, to a different amplitude than before to excite and rephase the next slice. This is equivalent to walking up to another chest of drawers (not shown in Figure 3.20).

The phase encoding gradient is applied again to the same polarity and amplitude as for slice 1, filling line +126 for chest of drawers or slice 2. The process is repeated for all slices, with line +126 being filled for each area of K space or each chest of drawers. All of this happens within the TR period. This is why the TR determines how many slices are permitted. Longer TRs result in more time to individually excite, rephase, phase and frequency encode slices. If the TR is short there is less time so fewer slices are possible.

Once line +126 has been filled for all slices, the TR is repeated. The slice gradient again selects chest of drawers 1, but this time a different line of K space or a different drawer is filled from that filled in the previous TR period. If the linear K space filling model is utilized, line +125 is filled (or the next drawer down from line +126). In order to do this, the phase encoding gradient must be switched on positively again but less steeply than in the previous TR period. This opens drawer +125 and when read-out occurs, data points are laid out in that drawer during application of the frequency encoding gradient. When this has been completed, the slice select gradient is applied again to select slice 2. The same amplitude and polarity of phase gradient is applied to open drawer +125 for slice or chest of drawers 2. This process is repeated for all slices.

As the pulse sequence continues, every TR the phase encoding amplitude is gradually decreased to step down through the lines of K space. To fill the bottom lines the phase gradient is switched negatively and gradually increased every TR to progressively fill the outer lines. If a 256 phase matrix has been selected, once lines +128 to −128 have been filled the scan is over. This is the most common type of K space filling method, although there are many others. These are discussed later. The process of data acquisition results in a grid of data points. The number of data points horizontally in each line equals the frequency matrix, e.g. 512 or 256; the number of data points vertically corresponds to the phase matrix selected e.g. 64, 128, 256, 384 or 512 (Figure 3.21).

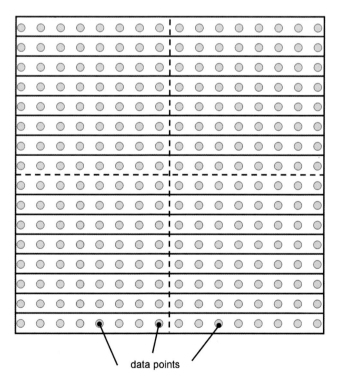

Figure 3.21 Data points.

data points

Learning point: an important fact about K space

It is very important to understand that K space is not the image. That is to say, data stored in the top line do not end up being the top of the image. Each data point contains information for the *whole* slice as the frequencies that represent it come from the *whole* echo and the echo comes from the whole slice.

To produce an image from the acquired data points we need to complete a mathematical process called **Fast Fourier transform** *or* **FFT**.

Fast Fourier transform (FFT)

The mathematics of FFT are well beyond the scope of this book but are described in its basic context here. An MR image consists of a matrix of pixels, the number of which is determined by the number of lines filled in K space (phase matrix) and the number of data points in each line (frequency matrix). As a result of FFT, each pixel is allocated a color on a grayscale corresponding to the amplitude of specific frequencies coming from the same spatial location as represented by that pixel. Each data point contains phase and frequency information from the whole slice at a particular moment in time during readout. In other words, frequency amplitudes are represented in the time domain. The FFT process mathematically converts this to frequency amplitudes in the frequency domain. This is necessary because gradients spatially locate signal according to their frequency, not their time.

Learning point: FFT and the keyboard analogy

Look at Figure 3.22. In the top diagram there is one frequency represented decaying over *time*. The FFT process converts this single frequency to show its *amplitude*. In the bottom diagram two frequencies are represented and FFT converts them into their separate amplitudes. The MR signal contains many different frequencies. In addition to this, each frequency has a different amplitude depending on whether the tissue it comes from is returning high or low signal intensity. Using the keyboard analogy previously described, an MR signal is a chord where several frequencies or notes are played at once. In addition each key is pressed to a different degree – some are pressed softly, others are pressed hard. The soft keys are analogous to frequencies in tissues returning a low signal, the hard keys to frequencies returning a high signal. By sampling the frequencies in the MR signal and performing FFT, the MR system can tell exactly which keys have been pressed and how hard they have been pressed. In other words, it has converted frequencies in the echo decaying over time into different frequencies and their relative amplitudes.

As the FFT process deals in frequencies the system must be able to convert the phase shift information produced as a result of applying the phase encoding gradient into a frequency. This is not as difficult as it sounds. The watch analogy explains how frequency is a change of phase over time or distance. By applying the phase encoding gradient over a distance across the bore of the magnet, a change of phase over distance is produced. This is extrapolated as a frequency by creating a sine wave formed by connecting all the phase values associated with a certain phase shift (Figure 3.23). This sine wave has a frequency or **pseudo-frequency**

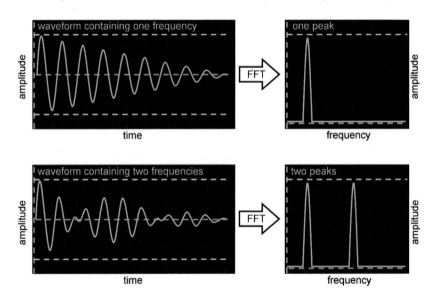

Figure 3.22 Fast Fourier transform.

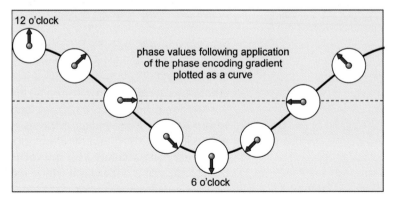

Figure 3.23 The phase curve.

steep phase encoding gradient, pseudo-frequency 1

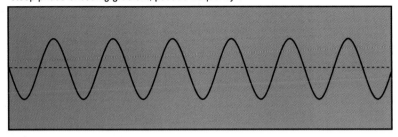

shallow phase encoding gradient, pseudo-frequency 2

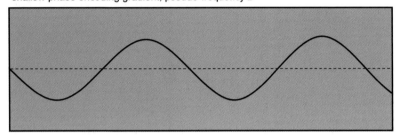

Figure 3.24
Pseudo-frequencies.

3

(as it has been indirectly obtained) that depends on the degree of phase shift produced by the gradient. Steep phase encoding gradients produce large phase shifts across a given distance in the patient and result in high pseudo-frequencies, while low amplitude phase gradients produce small phase shifts across the same distance and result in low pseudo-frequencies (Figure 3.24). There are some significant implications from this in optimizing image quality. These are discussed later.

Learning point: why does the phase gradient have to change?

You will remember that we need to change the amplitude of the phase encoding gradient to fill different lines of K space and therefore give resolution to our image. Another way of looking at this is that by changing the phase gradient and therefore the pseudo-frequency, the data 'look different' than in the previous TR period. This is how the system knows to place these data points in a new line of K space. If the data looked the same every TR, then the system would place the data in the same line every TR and the resultant image would have a resolution of only 1 pixel in the phase direction.

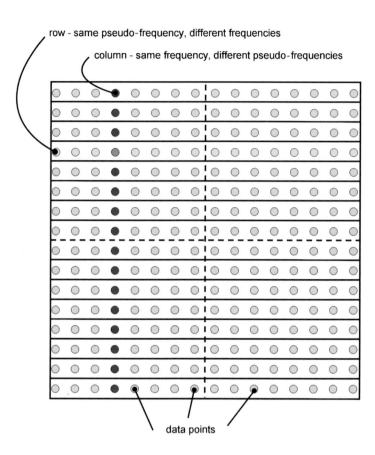

row - same pseudo-frequency, different frequencies

column - same frequency, different pseudo-frequencies

data points

Figure 3.25 Columns and rows in K space.

Therefore before FFT each data point contains frequency information from frequency encoding and pseudo-frequency information from phase encoding.

- In each *line* of K space the pseudo-frequency data in each data point are unchanged because they result from a particular slope of phase encoding gradient. The frequency data, however, are different in each data point as each data point was acquired at a different time during readout when the frequency encoding gradient was on.
- In each *column* of K space the frequency data are unchanged because each data point in the column was acquired at the same time during readout. The pseudo-frequency data, however, are different because each data point was acquired with a different slope of phase encoding gradient (Figure 3.25).

The FFT process differentiates these different types of data in two dimensions (i.e. horizontally across each line and vertically down each column). It then converts the data into signal amplitude vs its frequency and is therefore able to calculate the grayscale associated with every pixel in the two-dimensional matrix of the image, i.e. if a signal with a discrete value of frequency and pseudo-frequency at a certain spatial location has a high amplitude it is allocated a bright pixel. If a signal with a discrete value of frequency and pseudo-frequency at a certain spatial location has a low amplitude it is allocated a dark pixel. This process is completed for every area of K space, chest of drawers or slice and displays the image on the operator's monitor (Figure 3.25).

Important facts about K space

(1) *K space is not the image.* In other words, data points in the top line of K space do not result in the top of the image. In fact every data point contains information from the whole slice.

(2) *Data are symmetrical in K space.* This means that data in the top half of K space are identical to those in the bottom half. This is because the slope of phase gradient required to select a particular line in one half of K space is identical to that required to select the same line on the opposite side of K space. Although the polarity of the gradient is different, because the slope is the same, the pseudo-frequency in each line is also the same (Figure 3.26). In addition, data on the left side of K space are identical to those on the right. This is because as data points are laid out in a line during readout they are placed sequentially from left to right as the echo is rephasing, reaching its peak and dephasing, with the peak of the echo corresponding to the central vertical axis of K space. As echoes are symmetrical features, frequency data digitized from the echo are the same on one side as they are on the other (Figure 3.27). The resultant symmetry is called **conjugate symmetry** and is used to reduce scan times in many imaging options (see later).

3

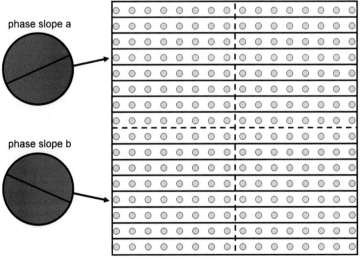

phase slope a

positive

phase slope b

negative

phase slope and therefore
pseudo-frequency the same
for these two lines of data

Figure 3.26 K space symmetry – phase.

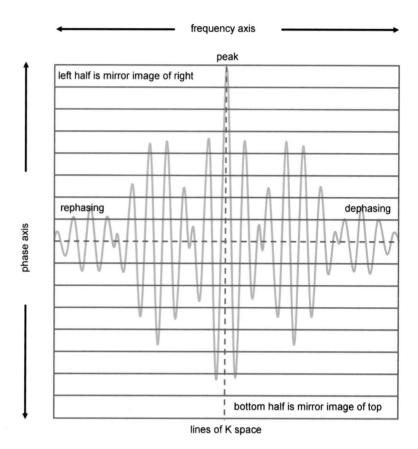

Figure 3.27 K space symmetry – frequency.

(3) Data acquired in the central lines contribute signal and contrast while data acquired in the outer lines contribute resolution. As previously described, the central lines of K space are filled using shallow phase encoding slopes and the outer lines are filled using steep phase encoding slopes. Shallow slopes result in low pseudo-frequencies because of small phase shifts. To produce signal the magnetic moments of nuclei must be coherent or in phase. By minimizing phase shifts, the resultant signal has a high signal amplitude and contributes largely to signal and contrast in the image. Steep slopes result in high pseudo-frequencies because of large phase shifts. The resultant signal therefore has relatively low signal amplitude and does not contribute signal and contrast in the image (Figure 3.28). However, large phase shifts mean that two points close together in the patient are likely to have a phase difference and will therefore be differentiated from each other. Therefore outer lines of K space, while not contributing signal, provide resolution. Conversely, central lines, which are filled as a result of small phase shifts, do not provide resolution as two points close together in the patient are unlikely to have different phase values and therefore cannot be differentiated from each other.

To summarize:

- The *central* portion of K space contains data that have *high signal* amplitude and *low resolution*.

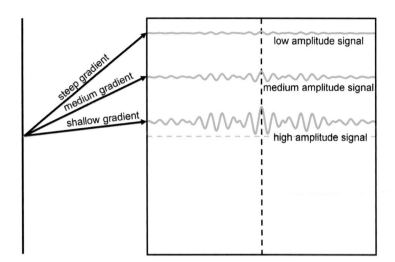

Figure 3.28 Phase gradient amplitude versus signal amplitude.

- The *outer* portion of K space contains data that have *low signal amplitude* and *high resolution*.

Signal and resolution are important image quality factors and are discussed in Chapter 4. If all K space is filled during an acquisition then both signal and resolution are obtained and displayed in the image. However, as we will see later, there are many different permutations of K space filling whereby the relative proportion of central to outer lines filled is altered. Under these circumstances image quality can be significantly affected. It is also worth noting that when the phase matrix is reduced the outer lines are dropped and the central lines of K space are still filled with data. For example, if the phase matrix is reduced to 128 then lines +64 to −64 are filled which are the signal producing lines of K space, rather than fill lines +128 to zero (Figure 3.29). This is because as a general rule signal is more important than resolution in the image. When resolution is also required, this is achieved by increasing the proportion of outer lines that contain resolution data.

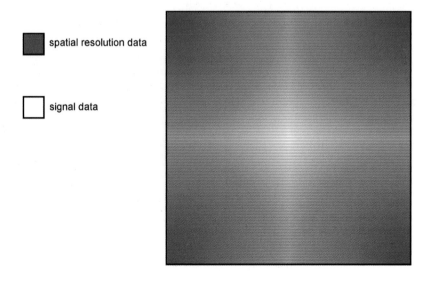

Figure 3.29 K space – signal and resolution.

Learning point: K space, resolution and signal

Figure 3.30 shows an image acquired using all K space. Both resolution and signal are seen on the image. Figure 3.31 illustrates what happens if an image is created out of data from the outer edges of K space. This image has good resolution in that the detail of the hair and eyes are well shown but there is very little signal. Figure 3.32 shows what happens if an image is created from data in the center of K space only. The resultant image has excellent signal but poor resolution. This example also demonstrates that K space is not the image. If it were, the image in Figure 3.31 would lose its nose and Figure 3.32 would show only the nose. Both images, however, show all the image, even though only a small percentage of the total number of data points in K space was used in their creation.

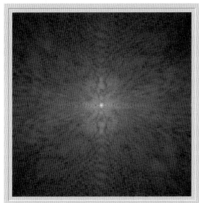 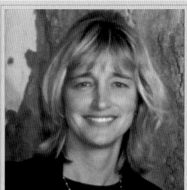

Figure 3.30   K space using all data.

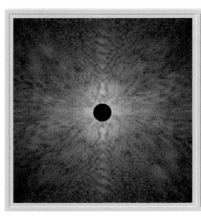 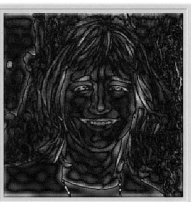

Figure 3.31   K space using resolution data only.

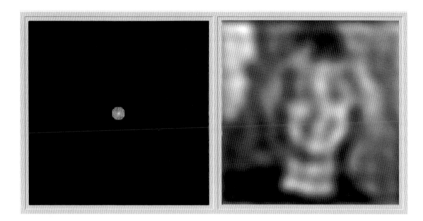

Figure 3.32 K space using signal data only.

(4) *The scan time is the time to fill K space.* The parameters that affect scan time in a typical acquisition are:

- repetition time (TR)
- phase matrix
- number of excitations (NEX).

Repetition time. Every *TR* each slice is selected, phase encoded and frequency encoded. Slices are not selected together but sequentially, i.e. slice 1 is selected and encoded and frequencies from its echo digitized. Then the next slice is selected, encoded and digitized and so on. This is why the maximum number of slices available depends on the TR. Longer TRs allow more slices to be selected, encoded and digitized than short TRs. A TR of, say, 500 ms may allow for 15 slices, while a TR of 2000 ms may allow for 40 slices.

3

Learning point: what is the TR?

It is important to understand that although the TR is defined as the time between excitation pulses it is NOT the time between each excitation pulse, i.e. the time between exciting slice 1 and 2, etc. It is the time between exciting a particular slice and then exciting it again to fill another line of K space. In other words, it is the time between filling 1 line of K space for a particular slice and filling the next line down in the same area of K space (Figure 3.33). This is why the TR is one of the parameters that governs scan time.

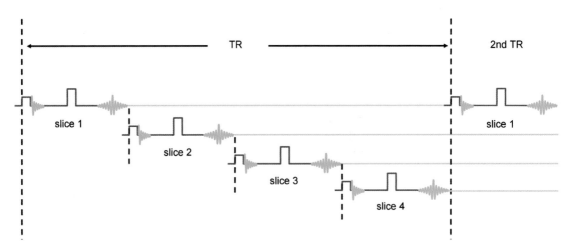

Figure 3.33 TR versus number of slices.

3

The *phase matrix* determines the number of lines that must be filled to complete the scan. As one line is filled per TR (in a typical pulse sequence) then if:

- A phase matrix of 128 is selected, 128 lines are filled and 128 TRs must be completed to finish the scan.
- A phase matrix of 256 is selected, 256 lines are filled and 256 TRs must be completed to finish the scan.

The *number of excitations* or *NEX* (also known as the **number of signal averages** or acquisitions, depending on manufacturer) is the number of times each line is filled with data. The signal can be sampled more than once by maintaining the same slope of phase gradient over several TRs instead of changing it every TR. In this way the same line of K space is filled several times, so that each line of K space contains more data. As there are more data in each line, the resultant image has a higher signal to noise ratio (see Chapter 4) but the scan time is proportionally longer.

For example:

TR 1000 ms, phase matrix 256, 1 NEX scan time = 256 s
TR 1000 ms, phase matrix 256, 2 NEX scan time = 512 s

Usually to fill each line more than once, the same slope of phase encoding gradient is used over two or more successive TRs, rather than filling all the lines once from +128 to −128 and then returning to repeat the process again.

Learning point: K space and scan time

Using the chest of drawers analogy:

- The TR is the time between filling the top drawer of a chest of drawers 1 and filling the next drawer down in a chest of drawers 1. During that time the top drawer in chest of drawers, 2, 3, 4, etc. are filled sequentially.
- The phase matrix is the number of drawers in each chest of drawers.
- The NEX is the number of times each drawer is filled e.g. once, twice, three times, etc.
- The scan is over when all the drawers in all the chest of drawers are full with the required amount of data.

K space traversal and gradients

3

The way in which K space is traversed and filled depends on a combination of the polarity and amplitude of both the frequency and phase encoding gradients.

- The amplitude of the *frequency* encoding gradient determines how far to the *left and right* K space is traversed (or how wide the chest of drawers are) and this in turn determines the size of the FOV in the frequency direction of the image.
- The amplitude of the *phase* encoding gradient determines how far *up and down* a line of K space is filled (or how high the chest of drawers are) and in turn determines the size of the FOV in the phase direction of the image (or the spatial resolution when the FOV is square).

The polarity of each gradient defines the direction traveled through K space as follows:

- *frequency* encoding gradient *positive*, K space traversed from *left to right*
- *frequency* encoding gradient *negative*, K space traversed from *right to left*
- *phase* encoding gradient *positive*, fills *top half* of K space
- *phase* encoding gradient *negative*, fills *bottom half* of K space.

In addition, the RF pulse portion of a pulse sequence also defines movement through K space. For example, an excitation pulse always takes us to the center of K space.

K space filling and gradients are best described using an illustration of a typical gradient echo sequence (Figure 3.34). In a gradient echo sequence the frequency encoding gradient switches negatively to forcibly dephase the FID and then positively to rephase and produce a gradient echo (*see*

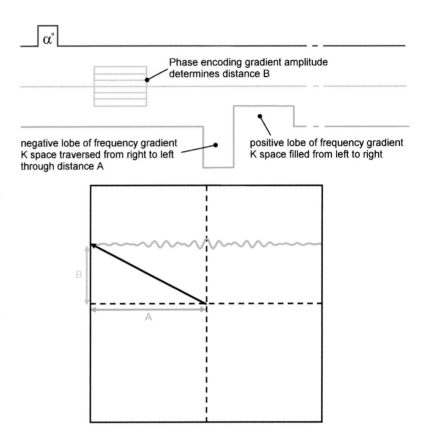

Figure 3.34 How gradients traverse K space.

Phase encoding gradient amplitude determines distance B

negative lobe of frequency gradient K space traversed from right to left through distance A

positive lobe of frequency gradient K space filled from left to right

Figure 5.22). When the frequency encoding gradient is negative, K space is traversed from right to left. The starting point of K space filling is at the center because the pulse sequence begins with an excitation pulse.

K space is traversed from the center to the left, to a distance (A) that depends on the amplitude of the negative lobe of the frequency encoding gradient. The phase encode in this example is positive and therefore a line in the top half of K space is filled. The amplitude of this gradient determines the distance traveled (B). The larger the amplitude of the phase gradient, the higher up in K space is the line that is filled with data from the echo. Therefore the combination of the phase gradient and the negative lobe of the frequency gradient determine at what point in K space data storage begins.

The frequency encoding gradient is then switched positively and during its application data are sampled from the echo. As the frequency encoding gradient is positive, data are placed in a line of K space from left to right. The distance traveled depends on the amplitude of the positive lobe of the gradient and determines the size of the FOV. This is only one example of how K space may be filled. If the phase gradient is negative then a line in the bottom half of K space is filled in exactly the same manner as above. K space traversal in spin echo sequences is more complex as the 180° RF pulse moves us through K space to the opposite side in both directions.

Options that fill K space

The way in which K space is filled depends on how the data are acquired and can be manipulated to suit the circumstances of the scan. This is especially true when reducing scan times. K space filling is manipulated in the following:

- rectangular field of view (Chapter 4)
- anti-aliasing (Chapter 7)
- fast spin echo sequences (Chapter 5)
- keyhole imaging (Chapter 5)
- respiratory compensation (Chapter 7)
- parallel imaging (Chapter 5)
- single shot and echo planar imaging (Chapter 5).

The K space filling associated with the above options is discussed in the relevant chapters and these are summarized in Table 3.4. However, it is appropriate here to describe two other options that use altered K space filling. These are:

- partial echo imaging
- partial or fractional averaging or half Fourier.

3

Partial echo imaging

Partial echo imaging is performed when only part of the signal or echo is read during application of the frequency encoding gradient. As previously described, the peak of the echo or signal is usually centered in the middle of the readout gradient. For example, if the frequency encoding gradient is switched on for 8 ms, frequencies are digitized during 4 ms of rephasing and 4 ms of dephasing. This signal is mapped relative to the frequency axis of K space and the left half of the frequency area of K space is the mirror image of the right half. Therefore, data placed in the left half of the frequency area of K space look like those in the right half. If the system only samples half the echo, only half of the frequency area of K space is filled. However, as the remaining is a mirror image, the system can calculate its amplitude accordingly. This filling of only half the area of K space along the frequency axis is called **partial or fractional echo.**

The echo no longer has to be centered on the middle of the frequency encoding gradient, as it can now occur at the beginning of the frequency encoding gradient application. In partial echo imaging the sampling window is shifted during readout so that only the peak and the dephasing part of the echo are sampled. As the peak of the echo occurs closer to the RF excitation pulse, the TE can be reduced when partial echo imaging is performed. In most systems, partial echo imaging is routinely used when a TE of less than 20 ms is selected. The use of a very short TE allows for maximum T1 and proton density weighting and slice number for a given TR (Figure 3.35).

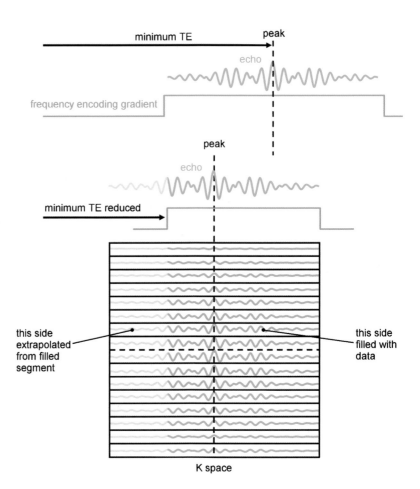

Figure 3.35   Partial echo.

Partial, fractional averaging or half Fourier

The negative and positive halves of K space on each side of the phase axis are symmetrical and a mirror image of each other. As long as at least half of the lines of K space that have been selected are filled during the acquisition, the system has enough data to produce an image. For example, if only 75% of K space is filled, only 75% of the phase encoding selected needs to be performed to complete the scan, and the remaining lines are filled with zeros (Figure 3.36). The scan time is therefore reduced.

256 phase encodings, 1 NEX and TR of 1 s are selected.

Scan time $= 256 \times 1 \times 1$
        $= 256$ s

256 phase encodings, 0.75 NEX and TR of 1 s are selected. Only 75% of K space is filled with data during the scan. The rest is filled with zeros.

Scan time $= 256 \times 0.75 \times 1$
        $= 192$ s

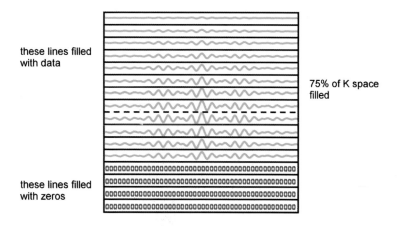

these lines filled with data

75% of K space filled

these lines filled with zeros

Figure 3.36 Partial Fourier.

Table 3.4 K space filling options.

Option	Resolution	SNR	Scan time	Purpose
Partial averaging	same	less	less	reduce time when SNR is good
Partial echo	same	same	same	automatic for a short TE
Rectangular FOV	same	less	less	reduce time when anatomy is rectangular
Anti-aliasing	same	same	same	to eliminate aliasing
Fast spin echo	same	same	less	reduce scan time
Keyhole imaging	same	same	less	for temporal resolution and SNR
Respiratory compensation	same	same	slightly more	reduce respiratory artefact
Parallel imaging	same	same	less	reduce scan time
	more	same	same	increase resolution

The scan time is reduced but fewer data are acquired so the image has less signal. **Partial averaging** can be used where a reduction in scan time is necessary, and where the resultant signal loss is not of paramount importance.

Types of acquisition

There are basically three ways of acquiring data:

- sequential
- two-dimensional volumetric
- three-dimensional volumetric.

Sequential acquisitions acquire all the data from slice 1 and then go on to acquire all the data from slice 2, (all the lines in K space are filled for slice 1 and then all the lines of K space are filled for slice 2, etc.). The slices are therefore displayed as they are acquired (not unlike computerized tomography scanning).

Two-dimensional volumetric acquisitions fill one line of K space for slice 1, and then go on to fill the same line of K space for slice 2, etc. When this line has been filled for all the slices, the next line of K space is filled for slice 1, 2, 3, etc. This is the most common type of data acquisition.

Learning point: acquisition type and the chest of drawers

Let us go back to the chest of drawers analogy to explain the different types of acquisition. Imagine three chest drawers representing three slices in our acquisition.

- Sequential acquisition is one in which we would fill all the drawers for chest of drawers 1 before going on to chest of drawers 2. This is a type of acquisition that might be used for breath-holding techniques.
- Two-dimensional volumetric acquisition is one where we would fill the top drawer in each of the three chests of drawers in one TR and then, in the next TR, fill the next drawer down in each of the three chests of drawers. This is the most typical type of acquisition and the one we have assumed for many explanations in this chapter (Figure 3.37).

Three-dimensional volumetric acquisition (volume imaging) acquires data from an entire volume of tissue, rather than in separate slices. The excitation pulse is not slice selective, and the whole prescribed imaging volume is excited. At the end of the acquisition the volume or slab is divided into discrete locations or partitions by the slice select gradient that, when switched on, separates the slices according to their phase value along the gradient. This process is now called **slice encoding**. Many slices can be obtained, (typically 28, 64 or 128) without a slice gap. In other words, the slices are contiguous. The advantages of volume imaging are discussed in more detail in Chapter 4.

This chapter has introduced the basic mechanisms of gradients. A more detailed discussion, including high-speed gradient systems and their applications, is to be found in Chapter 9.

As data acquisition and image formation have now been explored, the parameters available to the operator and how they interact with each other are described in the next chapter.

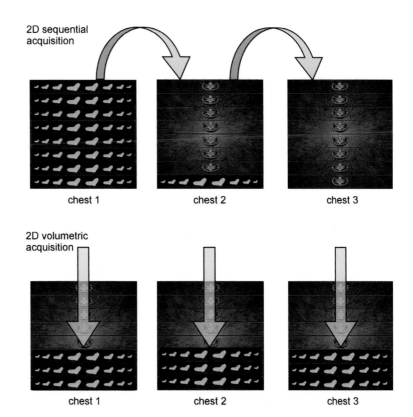

Figure 3.37 Data acquisition methods.

3

Questions

1 What controls the polarity of a gradient?

2 What factor does the frequency encoding gradient slope control?

3 What operator function alters the number of data points in K space?

4 What are the units of K space?

5 What happens if frequencies are insufficiently sampled?

6 Which area of K space contributes resolution?

7 In which direction is K space traversal when frequency encoding is positive?

4

Parameters and trade-offs

Introduction

There are many parameters available to the operator when setting up a sequence. The choice of pulse sequence determines the weighting and the quality of the images and their sensitivity to pathology. The timing parameters selected specifically determine the weighting of the images. As previously discussed:

- TR determines the amount of T1 and proton density weighting
- Flip angle controls the amount of T1 and proton density weighting
- TE controls the amount of T2 weighting.

The quality of the images is controlled by many factors. It is very important that the operator is aware of these factors and how they interrelate, so that the optimal image quality can always be obtained. The four main considerations determining image quality are:

- signal to noise ratio (SNR)
- contrast to noise ratio (CNR)
- spatial resolution
- scan time.

Signal to noise ratio (SNR)

The **signal to noise ratio** is the ratio of the amplitude of the signal received to the average amplitude of the noise.

- The **signal** is the voltage induced in the receiver coil by the precession of the NMV in the transverse plane.
- The **noise** represents frequencies that exist randomly in space and time. It is equivalent to the hiss on a radio when the station is not tuned in properly, and some of it is energy left over from the 'Big Bang'. In the MR context, noise is generated by the presence of the patient in the magnet, and the background electrical noise of the system. The noise is constant for every patient and depends on the build of the patient, the area under examination and the inherent noise of the system.

Noise occurs at all frequencies and is also random in time and space. The signal, however, is cumulative, occurs at time TE, depends on many factors and can be altered. The signal is therefore increased or decreased relative to the noise. Increasing the signal increases the SNR, while decreasing the signal decreases the SNR. Therefore, any factor that affects the signal amplitude in turn affects the SNR. The factors that affect the SNR include:

- magnetic field strength of the system
- proton density of the area under examination
- voxel volume
- TR, TE and flip angle
- NEX
- receive bandwidth
- coil type.

4

Magnetic field strength

The magnetic field strength plays an important part in determining SNR. As described in Chapter 1, as the field strength increases so does the energy gap between high- and low-energy nuclei. As the energy gap increases, fewer nuclei have enough energy to align their magnetic moments in opposition to B_0. Therefore the number of spin-up nuclei increases relative to the number of spin-down nuclei. The NMV therefore increases in size at higher field strengths and as a result there is more available magnetization to image the patient. SNR therefore increases. Although the magnetic field strength cannot be altered, when imaging with low field systems, SNR may be compromised and steps may have to be taken to boost the SNR that are not necessary when using high field systems. This usually manifests itself in longer scan times.

Proton density

The number of protons in the area under examination determines the amplitude of signal received. Areas of low proton density (such as the lungs) have low signal and therefore low SNR, while areas with a high proton density (such as the pelvis) have high signal and therefore high SNR. The proton density of a tissue is inherent to that tissue and cannot be changed (that is why it is an intrinsic contrast parameter, as discussed in Chapter 2). However, as the SNR is likely to be compromised when imaging areas of low proton density, steps may have to be taken to boost the SNR that are not necessary when scanning areas with a high proton density.

Voxel volume

The building unit of a digital image is a pixel. The brightness of the pixel represents the strength of the MRI signal generated by a unit volume of patient tissue (**voxel**). The voxel represents a volume of tissue within the patient, and is determined by the pixel area and the slice thickness (Figure 4.1). The pixel area is determined by the size of the FOV and the number of pixels in the FOV or matrix. Therefore:

pixel area = FOV dimensions ÷ matrix size

A **coarse matrix** is one with a low number of frequency encodings and/or phase encodings and results in a low number of pixels in the FOV. A

4

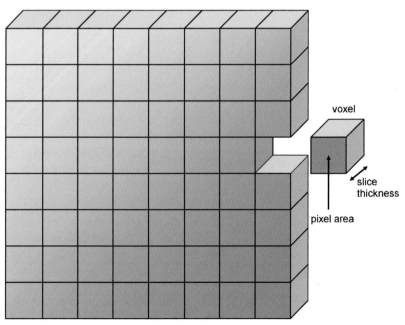

Figure 4.1 The voxel.
Note: the large green square is the FOV.

large voxel volume

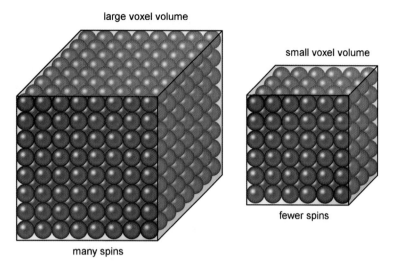

small voxel volume

fewer spins

Figure 4.2 Voxel volume and SNR (spin numbers are not representative).

many spins

coarse matrix results in large pixels and voxels (assuming a given square FOV). A **fine matrix** is one with a high number of frequency encodings and/or phase encodings, and results in a large number of pixels in the FOV. A fine matrix results in small pixels and voxels.

Large voxels contain more spins or nuclei than small voxels, and therefore have more nuclei within them to contribute towards the signal. Large voxels have a higher SNR than small voxels (Figure 4.2).

The SNR is therefore proportional to the voxel volume and any parameter that alters the size of the voxel changes the SNR. Any selection that decreases the size of the voxel decreases the SNR, and vice versa. This is achieved in three ways:

Changing the slice thickness. Look at Figures 4.3, 4.4 and 4.5. In this example the voxel size is altered by halving the slice thickness from 10 mm to 5 mm. Doing this halves the voxel volume from 1000 mm^3 to 500 mm^3 and hence the SNR. Comparing Figure 4.4 with 4.5, it is clear that the thicker slice has a better SNR than the thin slice.

Changing the image matrix. The image matrix is the number of pixels in the image. It is identified by two numbers: one denotes the number of pixels there are in the frequency direction (usually the long axis of the image), the other the number of phase pixels (usually the short axis of the image) (Figure 4.6). Look at Figures 4.7 and 4.8 where the phase matrix has been increased from 128 (Figure 4.7) to 256 (Figure 4.8). As the FOV has remained unchanged, there are smaller pixels and therefore voxels in Figure 4.8 than Figure 4.7. Therefore as the voxel volume has been halved in this example, the SNR is also halved. In addition, as the phase matrix affects scan time, increasing the phase matrix from 128 to 256 doubles the scan time.

Changing the FOV. Look at Figures 4.9, 4.10 and 4.11. The FOV has been halved, which has halved the pixel dimension along both axes. Therefore the voxel volume and SNR are reduced to one quarter of the original value (from 1000 mm^3 to 250 mm^3). When comparing Figure 4.10 with 4.11 it is evident that the SNR is significantly reduced in

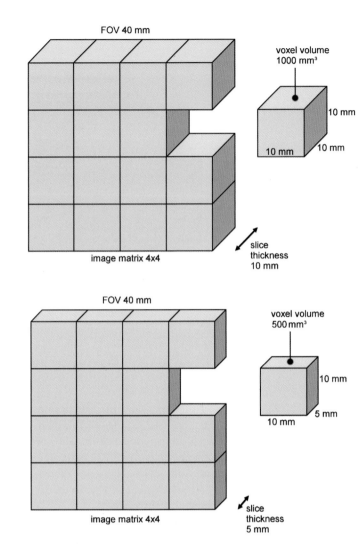

Figure 4.3 Slice thickness versus SNR.

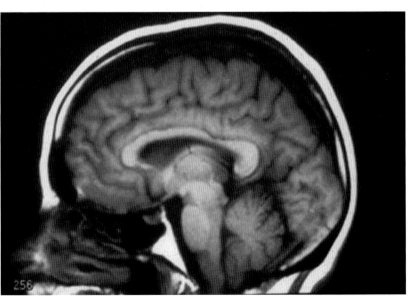

Figure 4.4 Sagittal T1 weighted image of the brain acquired with a slice thickness of 10 mm.

FOV 40 mm

voxel volume 1000 mm³

10 mm

10 mm

10 mm

image matrix 4x4

slice thickness 10 mm

FOV 40 mm

voxel volume 500 mm³

10 mm

10 mm

5 mm

image matrix 4x4

slice thickness 5 mm

4

256

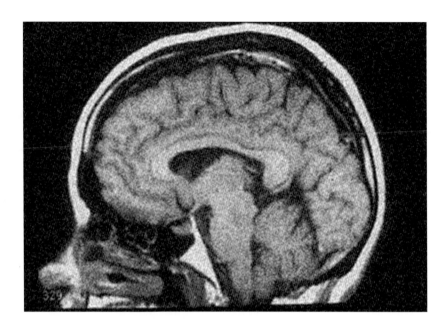

Figure 4.5 Sagittal T1 weighted image of the brain acquired with a slice thickness of 5 mm.

4

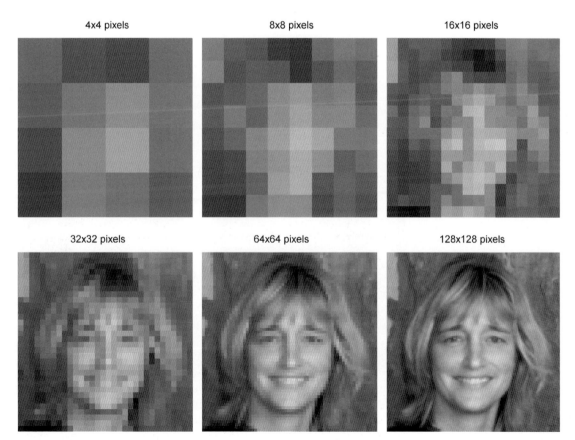

Figure 4.6 Changing the image matrix. Note how resolution changes.

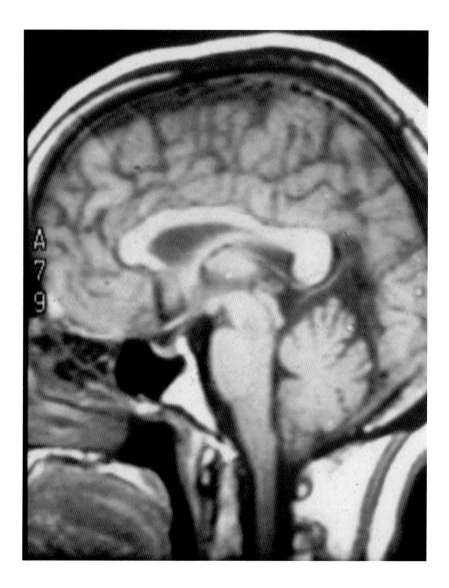

Figure 4.7 Sagittal T1 weighted image of the brain acquired with a 128 phase matrix.

Figure 4.11 but the resolution is increased. Depending on the area being imaged and the receiver coil used, it is sometimes necessary to take steps to increase the SNR when using a small FOV.

TR, TE and flip angle

Although TR, TE and flip angle are usually considered parameters that influence image contrast, they also influence the SNR and therefore overall image quality. Spin echo pulse sequences generally have more signal than gradient echo sequences, as all the longitudinal magnetization is converted into transverse magnetization by the 90° flip angle. Gradient echo pulse

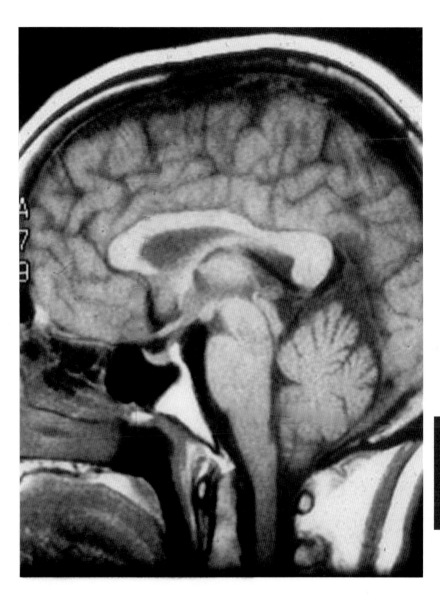

Figure 4.8 Sagittal T1 weighted image of the brain acquired with a 256 phase matrix.

4

sequences only convert a proportion of the longitudinal magnetization into transverse magnetization, as they use flip angles other than 90°. In addition, the 180° rephasing pulse is more efficient at rephasing than the rephasing gradient of gradient echo sequences, and so the resultant echo has greater signal amplitude.

- The flip angle controls the amount of transverse magnetization that is created which induces a signal in the coil (Figures. 4.12, 4.13 and 4.14). The maximum signal amplitude is created with flip angles of 90°. Look at Figures 4.13 and 4.14 in which the flip angle has been altered from 90° to 10°. The resultant SNR is significantly reduced so that steps are necessary to increase it to improve image quality.

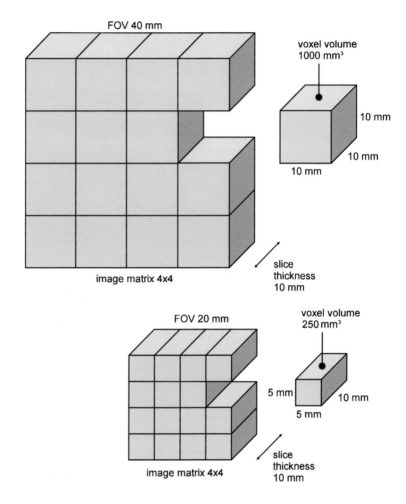

Figure 4.9   FOV vs SNR.

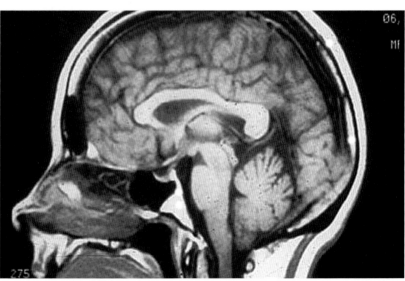

Figure 4.10   Sagittal T1 weighted image of the brain acquired with a FOV of 24 cm.

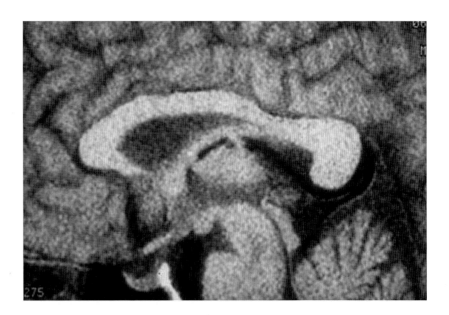

Figure 4.11 Sagittal T1 weighted image of the brain acquired with a FOV of 12 cm.

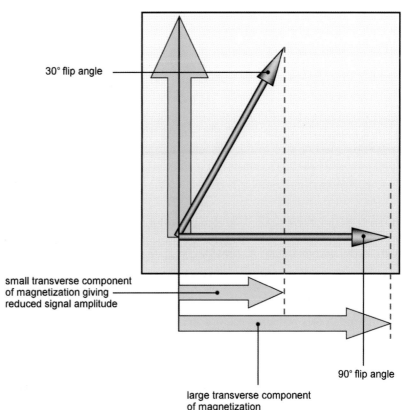

30° flip angle

small transverse component of magnetization giving reduced signal amplitude

90° flip angle

large transverse component of magnetization giving maximum signal

Figure 4.12 Flip angle vs SNR.

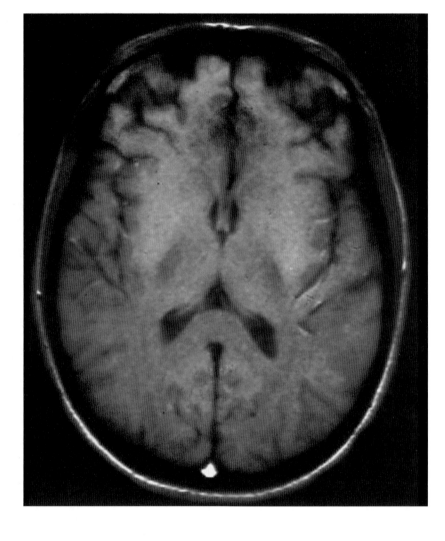

Figure 4.13 Axial gradient echo image through the brain using a flip angle of 90°.

- The TR controls the amount of longitudinal magnetization that is allowed to recover before the next excitation pulse is applied. A long TR allows full recovery of the longitudinal magnetization so that more is available to be flipped in the next repetition. A short TR does not allow full recovery of longitudinal magnetization, so less is available to be flipped (*see* Figure 2.8). Look at Figures 4.15, 4.16, 4.17 and 4.18 where the TR has been increased from 140 ms to 700 ms. It is easy to see how the SNR has improved as the TR increases. This is because as the TR increases more longitudinal magnetization is available to create transverse magnetization after excitation. However, as the TR is one of factors that affects scan time (*see* Chapter 3),

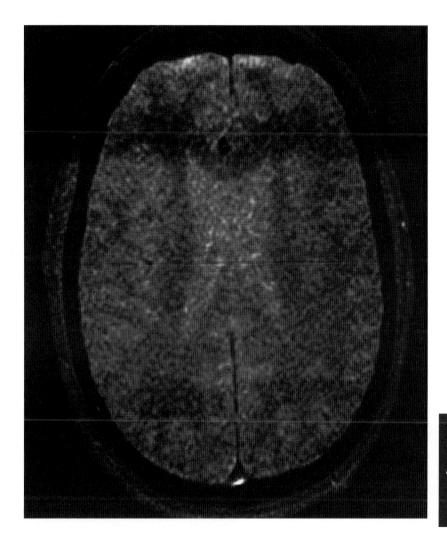

Figure 4.14 Axial gradient echo image through the brain using a flip angle of 10°.

4

increasing the TR also increases scan time and the chance of patient movement.

- The TE controls the amount of transverse magnetization that is allowed to decay before an echo is collected. A long TE allows considerable decay of the transverse magnetization to occur before the echo is collected, while a short TE does not (Figure 4.23). Look at Figures 4.19, 4.20, 4.21 and 4.22 where the TE has been increased from 11 ms to 80 ms. The SNR dramatically decreases as the TE increases, because there is less transverse magnetization available to be rephased and produce an echo. This is why T2 weighted sequences that use a long TE usually have a lower SNR than T1 or PD weighted sequences that use a short TE.

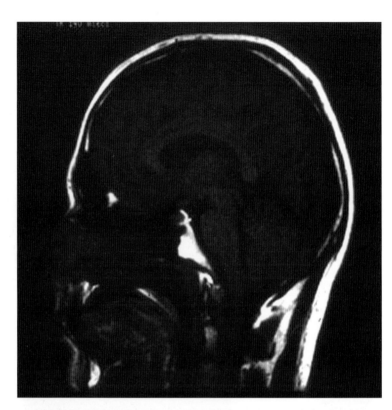

Figure 4.15 Sagittal T1 weighted image through the brain using a TR of 140 ms.

4

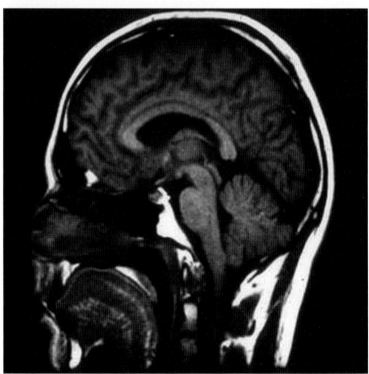

Figure 4.16 Sagittal T1 weighted image through the brain using a TR of 300 ms.

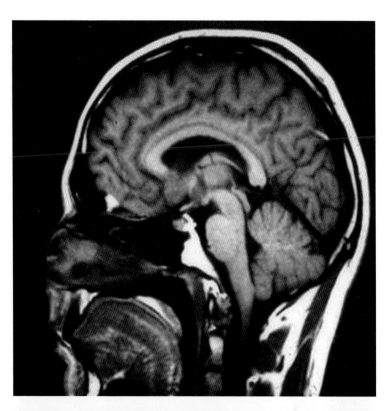

Figure 4.17 Sagittal T1 weighted image through the brain using a TR of 500 ms.

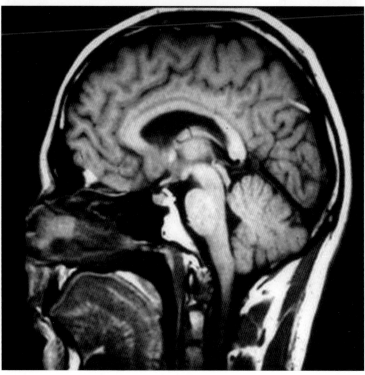

Figure 4.18 Sagittal T1 weighted image through the brain using a TR of 700 ms.

4

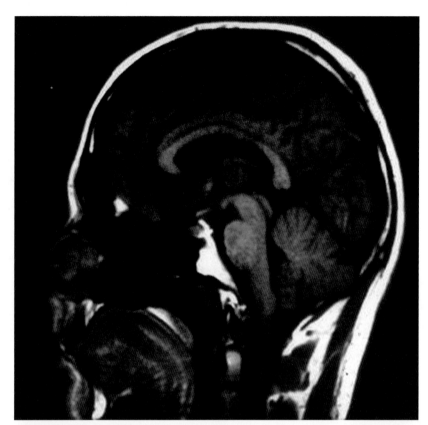

Figure 4.19 Sagittal T1 weighted image through the brain using a TE of 11 ms.

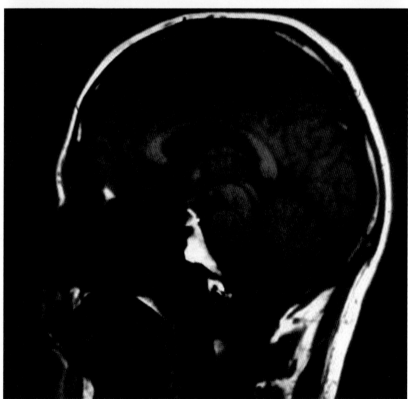

Figure 4.20 Sagittal T1 weighted image through the brain using a TE of 20 ms.

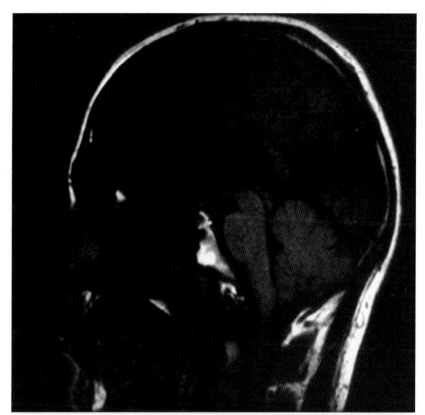

Figure 4.21 Sagittal T1 weighted image through the brain using a TE of 40 ms.

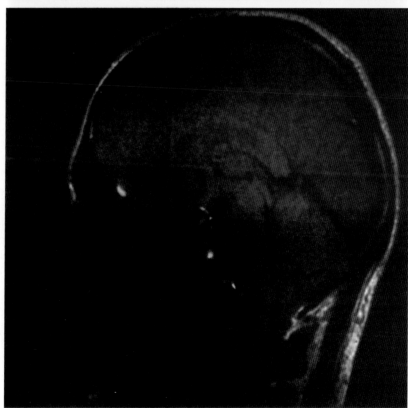

Figure 4.22 Sagittal T1 weighted image through the brain using a TE of 80 ms.

4

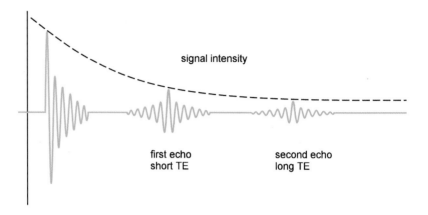

Figure 4.23 TE vs SNR.

Summary

- A long TR increases SNR and a short TR reduces SNR

- A long TE reduces SNR and a short TE increases SNR

- The lower the flip angle, the lower the SNR

Number of signal averages (NEX, NSA, Naq)

This is the number of times data are collected with the same amplitude of phase encoding slope. The NEX controls the amount of data that is stored in each line of K space (*see* Chapter 3). Referring to the chest of drawers analogy, the NEX is the number of times each drawer is filled with data. Doubling the NEX therefore doubles the amount of data that is stored in each line of K space, while halving the NEX halves the amount of data stored.

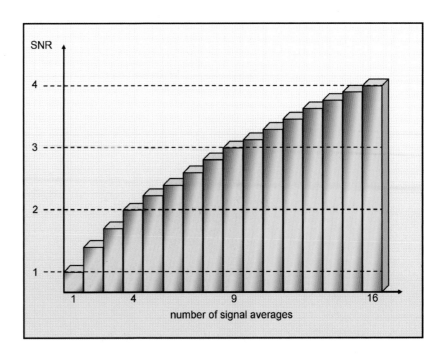

Figure 4.24 NEX vs SNR.

The data contain both signal and noise. Noise is random, as it is in a different position each time data are stored. Signal, however, is not random, as it always occurs at the same place when it is collected. The presence of random noise means that doubling the NEX only increases the SNR by $\sqrt{2}$ (=1.4). Therefore increasing the NEX is not necessarily the best way of increasing the SNR. This is demonstrated in Figure 4.24.

To double the SNR we need to increase the NEX and the scan time by a factor of four. To triple it requires a ninefold increase in NEX and scan time. Increasing the scan time increases the chances of patient movement. Look at Figures 4.25 and 4.26 where the NEX has been increased from 1 to 4. The SNR is undoubtedly greater in Figure 4.26 but took four times longer to acquire than in Figure 4.25. Increasing the NEX also reduces motion artefact. This is discussed later in Chapter 7.

Receive bandwidth

This is the range of frequencies that are sampled during the application of the readout gradient. Reducing the receive bandwidth results in less noise being sampled relative to signal because noise occurs at all frequencies and randomly in time. By applying a filter to the frequency encoding gradient, noise frequencies much higher and lower than signal frequencies are filtered out.

4

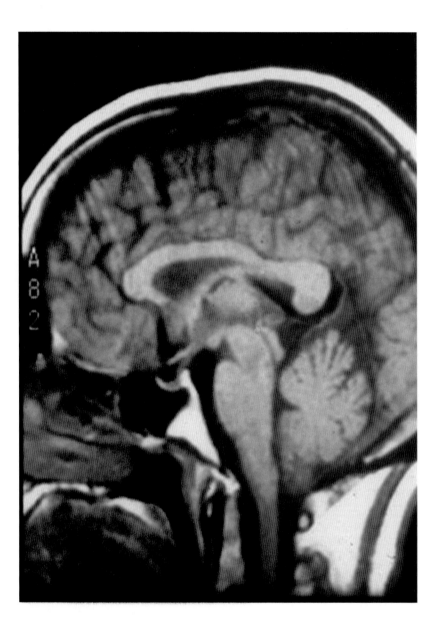

Figure 4.25 Sagittal T1 weighted image through the brain using a NEX of 1.

As less noise is sampled as a proportion of signal, the SNR increases as the receive bandwidth decreases (Figure 4.27). Halving the bandwidth increases the SNR by about 40%, but increases the sampling time. As a result, reducing the bandwidth increases the minimum TE available (*see* Chapter 3). Reducing the bandwidth also increases chemical shift artefact (*see* Chapter 7).

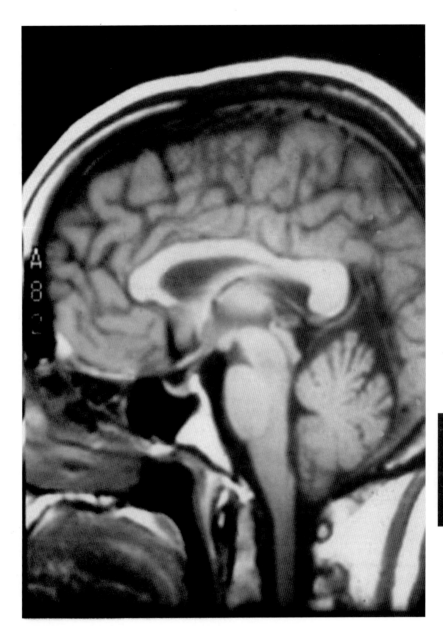

Figure 4.26 Sagittal T1 weighted image through the brain using a NEX of 4.

4

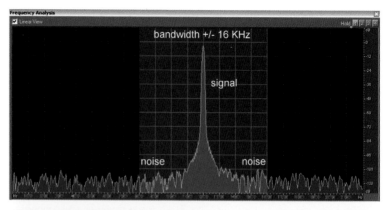

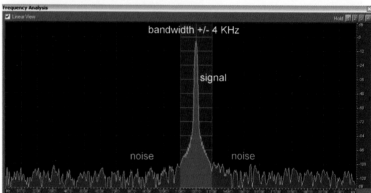

Figure 4.27   Bandwidth vs SNR.

4

Learning point: when to use a reduced receive bandwidth

Although these restrictions apply, there are some clinical situations where reducing the receive bandwidth is advantageous. Lengthening TEs are not important when a long TE is required for T2 weighting. In addition, chemical shift artefact only occurs when water and fat co-exist in the same voxel. Therefore reducing the receive bandwidth is a useful way of significantly improving SNR when performing T2 weighted images in conjunction with chemical saturation techniques (*see* Chapter 6) which remove signal from either fat or water and eliminate chemical shift artefact (*see* Chapter 7). Alternatively, lengthening the receive bandwidth is often necessary when very short TEs are required. Although this decreases SNR because more noise frequencies are sampled, to achieve very short TEs the sampling time must be significantly reduced. This is especially relevant in fast gradient echo imaging (*see* Chapter 5).

Type of coil

The type of coil used affects the amount of signal received and therefore the SNR. Coil types are discussed in Chapter 9. Quadrature coils increase SNR as two coils are used to receive signal. Phased array coils increase SNR even more as the data from several coils are added together. Surface coils placed close to the area under examination also increase the SNR. The use of the appropriate receiver coil plays an extremely important role in optimizing SNR. In general, the size of the receiver coil should be chosen such that the volume of tissue imaged optimally fills the sensitive volume of the coil. Large coils, however, increase the likelihood of aliasing, as tissue outside the FOV is more likely to produce signal. The position of the coil is also very important for maximizing SNR. To induce maximum signal, the coil must be positioned in the transverse plane perpendicular to B_0. Angling the coil, as sometimes happens when using surface coils, results in a reduction of SNR (Figure 4.28).

Summary

To optimize image quality the SNR must be the highest possible. To achieve this:

- use spin echo pulse sequences where possible (that use large flip angles)
- try not to use a very short TR and a very long TE
- use the correct coil and ensure that it is well tuned and positioned and immobilized correctly
- use a coarse matrix
- use a large FOV
- select thick slices
- use as many NEX as possible.

4

Contrast to noise ratio (CNR)

The **contrast to noise ratio** is defined as the difference in the SNR between two adjacent areas. It is controlled by the same factors that affect the SNR. The CNR is probably the most critical factor affecting image quality as it directly determines the eyes' ability to distinguish areas of high signal from areas of low signal. Image contrast depends on both intrinsic and extrinsic parameters as discussed in Chapter 2 and therefore these factors also affect the CNR. From a practical point of view the CNR is increased in the following ways:

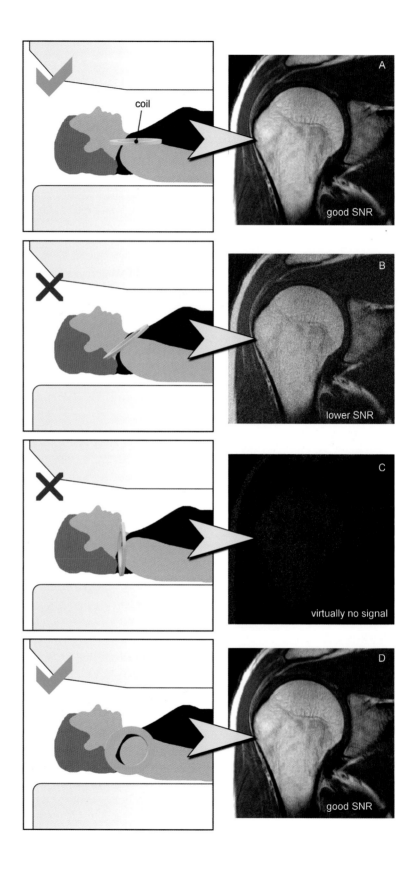

Figure 4.28 Coil position vs SNR.

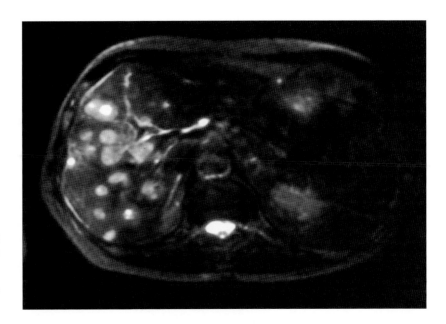

Figure 4.29 Axial T2 weighted image through the liver. Lesions within the liver have a much greater signal than normal liver. Hence the CNR is high and they are well seen.

Using a T2 weighted image. Although a T2 weighted image often has a much lower SNR than a T1 weighted image (due to the longer TE), the ability to distinguish tumor from normal tissue is often much greater because of the high signal of the tumor compared with the low signal of surrounding anatomy, i.e. the CNR is higher. This is shown in Figure 4.29 where, although overall image quality is poor, liver lesions are seen well because their signal intensity is very different from normal liver.

Using contrast agents. The purpose of administering contrast agents is to increase the CNR between pathology (which enhances) and normal anatomy (which does not) (*see* Chapter 11).

Using chemical pre-saturation technique: by saturating out normal anatomy, pathology is often seen more clearly (*see* Chapter 6 and Figure 6.19).

Using magnetization transfer contrast (MTC): In MRI, only protons that have a sufficiently long T2 time can be imaged. Other protons whose transverse components decay before the signal can be collected cannot be visualized adequately. These protons, mainly bound to large proteins, membranes, and other macromolecules are called bound protons. The protons that have longer T2 times can be visualized and are termed free protons. There is always a transfer of magnetization between the bound and the free protons, which causes a change in the T1 values of the free protons. This can be exploited by selectively saturating the bound protons, which reduces the intensity of the signal from the free protons due to **magnetization transfer contrast (MTC)**. The MTC saturation band is applied before the excitation pulse at a bandwidth that selectively destroys the transverse components of magnetization of the bound protons. The use of MTC increases the CNR between pathological and normal tissues and is useful in many areas, including angiography and joint imaging.

4

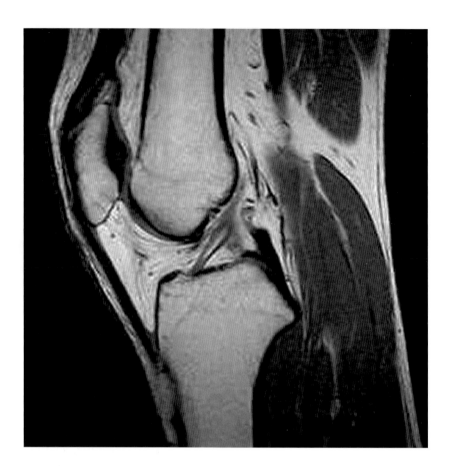

Figure 4.30 High resolution sagittal image of the knee.

4

Spatial resolution

The **spatial resolution** is the ability to distinguish between two points as separate and distinct, and is controlled by the voxel size. The voxel size is affected by:

- slice thickness
- FOV
- number of pixels or matrix (*see* Figure 4.1).

Small voxels result in good spatial resolution, as small structures can be easily differentiated (Figure 4.30). Large voxels, on the other hand, result in low spatial resolution, as small structures are not resolved so well. In large voxels, individual signal intensities are averaged together and are not represented as distinct within the voxel. This results in **partial voluming**.

- The thinner the slice, the greater the ability to resolve small structures in the slice select plane. Reducing the slice thickness therefore increases spatial resolution, while increasing the slice thickness reduces spatial resolution and increases partial voluming. However, thinner slices result in smaller voxels and reduced SNR (Figures 4.4 and 4.5).

- The matrix determines the number of pixels in the FOV. Small pixels increase spatial resolution as they increase the ability to distinguish between two structures close together in the patient. Increasing the matrix therefore increases the spatial resolution. However, fine matrices result in smaller voxels and therefore reduced SNR (Figures 4.7 and 4.8). In addition, the scan time increases as the phase matrix increases.
- The size of the FOV also determines the pixel dimensions. A large FOV results in large pixels, while a small FOV produces small pixels. Increasing the FOV size therefore decreases the spatial resolution. However, a small FOV results in smaller voxels and therefore reduced SNR (Figures 4.10 and 4.11).

Spatial resolution and pixel dimension

Square pixels always provide better spatial resolution than rectangular pixels as the image is equally resolved along both the frequency and phase axis. If the FOV is square, the pixels are also square if an even matrix is selected, e.g. 256×256. If the FOV is square and an uneven matrix is selected, for example, 256×128, the pixels are rectangular (Figure 4.31).

Usually, the frequency number of the matrix is the highest number and the phase number is altered to change the scan time and the resolution. If the phase number is less than the frequency number, the pixels are longer in the phase direction than in the frequency direction. The spatial resolution is therefore reduced along the phase axis. Some systems, however, automatically keep the pixels square regardless of the matrix selected. Therefore, if the number of phase encodings is half that of the frequency encodings, the FOV in the phase direction of the image is half the size that it is in the frequency direction, but the pixels remain square. This method maintains the spatial resolution regardless of the matrix selected (Figure 4.32).

However, the FOV should always cover the required anatomy along the phase axis. To increase the FOV in the phase direction, the number of phase encodings must be increased, and this increases the scan time. In addition, the SNR from the smaller square pixels is lower than with rectangular pixels. Systems that employ this method usually have the option of selecting rectangular pixels, which automatically keeps the FOV square, so that the anatomy in the phase direction is covered and the SNR increased. This is achieved without increasing the phase encoding number (and therefore the scan time), as the pixels are automatically made rectangular in the phase direction. Although the spatial resolution is reduced, the SNR increases as each pixel is now larger. Many systems always use this latter method of keeping the FOV square. In these systems, the matrix size governs the spatial resolution, SNR and scan time. These systems have an option called **rectangular FOV** to maintain spatial resolution with an uneven matrix.

4

even matrix square field of view

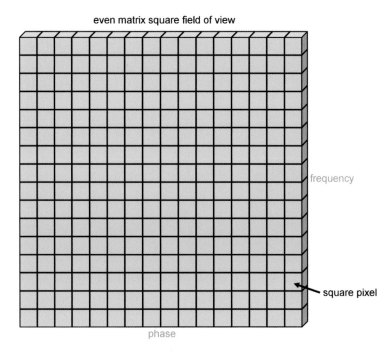

uneven matrix square field of view

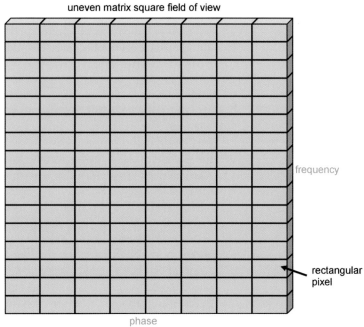

Figure 4.31 Pixel size versus matrix size.

even matrix square field of view

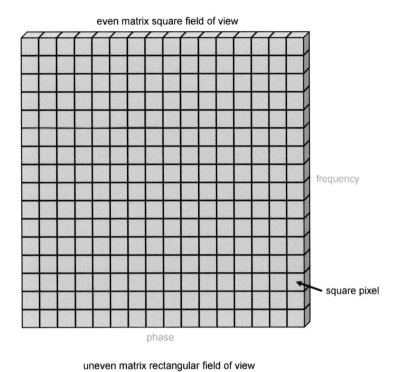

frequency

square pixel

phase

uneven matrix rectangular field of view

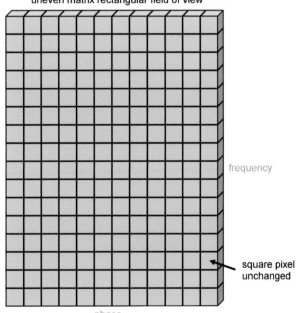

frequency

square pixel
unchanged

phase

Figure 4.32 Square pixels.

Rectangular FOV

In some cases, where the system allows for rectangular pixels but the anatomy does not fill a square FOV, a rectangular FOV may be desired. To acquire a square FOV, high-resolution image is costly in time. For this purpose many systems offer an option known as rectangular FOV. Rectangular FOV maintains spatial resolution but reduces the scan time as only a portion of the total number of phase encodings that are normally required are performed.

The dimension of the FOV in the phase direction is reduced compared to that in the frequency direction and so should be used when imaging anatomy that fits into a rectangle, for example, a sagittal lumbar spine image. For example, if rectangular FOV is selected with a 256 × 256 matrix and 24 cm frequency axis FOV with the requirement to halve the dimension of the phase axis FOV, the resolution of 256 × 256 is maintained, but the scan is completed after only 128 phase encodings. The FOV is 24 cm in the frequency direction and 12 cm in the phase direction and the scan time is halved (Figures 4.33 and 4.34).

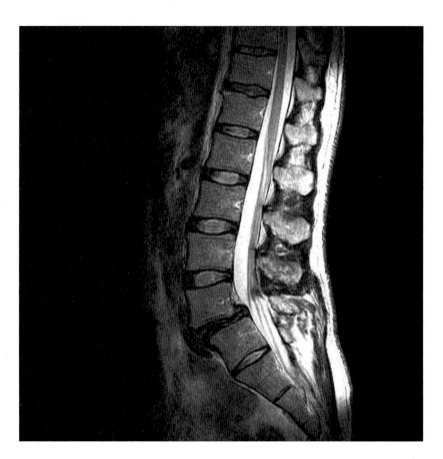

Figure 4.33 Sagittal T2 weighted image of the lumbar spine using a square FOV of 24 cm and image matrix of 256 x 256.

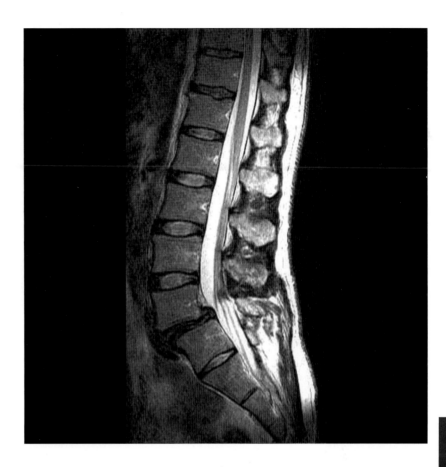

Figure 4.34 Sagittal T2 weighted image of the lumbar spine using a rectangular FOV of 12 cm in the phase direction. The scan time is half that of Figure 4.33 but the resolution remains unchanged.

4

Learning point: rectangular FOV and K space filling using the chest of drawers analogy

In rectangular FOV, the FOV in the phase direction is smaller than that in the frequency direction and the scan time is reduced but the resolution of the image remains unchanged. Using the chest of drawers analogy for K space described in Chapter 3, the height of the chest of drawers determines the top and bottom-most drawer that is filled with data. This in turn determines the resolution of the image. For example, if a 256 × 256 matrix is selected, lines +/–128 must be filled with data to achieve the required resolution (Figure 4.35).

To reduce the scan time, fewer phase encodes must be performed between these outer lines, or fewer drawers filled. To achieve this, the increment between each phase encoding step is increased. The phase increments are the difference in angle between successive phase encoding slopes and correspond to the depth of each drawer in

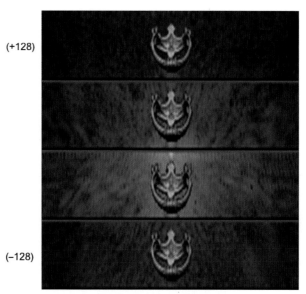

(+128)

each drawer
x2 normal height

(−128)

Figure 4.35 Rectangular FOV
and the chest of drawers.

4

the chest of drawers analogy. The size of the phase increment or the depth of the drawer is inversely proportional to the size of the FOV in the phase direction. Therefore deep drawers result in smaller dimension FOVs in the phase direction and shallow drawers, larger dimension FOVs in the phase direction. For example, if the phase increment is halved, the FOV in the phase direction doubles and vice versa. In rectangular FOV, the phase increment is increased so that fewer phase encodes are performed between lines +/−128. This reduces the scan time and at the same time reduces the size of the FOV in the phase direction producing a rectangular FOV. Using this analogy it is easy to see that some signal may be lost because fewer data are being acquired.

Summary

To improve image quality the spatial resolution must be optimized. The spatial resolution can be maintained by:

- selecting as thin a slice as possible
- selecting a fine matrix
- selecting a small FOV
- selecting rectangular FOV where possible

Learning point: how resolution affects the minimum TE

Resolution is controlled by the size of the voxel. To achieve a small voxel and therefore good resolution, we need to use thin slices, a small FOV and a fine matrix.

- The slice thickness is determined by the slope of the slice select gradient. Therefore to achieve *thin slices* the slice select gradient slope is *steep.*
- The size of the FOV is determined by the slope of the frequency encoding gradient. To achieve a *small FOV*, the frequency encoding gradient slope is *steep.*
- The matrix size in the phase direction is determined by the number of phase encodings performed. To achieve a *fine matrix* a high proportion of the phase encoding gradient slopes are *steep.*

If gradient slopes have to be steep during a pulse sequence because thin slices, fine matrices or a small FOV have been selected, their rise times are greater. The **rise time** of a gradient is the time required for it to achieve the correct slope (*see* Chapter 9). Steep gradient slopes result in a higher rise time for the gradient than shallow gradient slopes. Steep gradient slopes therefore stress the gradient coils more than shallow gradient slopes. This therefore increases the minimum TE as the system cannot collect the signal until all the gradient functions have been completed. A small FOV, thin slices and fine matrices increase the minimum TE and may result in fewer slices being available. If the TE increases, the selection and encoding of each slice takes longer, and therefore fewer slices can be excited in a given TR. Some systems compensate for this by increasing the TR so that all selected slices can be acquired; other systems keep the TR the same but put the slices into two acquisitions, or 'packages'.

4

Scan time

The scan time is the time to complete data acquisition or the time to fill K space (*see* Chapter 3). Scan times are important in maintaining image quality, as long scan times give the patient more chance to move during the acquisition. Any movement of the patient will probably degrade the images. As multiple slices are selected during a 2D and 3D volumetric acquisition, movement during these types of acquisition affects all the slices. During a sequential acquisition, movement of the patient only affects those slices that are acquired while the patient is moving. As discussed in Chapter 3, the factors that affect scan time are:

- *TR* – the time of each repetition or MR experiment, or the time between filling consecutive drawers. Doubling the TR doubles the scan time and vice versa.
- *Phase matrix* – the number of phase encodings determines the number of lines of K space or the number of drawers that are filled with data to complete the scan. If the number of phase encodings is doubled, the scan time also doubles.
- *NEX* – the number of times data are collected with the same slope of phase encoding gradient or the number of times each drawer is filled with data. Doubling the NEX doubles the scan time and vice versa.

Summary

To reduce the likelihood of patient movement, the scan time should always be as short as possible. To achieve the shortest scan time:

- use the shortest TR possible
- select the coarsest matrix possible
- reduce the NEX to a minimum

Summary

4

SNR is proportional to:

- pixel area/FOV^2
- slice thickness
- proton density
- $\sqrt{NEX}$
- $1/\sqrt{(number\ of\ phase\ encodings)}$
- 1/(number of frequency encodings)
- $1/\sqrt{(receive\ bandwidth)}$
- TR, TE and flip angle

Spatial resolution is determined by:

- FOV
- matrix size
- slice thickness

Scan time is proportional to:

- TR
- number of phase encodings
- NEX

Table 4.1 The results of optimizing image quality.

To optimize image	Adjusted parameter	Consequence
Maximize SNR	↑ NEX	↑ scan time
	↓ matrix	↓ scan time
	−	↓ resolution
	↑ slice thickness	↓ resolution
	↓ receive bandwidth	↑ minimum TE
	−	↑ chemical shift
	↑ FOV	↓ resolution
	↑ TR	↓ T1 weighting
	−	↑ number of slices
	↓ TE	↓ T2 weighting
Maximize resolution (assuming a square FOV)	↓ slice thickness	↓ SNR
	↑ matrix	↓ SNR
	−	↑ scan time
	↓ FOV	↓ SNR
Minimize scan time	↓ TR	↑ T1 weighting
	−	↓ SNR
	−	↓ number of slices
	↓ phase matrix	↓ resolution
	−	↑ SNR
	↓ NEX	↑ SNR
	−	↑ movement artefact
	↓ slice number in volume imaging	↓ SNR

Trade-offs

It is probably now obvious that there are many trade-offs when selecting parameters within a pulse sequence. Ideally an image has high SNR, good spatial resolution and is acquired in a very short scan time. However, this is rarely achievable as increasing one factor inevitably reduces one or both of the other two. It is vital that the user has a full understanding of all the parameters that affect each image quality parameter and the trade-offs involved. Table 4.1 gives the result of optimizing image quality. Table 4.2 gives the parameters and their associated trade-offs.

Decision making

The decisions made when setting up a pulse sequence depend on the area to be examined, the condition and co-operation of the patient and the clinical throughput required. There are really no rules in MRI. This can be very frustrating when trying to learn, but also makes the subject interesting and challenging. Every facility has protocols established with the

Table 4.2 Parameters and their associated trade-offs.

Parameter	Benefit	Limitation
TR ↑	↑ SNR ↑ number of slices	↑ scan time ↓ T1 weighting
TR ↓	↓ scan time ↑ T1 weighting	↓ SNR ↓ number of slices
TE ↑	↑ T2 weighting	↓ SNR
TE ↓	↑ SNR	↓ T2 weighting
NEX ↑	↑ SNR ↑ signal averaging	↑ scan time
NEX ↓	↓ scan time	↓ SNR ↓ signal averaging
Slice thickness ↑	↑ SNR ↑ coverage	↓ resolution ↑ partial voluming
Slice thickness ↓	↑ resolution ↓ partial voluming	↓ SNR ↓ coverage
FOV ↑	↑ SNR ↑ coverage	↓ resolution ↓ aliasing
FOV ↓	↑ resolution ↑ aliasing	↓ SNR ↓ coverage
Matrix ↑	↑ resolution	↑ scan time ↓ SNR if pixel small
Matrix ↓	↓ scan time ↑ SNR if pixel large	↑ resolution
Receive bandwidth ↑	↓ chemical shift ↓ minimum TE	↓ SNR
Receive bandwidth ↓	↑ SNR	↑ chemical shift ↑ minimum TE
Large coil	↑ area of received signal	↓ SNR sensitive to artefacts aliasing with small FOV
Small coil	↑ SNR less sensitive to artefacts less prone to aliasing with small FOV	↓ area of received signal

co-operation of the manufacturer and the radiologist. However, here are a few tips for optimizing image quality.

- Always choose the correct coil and position it correctly. This often makes the difference between a good and a bad quality examination.
- Make sure that the patient is comfortable. This is very important as a patient is more likely to move if he or she is uncomfortable. Immobilize the patient as much as possible to reduce the likelihood of movement.
- Try to ascertain from the radiologist exactly what sequences are required before the scan. This saves a lot of time as radiologists can be difficult to track down!
- The scan plane, pulse sequence type, and weighting required are usually (but not always) decided by the radiologist. In our view,

SNR is the most important image quality factor. There is no point in having an image with good spatial resolution if the SNR is poor. Sometimes, however, good spatial resolution is vital but if the SNR is low, the images will be of poor quality and the benefit of good spatial resolution is lost.

It is very important to keep the scan time as short as possible. Again, there is no point having an image with great SNR and spatial resolution if it took so long to acquire that the patient has moved during the scan. Remember, any patient can move – not just a restless one. The longer the patient is expected to lie on the table, the more likely it is that he or she will move.

As each system varies considerably, the following are only guidelines. The parameters given are not etched in stone but are only meant as indicators and are appropriate at most common clinical field strengths i.e. 0.5 T to 1.5 T. It is inadvisable to select:

- a very short TR (choose 400 ms not 200 ms)
- a very long TE (choose 100 ms not 200 ms)
- very low flip angles (choose 20° not 5°)
- very thin slices (choose 4 mm not 3 mm)
- a very small FOV (choose 12 cm not 8 cm), unless you are using a good local coil.

In most centers, the protocols selected work well and the radiologists are happy with the parameters set. However, it is worth remembering that, for example, a 1 mm difference in slice thickness can make all the difference in improving SNR, without noticeably reducing the spatial resolution. Also remember that as the FOV size decreases, the dimensions of the pixel along both axes are reduced (assuming that the system operates with a square FOV). Under these circumstances, the FOV is the most potent controller of SNR. Using a 16 cm FOV instead of an 8 cm FOV can be important in maintaining SNR.

If the area under examination has inherently good signal (for example, the brain), and the correct coil has been selected, it is usually possible for a fine matrix and fewer NEX to be used to achieve good quality images in terms of SNR and spatial resolution. However, when examining an area with inherently low signal (for example, the lungs), selection of more NEX and a coarser matrix may be necessary. Try to do all this and keep the scan time as low as possible. It is usually not practical to have sequences that last 30 minutes each!

Volume imaging

Volume imaging is advantageous in that very small lesions can be demonstrated, as the slice thickness can be drastically reduced compared with conventional imaging, and there is no slice gap. In conventional imaging

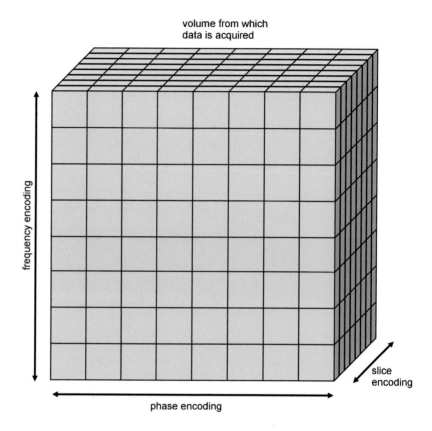

volume from which
data is acquired

frequency encoding

slice
encoding

phase encoding

Figure 4.36 Encoding in a
volume acquisition.

4

the slice thickness affects the SNR. In volume imaging the entire volume of
tissue is excited and the volume contains no gap, the SNR is superior, and
so fewer NEX can be used. The other main advantage of volumes is that as
data are collected from a slab, the slab can be manipulated to look at the
anatomy within the volume in any plane and at any angle of obliquity.

The disadvantages of volume imaging are that, in general, the scan times
associated with it is relatively long. For this reason, it is usually used in
conjunction with faster pulse sequences. In volume imaging, slices are
sectioned out by a technique known as slice encoding (Figure 4.36). This is
another series of phase encoding steps along the slice select axis. Therefore, just as the number of phase encoding steps increases the scan time in
conventional sequencing, the number of slices also affects the scan time in
volume imaging. Therefore:

$$\text{scan time} = \text{TR} \times \text{NEX} \times \text{number of phase encodings} \times \text{number of slice encodings}$$

The greater the number of slices prescribed, the longer the scan time.
However, this is offset somewhat by the fact that the greater the slice
number the greater the SNR, and so the NEX can be reduced.

Volume imaging and resolution

To obtain equal resolution in every plane and at every angle of obliquity, each voxel should be symmetrical (**isotropic**). That is to say, the voxel should have equal dimensions in every plane. If this is not true, the volume has poorer resolution in the planes other than the one in which it was acquired. For example, if a FOV of 24 cm and matrix of 256×256 is used, each pixel has a dimension of 0.9 mm (FOV/matrix). If the slice thickness selected is 3 mm, resolution is worse when the voxel is viewed from the side. Under these conditions, the voxel is **anisotropic**.

Sometimes volumes are acquired purely because the slices are contiguous and not because they are to be viewed in another plane, for example, coronal volumes of the brain can be very useful in detecting small temporal lobe lesions. However, they are not generally used to look at the brain axially or coronally. In this instance, 3 mm slices at 64 locations will cover the head adequately. In volume imaging of a joint, on the other hand, reformatting in other planes may be paramount. Under these circumstances it is important to obtain **isotropic** voxels, so thinner slices (1 mm or less) are required, although the number of slice locations may have to be increased to cover the anatomy.

The uses of volume imaging

Volume imaging has many potential applications, but it is widely used for imaging of joints, especially the knee, where anatomy is often confusing and not strictly in plane. Volumes can be very useful for following ligaments or other structures that cross over the imaging plane. Volumes should also be used when looking for very small lesions. The slice thickness can be lowered to less than 1 mm in most systems, and so extremely good resolution can be achieved. Lesions in the temporal lobes or posterior fossa especially lend themselves to volume imaging.

4

Summary

- Volume imaging allows reformatting in any plane
- Isotropic voxels give equal resolution in every plane
- The scan time depends on the slice number and the TR, phase encoding number and the NEX
- Increasing the slice number increases the SNR, but also increases the scan time
- Volume imaging increases the SNR as a whole volume of tissue is excited

Manipulating SNR, image contrast, spatial resolution and scan time is a real art and takes some time and experience. Even after many years the operator will probably get things wrong occasionally! However, perseverance is important, and eventually results in good image quality. As image quality factors and trade-offs have been explored, it is now important to understand pulse sequences and their individual uses. These are discussed in Chapter 5.

Questions

1   Of the following parameters which would give:
    (a) the best spatial resolution?
    (b) the highest SNR?
    256×256, 3 mm slice thickness, 12 cm FOV, 1 NEX,
    256×128, 8 mm slice thickness, 40 cm FOV, 4 NEX,
    512×256, 4 mm slice thickness, 8 cm FOV, 2 NEX.

2   List the factors that affect SNR.

3   Which could you change without affecting image contrast or scan time?

4   List three ways of improving the CNR between pathology and normal tissue.

5   How is K space filling altered in rectangular FOV?

6   How would you achieve equal resolution in all reformatting planes in a volume acquisition?

7   Define spatial resolution.

5

Pulse sequences

Introduction

Understanding pulse sequences forms an integral part of learning MRI. Pulse sequences enable us to control the way in which the system applies pulses and gradients. In this way, image weighting and quality is determined. There are many different pulse sequences available, and each is designed for a specific purpose. This chapter discusses the mechanisms, uses and parameters for each of the common pulse sequences, and their advantages and disadvantages. Each manufacturer uses different acronyms to distinguish between individual pulse sequences, which can be very confusing to the user.

A table comparing the common acronyms for each of the main manufacturers is included. This is provided as a guide only; it is not in any way meant to compare the performance or specification of each system. An omission from the table indicates only that information about a certain factor was unavailable, not necessarily that it is not an option. The parameters given are general as they depend on field strength. However, the parameters given should be suitable for most current clinical field strengths.

Learning point: what is a pulse sequence?

The definition of a pulse sequence is a series of RF pulses, gradient applications and intervening time periods. The RF pulses are applied for excitation purposes and, in the case of spin echo, for rephasing purposes. The gradients are applied to spatially encode signal (*see* Chapter 3) and to rephase and dephase spins depending on the type of pulse sequence and imaging option selected. The intervening time periods refer to the time intervals between these various functions, some of which are extrinsic contrast parameters that are selected at the console (*see* Chapter 2). Therefore a pulse sequence is a carefully co-ordinated and timed sequence of events to generate a particular type of image contrast. They can be thought of like dances. All dances involve movement of the feet as a series of steps, just as all pulse sequences involve RF pulses and gradients. However, just as the timing and the co-ordination of steps determines the type of dance, e.g. tango, foxtrot, etc., so the timing and co-ordination of elements within a pulse sequence determines the resultant image contrast.

Pulse sequences can generally be categorized as follows:

Spin echo pulse sequences (echoes are rephased by a 180° rephasing pulse)

- conventional spin echo
- fast or turbo spin echo
- inversion recovery

Gradient echo pulse sequences (echoes are rephased by a gradient)

- coherent gradient echo
- incoherent gradient echo
- steady state free precession
- balanced gradient echo
- fast gradient echo
- echo planar imaging

5

SPIN ECHO PULSE SEQUENCES

Conventional spin echo

Mechanism

This pulse sequence has previously been discussed in Chapter 2. To recap, spin echo uses a 90° excitation pulse followed by one or more 180° rephasing pulses to generate a spin echo. If only one echo is generated, a T1 weighted image can be obtained using a short TE and a short TR. For proton density and T2 weighting, two RF rephasing pulses, generating two spin echoes, are applied. The first echo has a short TE and a long TR to achieve proton density weighting, and the second has a long TE and a long TR to achieve T2 weighting (*see* Figures 2.23, 2.24 and 2.25).

Uses

Spin echo pulse sequences are the gold standard for most imaging. They may be used for almost every examination. T1 weighted images are useful for demonstrating anatomy because they have a high SNR. In conjunction with contrast enhancement, however, they can show pathology. T2 weighted images also demonstrate pathology. Tissues that are diseased are generally more edematous and/or vascular. They have increased water content and consequently have a high signal on T2 weighted images and can therefore be easily identified (*see* Figures 2.23 to 2.26).

Parameters

T1 weighting

Short TE 10–20 ms
Short TR 300–700 ms
Typical scan time 4–6 min

Proton density/T2 weighting

Short TE 20 ms/long TE 80 ms+
Long TR 2000 ms+
Typical scan time 7–15 min

5

Advantages

- good image quality
- very versatile
- true T2 weighting sensitive to pathology

Disadvantages

- scan times relatively long

Fast or turbo spin echo

Mechanism

As the name suggests, fast or turbo spin echo is a spin echo pulse sequence, but with scan times that are much shorter than conventional spin echo. To understand how fast spin echo achieves this, it is important to recap on data acquisition in conventional spin echo (*see* Chapter 3). A 90° excitation pulse is followed by a 180° rephasing pulse. Only one phase encoding step is applied per TR on each slice and therefore only one line of K space is filled per TR (Figure 5.1).

As the scan time is a function of the TR, NEX and number of phase encodings, to reduce the scan time, one or more of these factors should be reduced. Decreasing the TR and the NEX affects image weighting and SNR, which is undesirable. Reducing the number of phase encodings reduces the spatial resolution, which is also a disadvantage (*see* Chapter 4). In fast spin echo, the scan time is reduced by performing more than one phase encoding step and subsequently filling more than one line of K space per TR. This is achieved by using an echo train that consists of several 180° rephasing pulses (Figure 5.2). At each rephasing, an echo is produced and a different phase encoding step is performed.

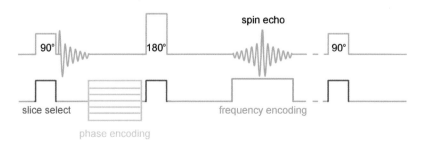

Figure 5.1 Spatial encoding in conventional spin echo.

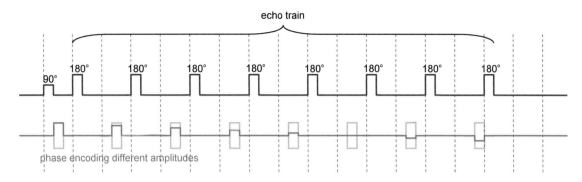

Figure 5.2 The echo train.

In conventional spin echo, raw image data from each echo are stored in K space, and the number of 180° rephasing pulses applied corresponds to the number of echoes produced per TR. Each echo is used to produce a separate image (usually proton density and T2). In fast spin echo, data from each echo are placed into *one* image. The number of 180° rephasing pulses performed per TR corresponds to the number of echoes produced and the number of lines of K space filled. This number is called the **turbo factor** or the **echo train length**. The higher the turbo factor, the shorter the scan time as more phase encoding steps are performed per TR.

For example:

- In conventional spin echo, if a 256 phase matrix is selected, 256 phase encodings must be applied. Assuming 1 NEX has been selected, 256 TR times elapse to complete the scan.
- In fast spin echo, using the same parameters but selecting a turbo factor of 16, 16 phase encoding steps are performed every TR. Therefore 256 ÷ 16 (16) TR times elapse to complete the scan. The scan time is therefore reduced to 1/16 of the original.

At each 180°/phase encoding combination, a different amplitude of phase encoding gradient slope is applied to fill out a different line of K space. In conventional spin echo only one line is filled per TR, while in fast spin echo several lines corresponding to the turbo factor are filled (Figure 5.2). Therefore K space is filled more rapidly and the scan time is reduced.

5

Learning point: the chest of drawers and fast spin echo

Using the chest of drawers analogy from Chapter 3, in conventional spin echo one drawer is opened per TR to fill one line of K space with data points. In fast spin echo, to decrease the scan time but maintain resolution, all the drawers must be filled (resolution) but more than one drawer must be opened per TR to fill K space more quickly, reducing the scan time. This is achieved by performing more than one application of the phase encoding gradient per TR, each one to a different slope to open a different drawer.

For example, if 10 drawers are to be opened per TR, then the phase encoding gradient must be applied 10 different times to 10 different amplitudes per TR to open 10 different drawers. Once the drawers are opened, there must be data to put into them. This requires producing 10 echoes, one for each drawer. To do this, 10 different 180° pulses must be applied. The number of RF pulses corresponds to the number of echoes and the number of drawers opened per TR. This is called the echo train length or turbo factor and indicates how much faster the scan is compared with conventional spin echo, i.e. a turbo factor of 16 indicates 16 drawers are opened per TR and the scan time is 16 times faster than for conventional spin echo.

Weighting in fast spin echo

The echoes are generated at different TE times and therefore data collected from them have variable weighting. All these data are stored and placed into one image. So how is a fast spin echo sequence weighted correctly? The TE selected is only an **effective TE**. In other words, it is the TE at which the operator wishes to weight the resultant image. To achieve this weighting, the system orders the phase encoding steps so that steep or shallow slopes are applied to the various echoes produced. As described in Chapter 3, each phase encoding step applies a different slope of gradient to phase shift the signal by a different amount. If 256 phase encodings are performed, the phase encoding gradient is switched on to varying degrees from +128 to −128 (Figure 5.3).

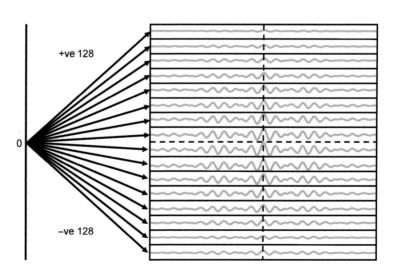

Figure 5.3   Phase encoding gradient slopes.

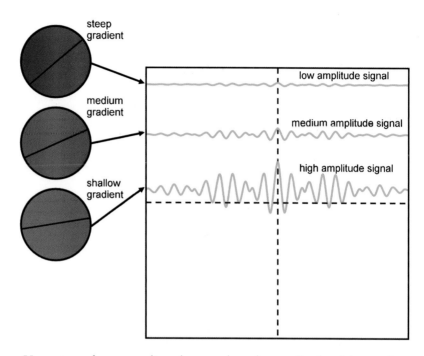

Figure 5.4 Phase encoding versus signal amplitude.

Very steep phase encoding slopes reduce the amplitude of the resultant echo. Shallow phase encoding slopes result in an echo that has maximum signal amplitude (Figure 5.4) (*see* Chapter 3). The system orders the phase encodings so that the shallow slopes that produce maximum signal are centered on the effective TE selected. The steep slopes that produce much smaller signal amplitude are placed away from the effective TE. The resultant image contains data from all the echoes in the echo train, but data from echoes collected around the effective TE have more impact on image contrast as they fill the central lines of K space, which produce the greatest signal amplitude. Data from echoes collected at the wrong weighting (other TEs), have much less of an effect on the contrast, as they fill the outer lines of K space and therefore have a smaller signal amplitude and a greater spatial resolution (Figure 5.5).

If a TE of 100 ms is selected, with a TR of 3000 ms and a turbo factor of 16, T2 weighting is required. The shallowest phase encodings are performed on echoes occurring around 100 ms. Data acquired from these phase encodings have a TE at or close to 100 ms. Phase encodings performed at the very beginning and end of the echo train are steep, and the signal amplitude of these echoes is small. They contain either proton density or very heavily T2 weighted data, which are present in the image but whose impact is less predominant.

Uses

Generally speaking, the contrast seen in fast spin echo images is similar to that in spin echo and, therefore, these sequences are useful in most clinical

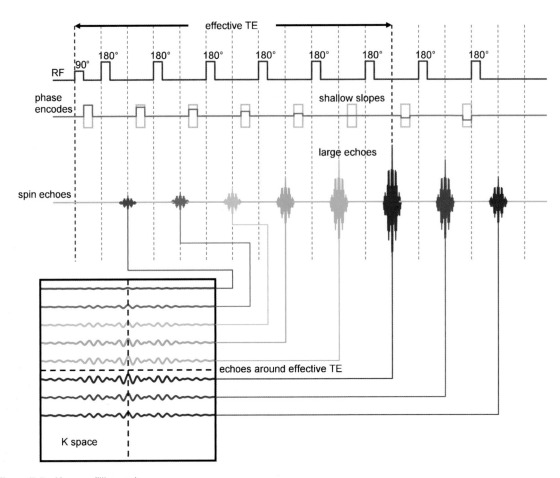

Figure 5.5 K space filling and phase re-ordering.

applications. In the central nervous system, pelvis and musculoskeletal regions, fast spin echo has now largely replaced spin echo. In the chest and abdomen, however, respiratory artefact is sometimes troublesome if respiratory compensation techniques are not compatible with fast spin echo software. This is offset somewhat by the fact that the shorter scan times of fast spin echo enable images to be produced while patients hold their breath.

There are, however, two contrast differences between spin echo and fast spin echo, both of which are due to the repeated, closely-spaced 180° pulses of the echo train. First, fat remains bright on T2 weighted images due to the multiple RF pulses which reduce the effects of spin–spin interactions in fat (**J coupling**) (Figure 5.6). However, fat saturation techniques can be used to compensate for this (*see* Chapter 6). Second, the repeated 180° pulses can increase magnetization transfer effects so that muscle, for example, appears darker on fast spin echo images than in conventional spin echo. In addition, the multiple 180° pulses reduce magnetic susceptibility effects, which can be detrimental when looking for small hemorrhages.

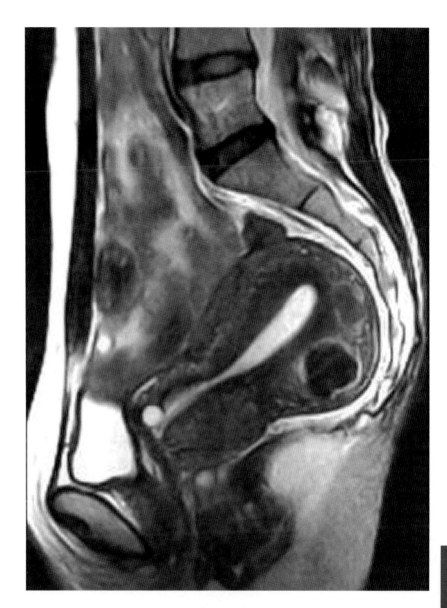

Figure 5.6 Sagittal T2 weighted fast spin echo sequence through the pelvis. Note that both fat and water have high signal intensity.

5

Image blurring occurs in fast spin echo images at the edges of tissues with different T2 decay values. This occurs because each line of K space filled during an echo train contains data from echoes with a different TE. When using long echo trains, late echoes that have a low signal amplitude contribute to the resolution of K space. If these echoes are negligible, then resolution is lost from the image and blurring occurs. The plus side, however, is that artefact from metal implants is significantly reduced when using fast spin echo because the repeated 180° RF pulses compensate for field inhomogeneity (*see* Chapter 7).

Parameters

These are similar to conventional spin echo. However, the turbo factor now plays an important role in image weighting. The higher the turbo factor, the shorter the scan time, but the resultant image has more of a mixture of weighting because there are more data collected at the wrong TE. This is not as important in T2 weighted scans, as the proton density data are offset somewhat by the heavily T2 weighted data. In T1 and proton density weighting, on the other hand, larger turbo factors place too much T2 weighting in the image and hence shorter turbo factors must be used. The scan time savings in T1 weighted imaging are therefore not as great as with T2 weighting.

For T1 weighting (Figure 5.7):

TR	300 ms to 700 ms
effective TE	minimum
turbo factor	2 to 8

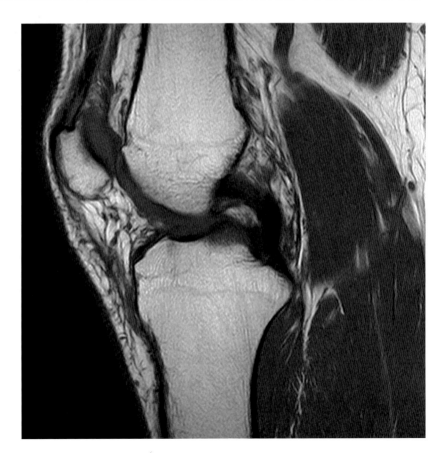

Figure 5.7   Sagittal T1 weighted fast spin echo image of the knee.

5

For PD weighting (Figure 5.8):

TR	3000 ms to 10 000 ms (depending on required slice number)
effective TE	minimum
turbo factor	2 to 8

For T2 weighting (Figure 5.9)

TR	3000 ms to 10 000 ms (depending on required slice number)
effective TE	80 to 140 ms
turbo factor	12 to 30

The TR of fast spin echo is often much longer than that used in conventional spin echo. The 180° RF pulses take time to perform and so fewer slices are available for a given TR. As the turbo factor increases, the number of slices available per TR decreases, and sometimes the TR has to be significantly increased to achieve the required slice number. In T1 weighting, increasing the TR reduces the weighting, and so in these circumstances we need to keep the TR short and to perform several acquisitions to obtain coverage of anatomy. The longer TR associated with fast spin echo somewhat offsets the reduction in scan time achieved, but is far less significant than the huge scan time savings produced by long echo trains.

Summary

Short turbo factor

- decreased effective TE
- increased T1 weighting
- longer scan time
- more slices per TR
- reduced image blurring

Long turbo factor

- increased effective TE
- increased T2 weighting
- reduced scan time
- reduced slice number per TR
- increased image blurring

5

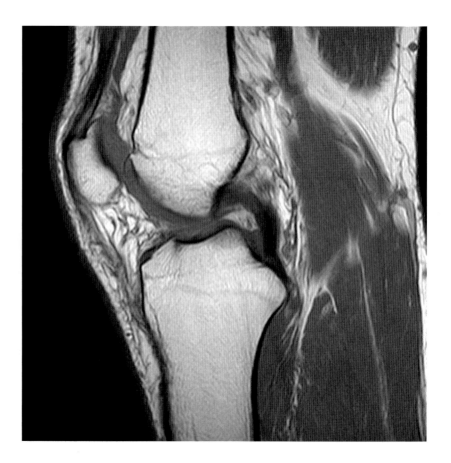

Figure 5.8   Sagittal PD weighted fast spin echo image of the knee.

Advantages

- scan times greatly reduced
- high-resolution matrices and multiple NEX can be used
- image quality improved
- increased T2 information

Disadvantages

- some flow and motion affects increased
- incompatible with some imaging options
- fat bright on T2 weighted images
- image blurring

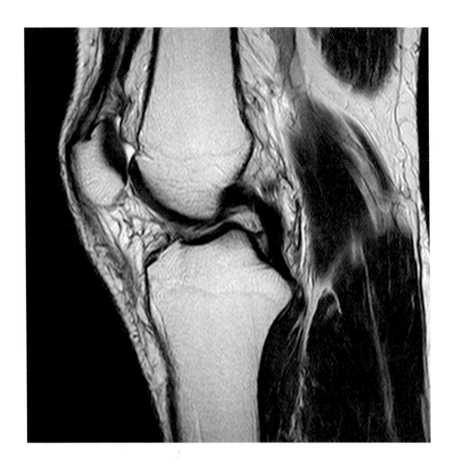

Figure 5.9 Sagittal T2 weighted fast spin echo image of the knee.

Single shot fast spin echo (SS-FSE)

It is possible to acquire fast spin echo images in even shorter scan times by using a technique known as **single shot fast spin echo (SS-FSE)**. In this technique all the lines of K space are acquired in one TR (*see* later). SS-FSE combines a partial Fourier technique with fast spin echo. Half of the lines of K space are acquired in one TR and the other half are transposed. This technique yields a reduction in imaging time as all the image data are acquired in one TR. However, there is an SNR penalty.

DRIVE

In another modification of FSE (which some manufacturers call **DRIVE**) a reverse flip angle excitation pulse is applied at the end of the echo train. This drives any transverse magnetization into the longitudinal plane so that it is available for excitation at the beginning of the next TR period. As water has the longest T1 and T2 times, most of this magnetization is composed of water and therefore this has a higher signal intensity on the

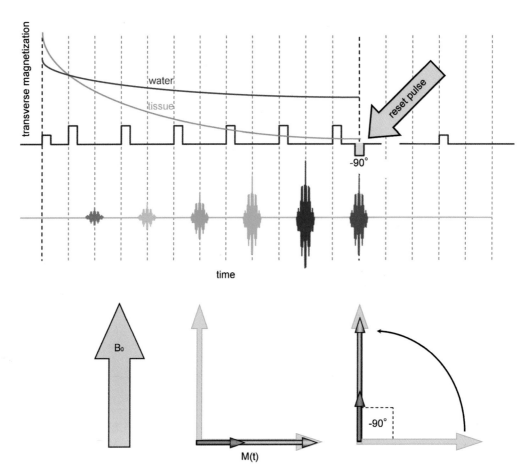

Figure 5.10 The DRIVE pulse sequence.

resultant images. This sequence produces an increase in signal intensity in fluid-based structures such as cerebrospinal fluid when using shorter TRs than normal in FSE (Figures 5.10 and 5.11).

Inversion recovery

Mechanism

Inversion recovery was developed in the early days of MRI to provide good T1 contrast on low field systems. However, the scan times were relatively long and when high field superconducting systems were widely used, this sequence became somewhat redundant. However, it has re-emerged

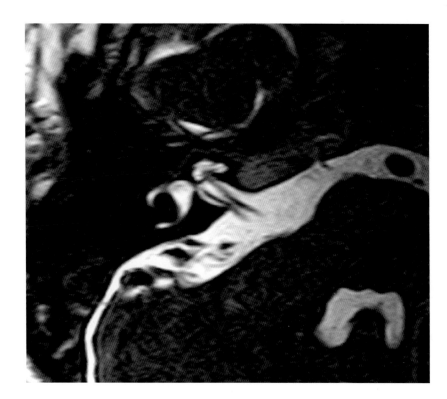

Figure 5.11 Axial DRIVE image through the right internal auditory meatus. Note high signal intensity in CSF.

combined with fast spin echo to produce images in a few minutes. It is usually used to suppress the signal from certain tissues in conjunction with long TEs and T2 weighting, although at low field it is still used for T1 contrast. All varieties are discussed here.

Inversion recovery is a pulse sequence that begins with a 180° inverting pulse. This inverts the NMV through 180° into full saturation. When the inverting pulse is removed, the NMV begins to relax back to B_0. A 90° excitation pulse is then applied at a time from the 180° inverting pulse known as the **TI (time from inversion)**(Figure 5.12). The resultant FID is then rephased by a 180° pulse to produce a spin echo at time TE (Figure 5.13).

The contrast of the resultant image depends primarily on the length of the TI. If the 90° excitation pulse is applied while the NMV is recovering from inversion, through the transverse plane, the contrast in the image depends on the amount of longitudinal recovery of each vector (as in spin echo). The resultant image is heavily T1 weighted, as the 180° inverting pulse achieves full saturation and ensures a large contrast difference between fat and water (Figure 5.14). If the 90° excitation pulse is not applied until the NMV has reached full recovery, a proton density weighted image results, as both fat and water have fully relaxed (Figure 5.15).

5

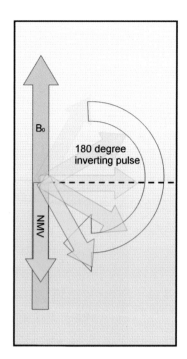

Figure 5.12 The 180°
inverting pulse in an inversion
recovery sequence.

5

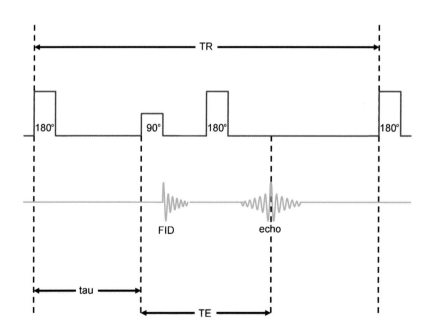

Figure 5.13 The inversion
recovery sequence.

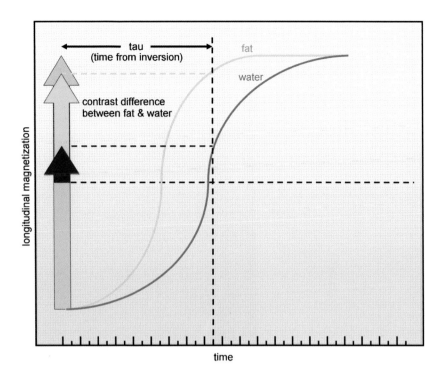

Figure 5.14 T1 weighting in inversion recovery.

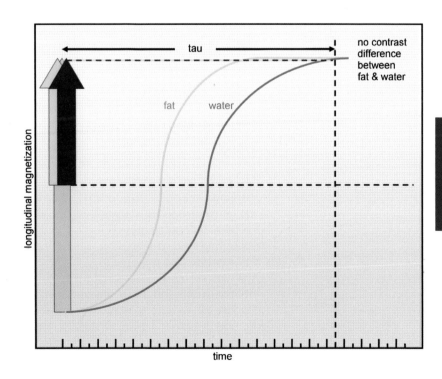

Figure 5.15 PD weighting in inversion recovery.

5

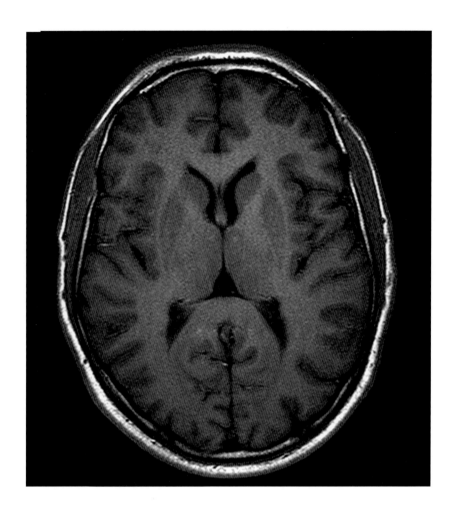

Figure 5.16 Axial T1 weighted inversion recovery sequence through the brain. A TI of 700 ms was used.

5

Uses

Inversion recovery was conventionally used to produce heavily T1 weighted images to demonstrate anatomy (Figure 5.16). The 180° inverting pulse produces a large contrast difference between fat and water because full saturation of the fat and water vectors is achieved at the beginning of each repetition. Therefore tissues begin their recovery from full saturation as opposed to from the transverse plane as in conventional spin echo. This allows more time for differences in the T1 recovery times between tissues to show up, and therefore IR pulse sequences produce heavier T1 weighting than conventional spin echo. As the use of gadolinium primarily shortens the T1 times of certain tissues, IR pulse sequences increase the signal from structures that have enhanced as a result of a contrast injection.

Parameters

When inversion recovery is used to produce predominantly heavily T1 weighted images at low field, the TE controls the amount of T2 decay, and so it is usually kept short to minimize T2 effects. However, it can be lengthened to give tissues with a long T2 a bright signal. This is called **pathology weighting** and produces an image that is predominantly T1 weighted, but where pathological processes appear bright. The TI is the most potent controller of contrast in the inversion recovery sequence. Medium TI values give T1 weighting but as this is lengthened, the image becomes more proton density weighted. The TR should always be long enough to allow full recovery of the NMV before the next inverting pulse is applied. If this is not so, individual vectors recover to different degrees, and the weighting is affected. For example, at 1 T to achieve full recovery of the NMV, the TR should be longer than 2000 ms. Most systems now use inversion recovery fast spin echo (*see* below).

T1 weighting

medium TI	400–800 ms (varies at different field strengths)
short TE	10–20 ms
long TR	2000 ms+
average scan time	5–15 min

Proton density weighting

long TI	1800 ms
short TE	10–20 ms
long TR	2000 ms+
average scan time	5–15 min

Pathology weighting

medium TI	400–800 ms
long TE	70 ms+
long TR	2000 ms+
average scan time	5–15 min

5

Advantages

- very good SNR as the TR is long
- excellent T1 contrast

Disadvantages

- long scan times unless used in conjunction with fast spin echo

Fast inversion recovery

In this sequence modification the 180° inverting pulse is followed after the TI time by the 90° excitation pulse and the train of 180° RF pulses to fill out multiple lines of K space as in fast spin echo. This greatly reduces the scan time and has enabled a re-emergence of this sequence in clinical imaging. However, instead of being used to produce T1 weighted images, fast inversion recovery is usually used to suppress signal from certain tissues in conjunction with T2 weighting so that water and pathology return a high signal. The two main sequences in this category are STIR and FLAIR.

STIR (short tau inversion recovery)

Mechanism

STIR is an inversion recovery pulse sequence that uses a TI (sometimes called **tau**) that corresponds to the time it takes fat to recover from full inversion to the transverse plane so that there is no longitudinal magnetization corresponding to fat. This is called the **null point** (Figure 5.17). When the 90° excitation pulse is applied, as there is no longitudinal

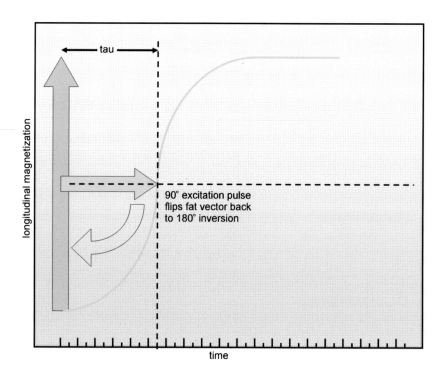

Figure 5.17 STIR.

component of fat, there is no transverse component after excitation and the signal from fat is nulled. A TI of 100–175 ms achieves fat suppression, although this value varies slightly at different field strengths. The TI required to null the signal from a tissue is 0.69 times its T1 relaxation time. It is important to note that STIR should not be used in conjunction with contrast enhancement, which shortens the T1 times of enhancing tissues, making them bright. The T1 times of these structures are shortened so that they approach the T1 time of fat. In a STIR sequence therefore, enhancing tissue may also be nulled.

Uses

STIR is an extremely important sequence in musculoskeletal imaging as normal bone, which contains fatty marrow, is suppressed and lesions within bone such as bone bruising and tumors are seen more clearly (Figure 5.18 and 5.19). It is also a very useful sequence for suppressing fat in general MR imaging (*see* Chapter 6).

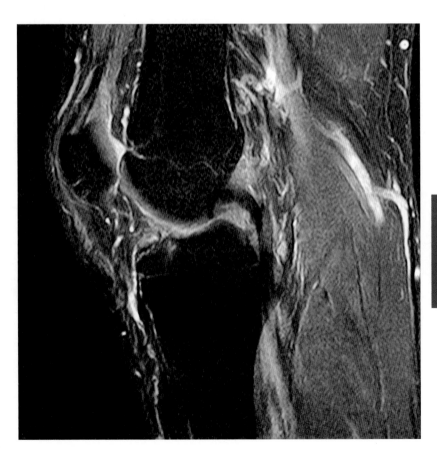

Figure 5.18 Sagittal STIR sequence of the knee. Normal bone marrow has been nulled. Synovial fluid in the joint has a high signal as the TE is long and the image is therefore T2 weighted.

5

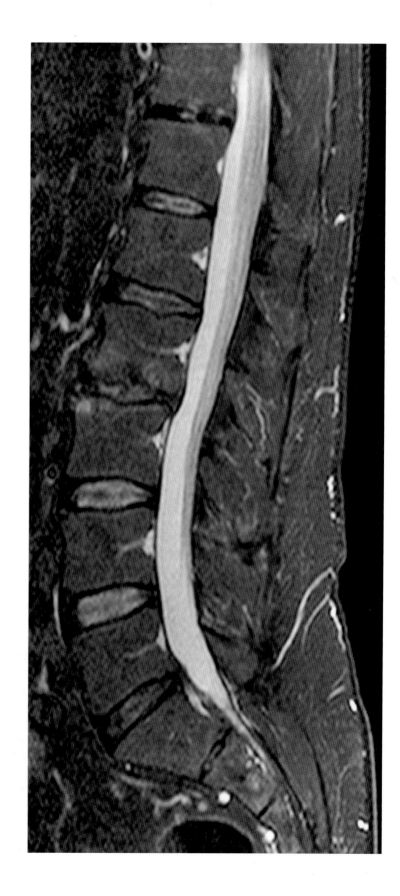

Figure 5.19 Sagittal STIR sequence of the lumbar spine using similar parameters to Figure 5.18.

Parameters

Short TI (tau)	150–175 ms (to suppress fat depending on field strength)
Long TE	50 ms+ (to enhance signal from pathology)
Long TR	4000 ms+ (to allow full recovery)
Long turbo factor	16–20 (to enhance signal from pathology)
Average scan time	5–15 min

FLAIR (fluid attenuated inversion recovery)

Mechanism

FLAIR is another variation of the inversion recovery sequence. In FLAIR, selecting a TI corresponding to the time of recovery of CSF from 180° to the transverse plane nulls the signal from CSF. There no longitudinal magnetization present in CSF. When the 90° excitation pulse is applied, as there is no longitudinal component of CSF, there is no transverse component after excitation and the signal from CSF is nulled. FLAIR is used to suppress the high CSF signal in T2 weighted images so that pathology adjacent to CSF is seen more clearly. A TI of 1700–2200 ms achieves CSF suppression (although this varies slightly at different field strengths and is calculated by multiplying the T1 relaxation time of CSF by 0.69).

Uses

FLAIR is used in brain and spine imaging to see periventricular and cord lesions more clearly, as the high signal from CSF that lies adjacent is nulled. It is especially useful in visualizing multiple sclerosis plaques, acute sub-arachnoid hemorrhage and meningitis (Figure 5.20). Sometimes gadolinium is given to enhance pathology. However, the contrast mechanism is not due to T1 shortening but to T2 prolongation. Another modification of this sequence in brain imaging is selecting a TI time that corresponds to the null point of white matter. This nulls the signal from normal white matter so that lesions within it appear much brighter by comparison. This sequence (which requires a TI of about 300 ms) is very useful for white matter lesions such as periventricular leukomalacia and for congenital gray/white matter abnormalities (Figure 5.21).

5

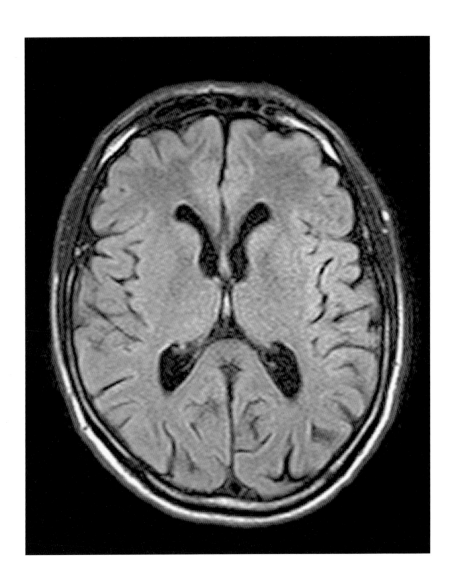

Figure 5.20   Axial FLAIR image through the brain.

5

Parameters

Long TI	1700–2200 ms (to suppress CSF depending on field strength)
Long TE	70 ms + (to enhance signal from pathology)
Long TR	6000 ms + (to allow full recovery)
Long turbo factor	16–20 (to enhance signal from pathology)
Average scan time	13–20 mins

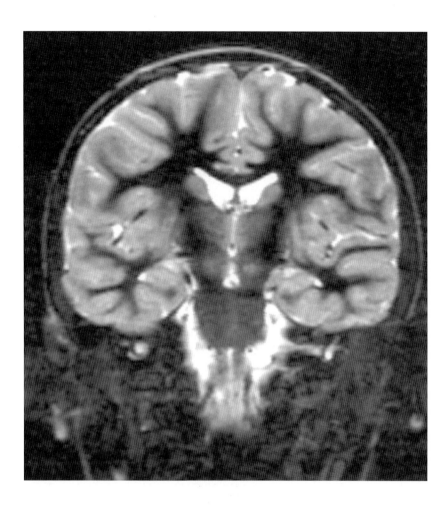

Figure 5.21 Coronal IR sequence using a TI that nulls white matter.

IR prep sequences

There are two further modifications of fast IR that were specifically developed to null blood in cardiac imaging (*see* Chapter 8). Double IR prep begins with two 180° pulses. One is non-slice selective and inverts all spins in the imaging volume, and the other is slice selective and re-inverts spins within a slice. A TI corresponding to the null point of blood (about 800 ms) completely nulls the signal from blood in the slice so that black blood imaging results. This is useful when looking at the morphology of the heart and great vessels. Triple IR prep adds a further inverting pulse at the TI of fat (about 150 ms) to null fat and blood together. This is useful when determining fatty infiltration of the heart walls (*see* Figure 8.3).

5

GRADIENT ECHO PULSE SEQUENCES

Conventional gradient echo

Mechanism

Gradient echo pulse sequences have been discussed in Chapter 2. To recap, gradient echo sequences use variable flip angles so that the TR and therefore the scan time can be reduced without producing saturation. A gradient rather than a 180° rephasing RF pulse is used to rephase the FID. The frequency encoding gradient is used for this purpose because it is quicker to apply than a 180° pulse and therefore the minimum TE can be reduced. The frequency encoding gradient is initially applied negatively to speed up the dephasing of the FID, and then its polarity is reversed, producing rephasing of the gradient echo. However, the gradient does not compensate for magnetic field inhomogeneities, so the resultant echo displays a great deal of T2* information (Figure 5.22).

Uses

Gradient echo pulse sequences can be used to acquire T2*, T1 and proton density weighting. However, there is always some degree of T2* weighting

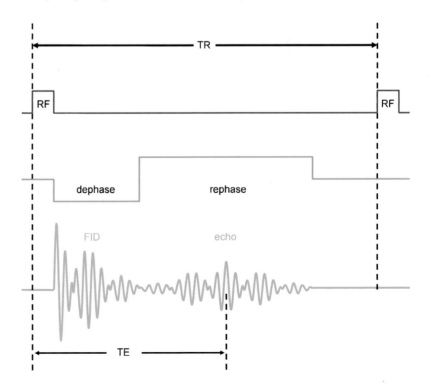

Figure 5.22 A basic gradient echo sequence showing how a bipolar application of the frequency encoding gradient produces a gradient echo.

present on any image due to the absence of a 180° rephasing pulse. Gradient echo sequences allow for a reduction in the scan time as the TR is greatly reduced. They can be used for single-slice breath-hold acquisitions in the abdomen, and for dynamic contrast enhancement. They are very sensitive to flow as gradient rephasing is not slice selective, so flowing nuclei always give a signal, as long as they have been previously excited (*see* Chapter 6). Because of this, gradient echo sequences may be used to produce angiographic-type images.

Parameters

The flip angle, in conjunction with the TR, determines the degree of saturation and therefore T1 weighting. To prevent saturation, the flip angles should be small and the TR long enough to permit full recovery. If saturation is required, the flip angle should be large and the TR short, so that full recovery cannot occur. The TE controls the amount of T2* dephasing. To minimize T2* the TE should be short. To maximize it, the TE should be long (*see* heat analogy in Chapter 2 and Figures 2.36 and 2.37).

T1 weighting

large flip angle	70°–110° (to maximize saturation)
short TR	less than 50 ms (to maximize saturation)
short TE	5–10 ms (to minimize T2*)
average scan time	several seconds to minutes

T2* weighting

small flip angle	5°–20° (to minimize saturation)
long TR	(to minimize saturation)
long TE	15–25 ms (to maximize T2*)
average scan time	several seconds to minutes

Proton density weighting

small flip angle	5°–20° (to minimize saturation)
long TR	(to minimize saturation)
short TE	5–10 ms (to minimize T2*)
average scan time	several seconds to minutes

In conventional gradient echo the TR does not always affect image contrast. Once a certain value of TR has been exceeded, the NMV recovers fully, regardless of the flip angle selected. Under these circumstances the flip angle and TE control the degree of saturation and dephasing respectively. In most systems, the conventional gradient echo sequence can be used to acquire slices in a 2D volumetric acquisition (*see* Chapter 3). The TR purely controls the number of slices that can be excited during the acquisition.

5

The steady state and echo formation

The **steady state** is a condition where the TR is shorter than the T1 and T2 relaxation times of the tissues. There is therefore no time for transverse magnetization to decay before the pulse sequence is repeated. In the steady state, there is co-existence of both longitudinal and transverse magnetization. To achieve this, energy given to hydrogen via the excitation pulse (as determined by the flip angle) should be similar to the energy hydrogen loses during the TR period. There are, therefore, critical values of flip angle and TR to maintain the steady state that holds the longitudinal and transverse components of magnetization steady during data acquisition (Figure 5.23). Generally, flip angles of 30° to 45° in conjunction with a TR of 20 to 50 ms achieve the steady state.

If the steady state is maintained, the transverse component of magnetization does not have time to decay during the pulse sequence, and therefore it affects image contrast as it induces a voltage in the receiver coil. This transverse magnetization, produced as a result of previous excitations, is called the **residual transverse magnetization**. It affects image contrast as it results in tissues with long T2 times (such as water) appearing bright on the image. Generally speaking, as the TR is so short, magnetization in tissues does not have time to reach its T1 or T2 relaxation times before the next excitation pulse is applied. Therefore in the steady state image

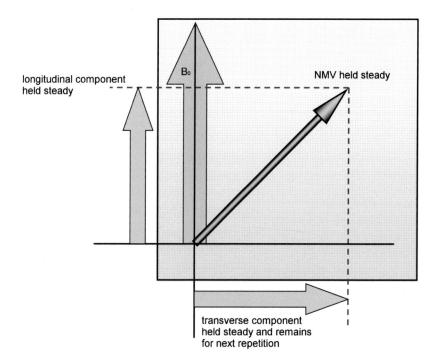

longitudinal component held steady

B₀

NMV held steady

transverse component held steady and remains for next repetition

Figure 5.23   The steady state.

5

Table 5.1   Tissue decay times and signal intensity in the steady state at 1 T.

Tissue	T1 Time (ms)	T2 Time (ms)	T1/T2	Signal intensity
Water	2500	2500	1	↑
Fat	200	100	0.5	↑
CSF	2000	300	0.15	↓
White matter	500	100	0.2	↓

contrast is not due to differences in the T1 and T2 relaxation times of tissues but rather to the ratio of T1 to T2, i.e. in tissues where T1 and T2 times are similar, the signal intensity is high.

In the human body, fat and water have this parity (fat, short T1 and T2 times; water, long T1 and T2 times) and therefore return high signal intensity in steady state sequences (Table 5.1). Most gradient echo sequences use the steady state as the shortest TR and, therefore, scan time is achieved. Gradient echo sequences are classified according to whether the residual transverse magnetization is in phase (**coherent**) or out of phase (**incoherent**).

Learning point: echo formation

The steady state involves repeatedly applying RF pulses at time intervals less than the T2 and T1 times of all the tissues. This train of RF pulses generates two signals:

- A *FID signal* which occurs as a result of the withdrawal of the RF pulse and, once rephased, contains either T2* or T1 information depending on the TE.
- A *spin echo* whose peak occurs at the same time as a subsequent RF pulse and contains T2* and T2 information.

This happens because every RF pulse (regardless of its net amplitude) contains energies that are sufficient to rephase transverse magnetization. These energies rephase the residual transverse magnetization left over from previous RF excitation pulses to form a spin echo. This occurs at exactly the same time as the next RF pulse as the residual transverse magnetization takes the same time to rephase as it took to dephase in the first place. Therefore, when utilizing the steady state, the TR equals the TAU of the spin echo.

Look at Figures 5.24 and 5.25. The first RF pulse (RF pulse 1 shown in red) produces a FID (also shown in red). The second RF

5

pulse (RF pulse 2, shown in orange) also produces a FID (also shown in orange). However, because the TR between RF pulses 1 and 2 is shorter than the relaxation times of the tissues, transverse magnetization is still present when the RF pulse 2 is applied. RF pulse 2 produces a FID and rephases the residual transverse magnetization still present from the first RF pulse. A spin echo is therefore produced. This occurs at the same time as the third RF pulse (RF pulse 3 shown in blue) because the time for rephasing this transverse magnetization is the same as it took to dephase. Therefore at RF pulse 3 there are two signals: a FID (shown in blue) produced as a result of the excitation properties of RF pulse 3 and a spin echo (shown in red) that was produced by RF pulse 1 and rephased by RF pulse 2.

Any two RF pulses produce a spin echo. The first RF pulse excites the nuclei regardless of its net amplitude; the second RF pulse rephases the FID and any residual magnetization present to produce a spin echo (Figures 5.24 and 5.25). These echoes are termed **Hahn** or **stimulated echoes** depending on the amplitude of the RF pulses involved. Any two 90° RF pulses produce a Hahn echo (after Edwin Hahn who discovered them). Any two RF pulses with varying amplitude, i.e. with flip angles other than 90°, are called stimulated echoes. This type of echo is used in steady state gradient echo sequences. Most gradient echo sequences contain data from FIDs and stimulated echoes. Their contrast is determined by which of these are digitized and used in the resultant image. In practice, echo production is so rapid that the tails of FID signals merge with stimulated echoes, resulting in a continuous signal of varying amplitude. However, in the interests of simplicity, the diagrams in this chapter show them separately.

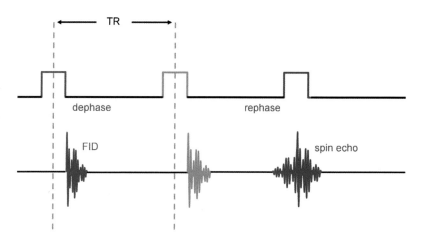

Figure 5.24   Echo formation in the steady state I.

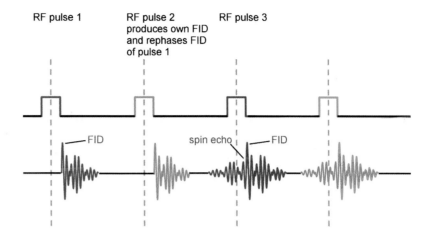

RF pulse 1   RF pulse 2 produces own FID and rephases FID of pulse 1   RF pulse 3

FID   spin echo   FID

Figure 5.25   Echo formation in the steady state II.

Summary

- The steady state is created when the TR is shorter than the relaxation times of tissues
- Residual magnetization therefore builds up in the transverse plane
- The residual transverse magnetization is rephased by subsequent RF pulses to produce stimulated echoes
- The resultant image contrast is due to the ratio of T1 to T2 in a particular tissue and depends on whether the FID and/or the stimulated echo are sampled

Coherent gradient echo

Mechanism

Coherent gradient echo pulse sequences use a variable flip angle excitation pulse followed by gradient rephasing to produce a gradient echo. The steady state is maintained by selecting a TR shorter than the T1 and T2 times of the tissues. There is therefore residual transverse magnetization left over when the next excitation pulse is delivered. These sequences keep this residual magnetization coherent by a process known as rewinding (*see* Chapter 2). Rewinding is achieved by reversing the slope of the phase encoding gradient after readout (Figure 5.26). This results in the residual magnetization rephasing, so that it is in phase at the beginning of the next repetition.

The rewinder gradient rephases all transverse magnetization regardless of when it was created. Therefore the resultant echo contains information from the FID and the stimulated echo. These sequences can therefore be

5

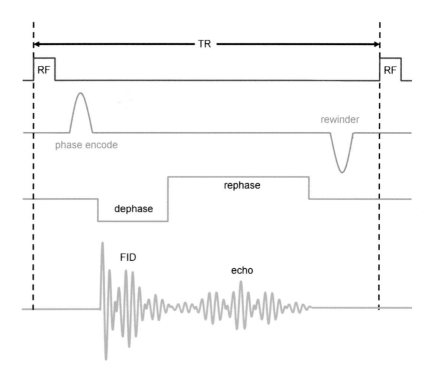

Figure 5.26 The coherent gradient echo sequence.

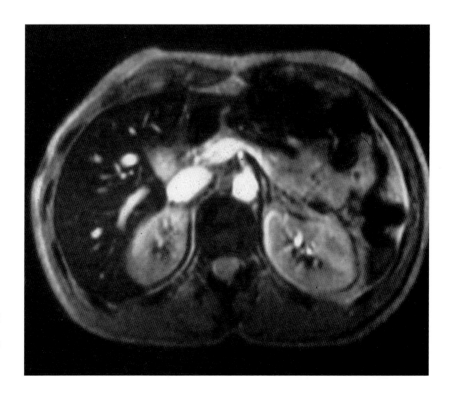

Figure 5.27 Axial, breath-hold coherent gradient echo sequence through the abdomen showing vessel patency in the aorta and IVC.

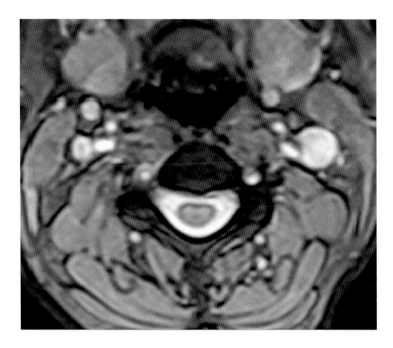

Figure 5.28 Axial coherent gradient echo sequence through the cervical spine. Note the high signal in the carotid arteries and jugular veins.

used to achieve T1 or T2* weighted images, although traditionally they are used in conjunction with a long TE to produce T2* weighting.

Uses

Coherent gradient echo pulse sequences usually produce rapid images that are T2* weighted (Figures 5.27 and 5.28). As water is bright they are often said to give an angiographic, myelographic or arthrographic effect. They can be used to determine whether a vessel is patent, or whether an area contains fluid. They can be acquired slice by slice, or in a 3D volume acquisition. As the TR is short, slices can be acquired in a single breath hold.

Parameters

5

To maintain the steady state:

    flip angles   30°–45°
    TR   20–50 ms

To maximize T2*:

    long TE   15–25 ms (although a short TE will maximize T1 effects)

Use gradient moment rephasing to accentuate T2* and reduce flow artefact (*see* Chapter 6)
Average scan time: seconds for single slice, 4–15 min for volumes

Advantages

- very fast scans, breath-holding possible
- very sensitive to flow so good for angiography
- can be acquired in a volume acquisition

Disadvantages

- poor SNR in 2D acquisitions
- magnetic susceptibility increases (*see* Chapter 7)
- loud gradient noise

Incoherent gradient echo (spoiled)

Mechanism

Incoherent gradient echo pulse sequences begin with a variable flip angle excitation pulse and use gradient rephasing to produce a gradient echo. The steady state is maintained, so that residual transverse magnetization is left over from previous repetitions. These sequences dephase or spoil this magnetization so that its effect on image contrast is minimal. Only transverse magnetization from the previous excitation is used, enabling T1 contrast to dominate. There are two ways to achieve spoiling. These are:

RF spoiling: In this sequence RF is transmitted at a particular frequency to excite a slice *and* at a specific phase. The receiver coil digitally communicates with the transmit coil and only frequencies from the echo that has just been created by the excitation pulse are digitized. Using the watch analogy from Chapter 1, disregard the precessional rotation of transverse magnetization for the purposes of this explanation and look at Figure 5.29. The first RF excitation pulse applied to a particular slice has a phase of 3 o'clock. This means that the resultant transverse magnetization is created at 3 o'clock in the transverse plane. Spins dephase and are rephased by a gradient to produce a gradient echo. The receiver coil, which is situated in the transverse plane, samples frequencies within this echo and data from them are sent to K space to produce the resultant image.

A short TR period later the process is repeated, but this time the RF excitation pulse creates transverse magnetization at a different phase such as 6 o'clock. Spins dephase and are rephased by a gradient to produce a second gradient echo. The receiver coil samples frequencies within this

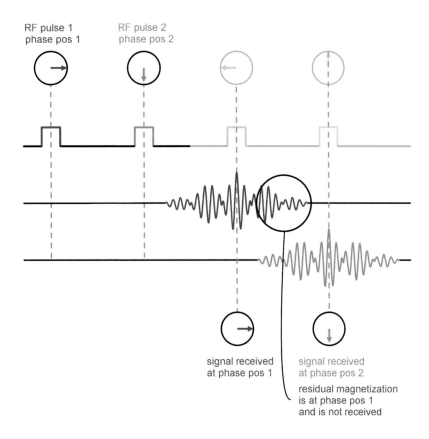

RF pulse 1
phase pos 1

RF pulse 2
phase pos 2

signal received
at phase pos 1

signal received
at phase pos 2

residual magnetization
is at phase pos 1
and is not received

Figure 5.29 RF spoiling in the incoherent gradient echo sequence.

echo and data from them are sent to K space to produce the resultant image. However, as the TR was so short, magnetization created at 3 o'clock is still present as it has not had time to decay. This is the residual transverse magnetization but, because it has a different phase to the transverse magnetization just created, it is not sampled and therefore does not impact image contrast. This is **RF spoiling** and enables only information from the most recently created magnetization to affect image contrast.

Gradient spoiling: Gradients can be used to dephase and rephase the residual magnetization (*see* Chapter 2). Gradient spoiling is the opposite of rewinding. In gradient spoiling, the slice select, phase encoding and frequency encoding gradients can be used to dephase the residual magnetization, so that it is incoherent at the beginning of the next repetition. In this way, T2* or T2 effects are reduced. Generally, the uses and parameters involved in these sequences are similar to those used in RF spoiling. However, most manufacturers use RF spoiling in incoherent gradient echo sequences.

Uses

As the stimulated echo that contains mainly T2* and T2 information is spoiled, RF spoiled pulse sequences produce T1 or proton density

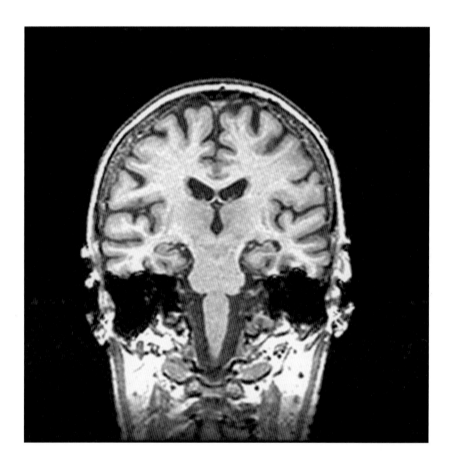

Figure 5.30 Coronal incoherent gradient echo sequence through the brain. This was acquired as part of a volume acquisition enabling T1 weighted high resolution imaging.

weighted images (Figure 5.30). They can be used for 2D and volume acquisitions and, as the TR is short, 2D acquisitions can be used to acquire T1 weighted breath-hold images. RF spoiled sequences demonstrate good T1 anatomy and pathology after gadolinium.

Parameters

To maintain the steady state:

flip angle	30°–45°
TR	20–50 ms

To maximize T1:

short TE	5–10 ms
average scan time	several seconds for single slice, 4–15 min for volumes

Advantages

- can be acquired in a volume or 2D
- breath-holding possible
- good SNR and anatomical detail in volume

Disadvantages

- SNR poor in 2D
- loud gradient noise

Steady state free precession (SSFP)

Mechanism

In gradient echo sequences the TE is not long enough to measure the T2 time of tissues as a TE of at least 70 ms is required for this. In addition, gradient rephasing is so inefficient that any echo is dominated by T2* effects and therefore true T2 weighting cannot be achieved. The SSFP sequence overcomes this problem to obtain images that have a sufficiently long TE and less T2* than in other steady state sequences. This is achieved in the following manner.

As previously described, every RF pulse, regardless of its net magnitude, contains energies that have sufficient magnitude to rephase spins and produce a stimulated echo. However, in SSFP we need to digitize frequencies only from this stimulated echo and not from the FID. To do this, the stimulated echo must be repositioned so that it does not occur at the same time as the subsequent excitation pulse. This is achieved by applying a rewinder gradient which speeds up the rephasing process initiated by the RF pulse so that the stimulated echo occurs sooner in the sequence (Figure 5.31).

The resultant echo demonstrates more true T2 weighting than conventional gradient echo sequences. This is because:

The TE is now longer than the TR. In SSFP, there are usually two TEs. The **actual TE** is the time between the echo and the next excitation pulse. The **effective TE** is the time from the echo to the excitation pulse that created its FID. Therefore:

effective TE = (2 × TR) − TE

If the TR is 50 ms and the TE is 10 ms, then:

effective TE = (2 × 50) − 10 = 90 ms

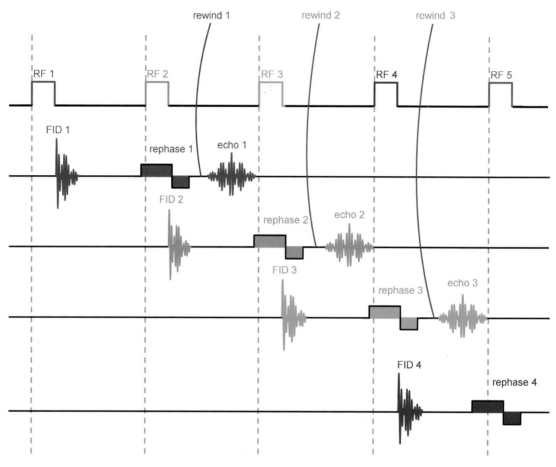

Figure 5.31   The SSFP sequence. Note how a rewinder gradient repositions each spin echo so that it no longer occurs at the same time as an excitation pulse but just before it. It can therefore be sampled on its own and the effects of the FID are eliminated.

This means that spins within the echo have had 90 ms to dephase between their excitation pulse and the regeneration of the echo. T2 weighting results.

Rephasing has been initiated by an RF pulse rather than a gradient so that more T2 information is present. The rewinder gradient merely repositions the stimulated echo at a time when it can be received.

Uses

SSFP sequences are used to acquire images that demonstrate true T2 weighting (Figure 5.32). They are especially useful in the brain and joints and on most systems can be used with both 2D and 3D volumetric acquisitions. However, FSE has now largely replaced this sequence as it produces better T2 weighting in short scan times.

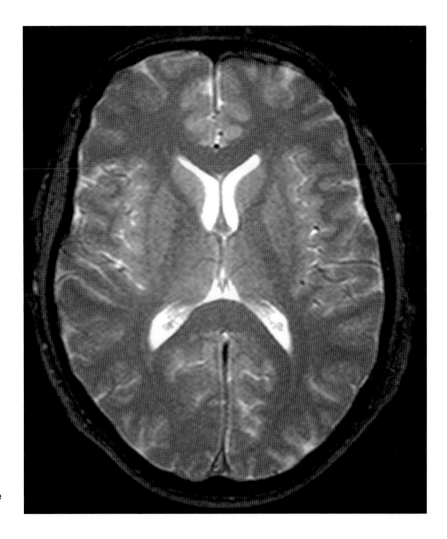

Figure 5.32 Axial SSFP image through the brain.

5

Learning point: T2* vs true T2

It is important to understand the difference between the terms true T2 and T2*. This is best demonstrated in imaging of the cervical spine. If the suspected pathology is a herniated disc, then using a T2* gradient echo sequence such as coherent gradient echo is appropriate. The disc will be demonstrated as a low signal intensity disc bulge into a high signal intensity CSF-filled thecal sac and produces a change in morphology (Figure 5.33). If, however, the pathology is more subtle, for example a small MS plaque within the cord, then we need to use a true T2 weighted sequence where the contrast seen depends on differences between the T2 times of the pathology and surrounding cord (Figure 5.34). In these circumstances it is better to use spin echo type sequences such as CSE, FSE or SSFP that use TEs long enough to measure the T2 decay times of tissues present.

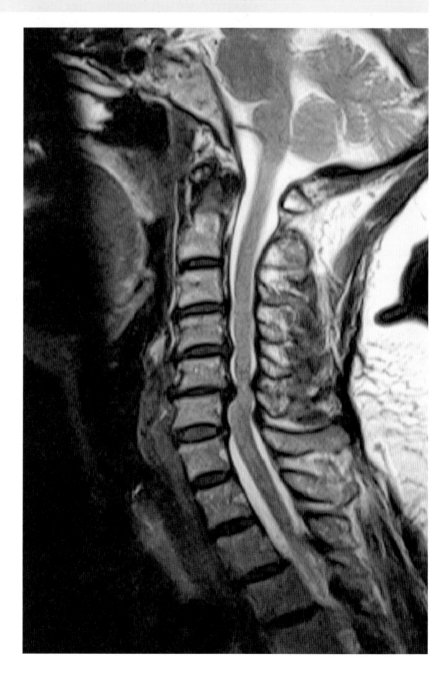

Figure 5.33 Sagittal T2* weighted coherent gradient echo sequence through the cervical cord. The prolapsed discs are well seen as they indent the thecal sac.

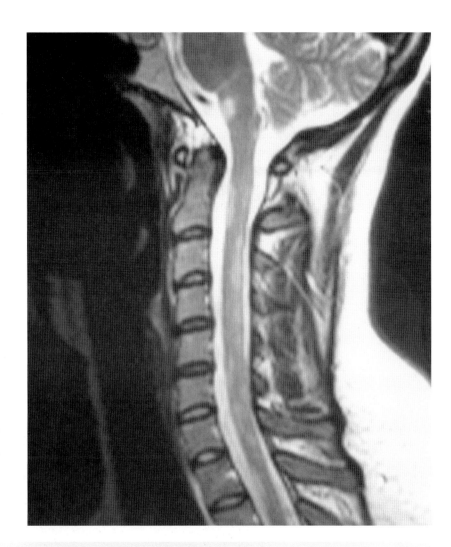

Figure 5.34 Sagittal T2 weighted FSE sequence through the cervical spine showing MS plaques within the cord. It is possible that these may have been missed in a T2* weighted sequence where the TE is not long enough to measure the T2 decay times of the pathology and surrounding cord.

Parameters

5

To maintain the steady state:

| flip angle | 30°–45° |
| TR | 20–50 ms |

The actual TE affects the effective TE. The longer the actual TE, the lower the effective TE. Actual TE should therefore be as short as possible.

Average scan time 4–15 min volume acquisition. Some manufacturers suggest decreasing the effective TE to reduce magnetic susceptibility, and increasing the flip angle to create more transverse magnetization, which results in higher SNR.

Advantages

- can be acquired in a volume and in 2D
- true T2 weighting achieved

Disadvantages

- susceptible to artefacts
- image quality can be poor
- loud gradient noise

Learning point: differentiating common steady state sequences

As previously explained, the steady state produces two signals:

- *a FID* made up of transverse magnetization that has just been created
- *a stimulated echo* made up of the residual transverse magnetization component.

Coherent gradient echo, incoherent gradient echo and SSFP pulse sequences can be differentiated according to whether they use one or both of these signals.

- Coherent gradient echo samples both the FID and the stimulated echo to produce either T1 or T2* weighted images depending on the TE used (Figure 5.35).
- Incoherent pulse sequences samples the FID only to produce mainly T1 weighted images (Figure 5.36).
- SSFP samples the stimulated echo only to produce images that are more T2 weighted (Figure 5.37).

Balanced gradient echo

Mechanism

This sequence is a modification of the coherent gradient echo sequence that uses a balanced gradient system to correct for phase errors in flowing blood and CSF and an alternating RF excitation scheme to enhance steady

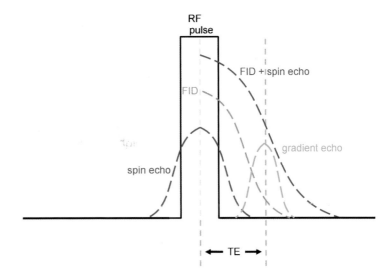

Figure 5.35 Echo formation in coherent gradient echo.

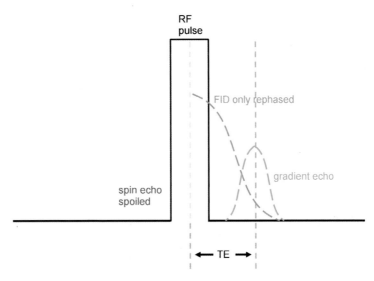

Figure 5.36 Echo formation in incoherent gradient echo.

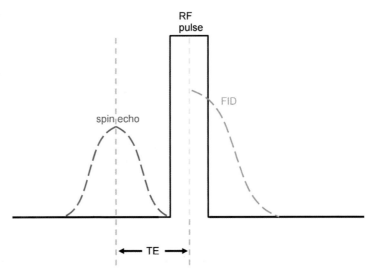

Figure 5.37 Echo formation in SSFP.

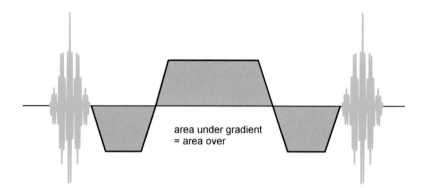

area under gradient
= area over

Figure 5.38   Balanced gradient system in balanced gradient echo.

state effects. In addition, both the FID and the spin echo are collected within a single readout. This results in images where fat and water produce a higher signal, greater SNR and fewer flow artefacts than coherent gradient echo in shorter scan times.

The balanced gradient system is shown in Figure 5.38. As the area of the gradient under the line equals that above the line, moving spins accumulate a zero phase change as they pass along the gradients. As a result, spins in blood and CSF are coherent and have a high signal intensity. This gradient formation is the same as flow compensation or gradient moment rephasing (*see* Chapter 6). In balanced gradient echo this gradient is applied in all three axes.

In addition, the steady state is maintained by using higher flip angles and shorter TRs than in coherent gradient echo, producing a higher SNR and shorter scan times. This is achieved by selecting a flip angle of 90°, for example, but in the first TR period only applying half of this, i.e. 45°. In successive TRs the full flip angle is applied but with alternating polarity so that the resultant transverse magnetization is created at a different phase every TR (i.e. 180° apart) (Figure 5.39). In this way fat and water, which have T1/T2 values approaching parity, return much higher signal than tissues that have not. The resultant images display high SNR, good CNR between fat, water and surrounding tissues, fewer flow voids and require very short scan times.

Uses

Balanced gradient echo was developed initially for imaging the heart and great vessels but it is now also used in spinal imaging, especially the

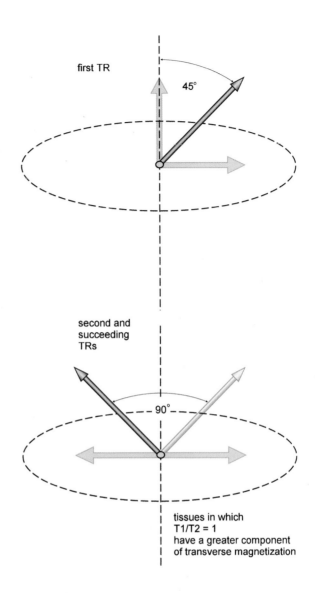

first TR

45°

second and
succeeding
TRs

90°

tissues in which
T1/T2 = 1
have a greater component
of transverse magnetization

Figure 5.39 Maintenance of
the steady state in balanced
gradient echo.

5

cervical spine and internal auditory meatus as CSF flow is reduced. It
is also sometimes used in joint and abdominal imaging (Figures 5.40
and 5.41).

Parameters

Large flip angle	90° (enhances SNR)
Short TR	10 ms (reduces scan time and flow artefact)
Long TE	15 ms (to enhance T2*)

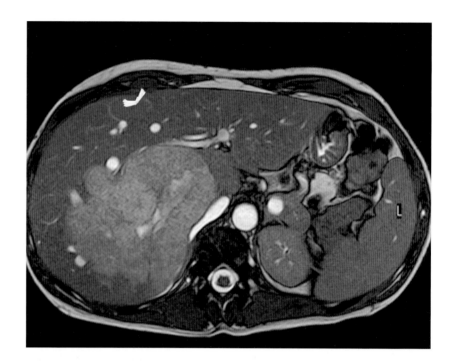

Figure 5.40   Axial balanced gradient echo image through the abdomen.

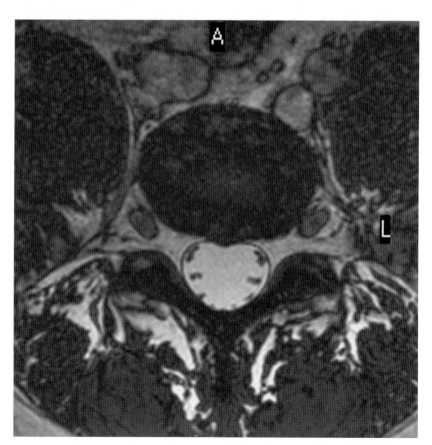

Figure 5.41   Axial balanced gradient echo image through the lumbar spine.

Fast gradient echo

Very fast pulse sequences have been developed that can acquire several slices or a volume in a single breath hold. These usually employ coherent or incoherent gradient echo sequences but the TE is significantly reduced. This is achieved by applying only a portion of the RF excitation pulse, so that it takes much less time to apply and switch off. Only a proportion of the echo is read (partial echo). These measures ensure that the TE is kept to a minimum, so that the TR and therefore the scan time can be reduced accordingly. In addition, many fast sequences use extra pulses applied before the pulse sequence begins, to pre-magnetize the tissue. In this way, certain contrast can be obtained. This pre-magnetization is achieved in the following two ways.

- A 180° pulse is applied before the pulse sequence begins. This inverts the NMV into full saturation and, at a specified delay time, the pulse sequence itself begins. This can be used to enhance T1 contrast or to null signal from certain organs and tissues, and is similar to inversion recovery.
- A 90°/180°/90° combination is applied before the pulse sequence begins. The first 90° pulse produces transverse magnetization. The 180° pulse rephases this, and at a specified time later the second 90° pulse is applied. This drives the coherent transverse magnetization into the longitudinal plane, so that it is available to be flipped when the pulse sequence begins. This is used to produce T2 contrast and is sometimes known as **driven equilibrium** (see also DRIVE which uses a similar principle).

Fast gradient systems permit multi-slice gradient echo sequences with TEs as short as 0.7 ms. Multiple images can therefore be acquired in a single breath hold and are free from respiratory motion artefacts. In addition, fast gradient echo acquisitions are useful when temporal resolution is required. This is especially important after the administration of contrast when the selection of fast gradient echo permits dynamic imaging of an enhancing lesion (*see* Chapter 8). This important technique has applications in many areas including the abdominal viscera and the breast.

5

K space filling in fast gradient echo sequences

To scan rapidly, it is usually necessary to fill K space in a different way to normal acquisitions. There are several permutations, most of which enhance signal and contrast and achieving rapid scan times.

Centric K space filling. This fills K space linearly (line by line) but instead of starting at an outer edge and working either upwards or downwards, it fills the central lines first. This is achieved by applying all the shallowest phase encoding gradients first, leaving the steep ones until the end of the pulse sequence. In this way, signal and contrast are maximized as the central lines are filled when echoes have their highest amplitude as

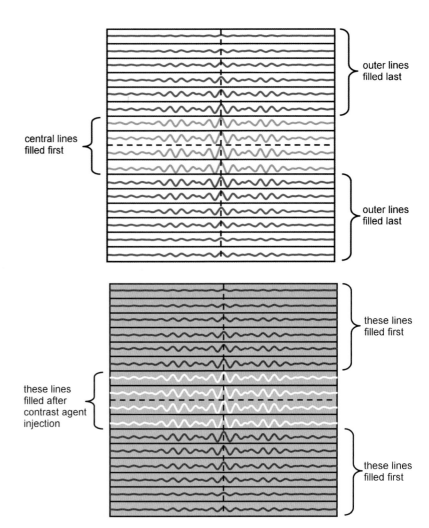

outer lines
filled last

central lines
filled first

outer lines
filled last

Figure 5.42 Centric K space filling.

these lines
filled first

these lines
filled after
contrast agent
injection

these lines
filled first

Figure 5.43 Keyhole imaging.

they have not yet decayed. This type of K space filling is important when using fast gradient echo techniques in which SNR and contrast is compromised (Figure 5.42).

Keyhole filling. This fills K space linearly and similarly to centric K space filling except that the central lines are only filled during a certain part of the sequence. This type of filling is used mainly in contrast enhanced angiography where we need to have a high temporal resolution for data acquired when gadolinium is present in the imaging volume (*see* Chapter 8). Before gadolinium arrives in the imaging volume, the system fills the outer resolution lines of K space. When gadolinium is in the imaging volume only a percentage of the central lines are filled. This means that acquisition times are short in this part of the sequence. At the end of the scan, the system 'stitches' the outer and central lines together to produce an image that has resolution and contrast. The contrast portion is acquired only when the gadolinium is present (Figure 5.43).

Echo planar imaging (EPI)

As shown in fast spin echo, the scan time is significantly reduced by filling more than one line of K space at once. Taking this concept to the limits, the fastest scan time possible would be one where all the lines are filled during one repetition. This forms the basis of EPI. EPI is an MR acquisition method that collects all the data required to fill all the lines of K space from a single echo train. To achieve this, multiple echoes are generated and each is phase encoded by a different slope of gradient to fill all the required lines of K space in a single TR period. For example, if a phase matrix of 128 is required then an echo train of 128 echoes is produced and individually phase encoded to fill 128 lines of K space in a single TR period. To fill all K space in one repetition, the readout and phase encode gradients must rapidly switch on and off and change direction (*see* Chapter 3). This forms the basis of single shot imaging (as used in single shot FSE) and EPI.

Filling K space in this way involves rapidly switching the readout gradient from positive to negative: positively to fill a line of K space from left to right and negatively to fill a line from right to left. This rapid change in gradient polarity also rephases the FID produced after the excitation pulse to generate the gradient echoes within the echo train. As the readout gradient switches its polarity so rapidly it is said to oscillate.

The phase gradient also has to switch on and off rapidly but its polarity does not need to change in this type of K space traversal. The first application of the phase gradient is maximum positive to fill the top line. The next application (to encode the next echo in the echo train) is still positive but its amplitude is slightly less so that the next line down is filled. This process is repeated until the center of K space is reached when the phase gradient switches negatively to fill the bottom lines. The amplitude is gradually increased until maximum negative polarity is achieved, filling the bottom line of K space. This type of gradient switching is called **blipping** (Figure 5.44). This type of single shot imaging is the simplest form in that, although all lines are filled in one TR, lines are filled linearly.

Spiral K space filling

A more complex type of K space traversal is shown in Figure 5.45. In this example both the readout and the phase gradient switch their polarity rapidly and oscillate. In this spiral form of K space traversal, the readout gradient oscillates to fill lines from left to right and then right to left, and K space filling begins at the center, the phase gradient must also oscillate to fill a line in the top half followed by a line in the bottom half. To understand this more clearly, place a pen at the center of K space on the diagram and work out the amplitude and polarity of each gradient as you move your pen along. In this example, the pen is never removed from the paper, indicating that there is no TR; all K space is filled in one go. Other

5

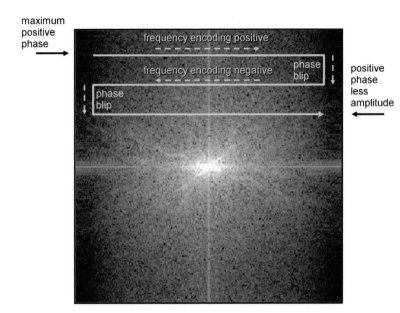

maximum
positive
phase

positive
phase
less
amplitude

Figure 5.44   K space filling
in EPI.

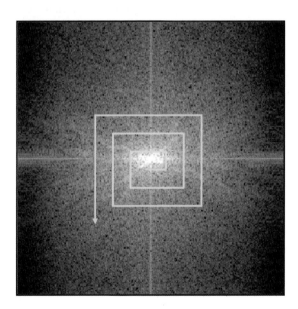

Figure 5.45   Spiral K space
filling.

5

modifications of spiral or radial K space filling ensure rapid filling of K space with enhanced filling of the central lines. These currently include:

- *elliptical K space filling*, where the central ellipse portion of K space is acquired as a 3D block
- *propeller K space filling*, where lines are acquired as a block but then rotated.

As all the echoes must be encoded before the transverse magnetization has decayed to zero, images contain a significant amount of T2* decay and the SNR is relatively poor. To compensate for this, K space may be acquired in segments. This is called **multi-shot** where data are acquired in several TR passes. In multi-shot EPI the effective time between echoes is dramatically reduced. As chemical shift, distortion and blurring are all proportional to echo spacing, artefacts in multi-shot EPI are reduced relative to single shot EPI. There are two multi-shot methods:

- *K space segmentation by acquisition* acquires a section of K space at a time (e.g. 4 quarters) so that there are four excitations and TR periods. If a 128 phase matrix is required then a turbo factor of 32, repeated four times, fills K space.
- *K space segmentation by echo* uses a turbo factor that is repeated several times (e.g. turbo factor of 4 repeated 32 times). Data from the first echoes are placed in the top quarter of K space, data from the second echoes in the next quarter, and so on.

Both methods increase the scan time compared to single shot imaging methods but produce images with improved quality.

EPI and single shot sequences place exceptional strains on the gradients and therefore gradient modifications are required at significant cost. The slew rates of the gradients must be about four times that of conventional gradients (*see* Chapter 9). Two types of gradient power supply modifications can be used:

- *Resonant power supplies* allow the readout and phase gradients to oscillate at the same frequency, reducing gradient requirements. The disadvantage is that they are only able to operate at a fixed frequency and amplitude. In practical terms this means that the gradients could only be used for EPI sequences so that the system would require two power supplies: one for EPI and one for conventional imaging.
- *Non-resonant power supplies* produce any gradient waveform so that both EPI and conventional sequences may be run off the same supply. This significantly reduces the cost but also the specifications of the gradients as they have to be able to cope with both types of sequence.

EPI contrast and parameters

In EPI, echoes are typically generated by oscillation of the readout gradient. However, different contrasts are achieved by either beginning the sequence variable RF excitation pulse termed **gradient echo EPI (GE-EPI)** or with 90° and 180° RF pulses termed **spin echo EPI (SE-EPI)**. GE-EPI begins with an excitation pulse of any flip angle and is followed by EPI readout of gradient echoes (Figure 5.46). In this scenario, images are acquired in one TR pass in milliseconds. Since gradient echoes are less time intensive than spin echoes, GE-EPI can be acquired faster than SE-EPI. Unfortunately GE-EPI images demonstrate the same detrimental artefacts that are found in conventional gradient echo images.

5

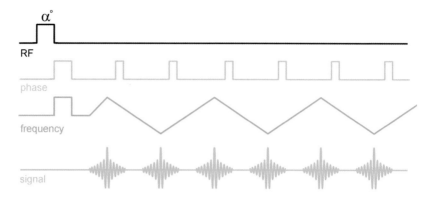

Figure 5.46 GE-EPI sequence.

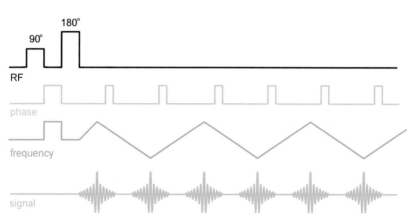

Figure 5.47 SE-EPI sequence.

In SE-EPI the sequence begins with a 90° excitation pulse followed by a 180° rephasing pulse followed by an EPI readout of gradient echoes (Figure 5.47). The application of the refocusing pulse helps to clean up some of the artefacts caused by magnetic field inhomogeneities and chemical shift. SE-EPI has longer scan times but generally better image quality than GE-EPI but the extra RF pulses increase RF deposition to the patient. EPI sequences may be preceded with any type of RF pulse. An example is EPI-FLAIR where CSF is nulled but the sequence is significantly faster than in conventional FLAIR sequencing (Figure 5.49)

Hybrid sequences, which combine gradient and spin echoes, such as **GRASE (gradient and spin echo)** are an effective compromise. Typically, a series of gradient rephasings is followed by an RF rephasing pulse (Figure 5.48). The hybrid sequence uses the benefits of both types of rephasing methods: the speed of the gradient and the ability of the RF pulse to compensate for T2* effects. These sequences increase the scan time to over 100 ms per image but the benefits in terms of image quality are significant.

In single shot imaging EPI techniques all K space is filled at once, the recovery rates of individual tissues are not critical. For this reason the TR is said to equal infinity (because it is infinitely long). Either proton density or T2 weighting is achieved by selecting either a short or long effective TE

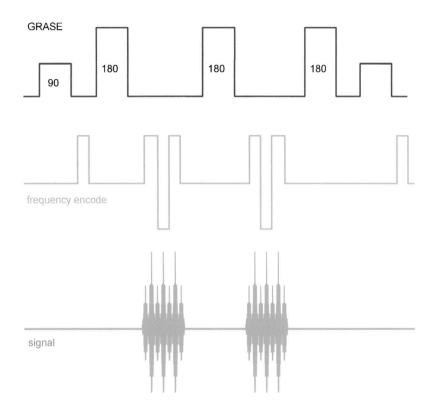

Figure 5.48 GRASE sequence.

which corresponds to the time interval between the excitation pulse and when the center of K space is filled. T1 weighting is possible by applying an inverting pulse before the excitation pulse to produce saturation.

Uses and limitations

Some typical EPI and GRASE images are shown in Figures 5.49, 5.50 and 5.51 and in Chapter 12. EPI and single shot techniques have increased the use of functional MRI (*see* Chapter 12). Scanning rapidly enables the freezing of physiological motion, which is advantageous when imaging the heart and coronary vessels (*see* Chapter 8) and when performing interventional techniques (*see* Chapter 12). Rapid imaging also enables visualization of physiology such as perfusion and blood oxygenation (*see* Chapter 12). Concerns over safety have, however, been expressed. The rapid switching of gradients causes nerve stimulation and gradient noise is severe, so acoustic insulation and ear protection are essential. In addition, many artefacts are seen in EPI including distortion and chemical shift.

As each echo is acquired rapidly, chemical shift in the frequency direction is relatively small. However, as the sampling in the phase direction is similar to a narrow readout bandwidth, there is a larger chemical shift along the phase axis. This phase directional chemical shift artefact does

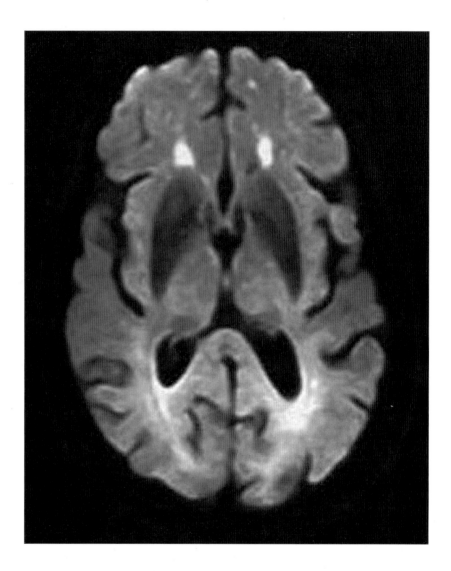

Figure 5.49 Axial EPI-FLAIR sequence through the brain. Note how the CSF signal is nulled.

5

not appear in standard spin or gradient echo acquisitions since echoes with different phase encodes are acquired at exactly the same time after excitation. The length of time required to acquire a train of phase encodes results in a small effective bandwidth of phase encode. For this reason, in EPI chemical shifts for fat are typically 10–20 pixels compared with the 1–2 pixel misregistration in spin echo imaging.

Other artefacts seen on EPI include blurring and ghosting. Blurring occurs as the result of T2* decay during the course of the EPI acquisition. If the train of echoes takes a similar time to decay, the signal from the end of the acquisition is reduced, resulting in a loss of resolution and blurring. Half of the FOV ghosts occur as the result of small errors in the timing and shape of readout gradients. This causes differences between echoes acquired with positive and negative readout gradients. These errors cause a ghost of the real image that appears shifted in the phase direction by one

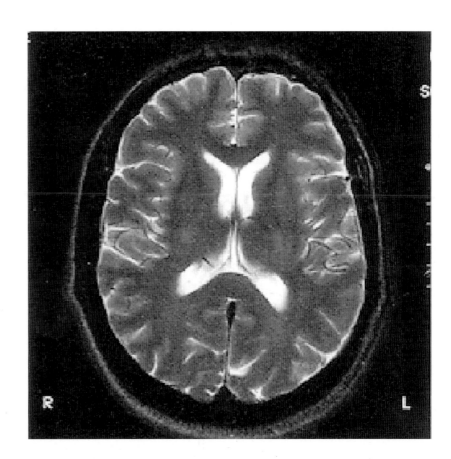

Figure 5.50 Axial GRASE image through the brain.

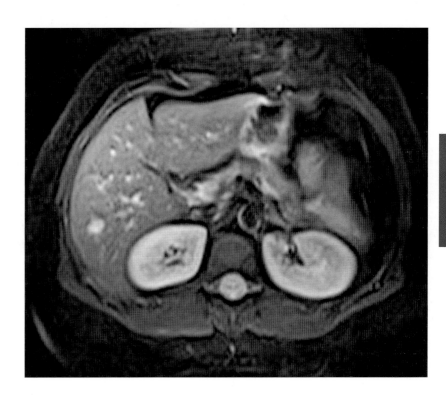

Figure 5.51 Axial SE-EPI image through the abdomen.

half of the FOV. Since it is difficult to eliminate these errors, a correction is usually performed during image reconstruction using information acquired during the reference scan. Despite these problems EPI and hybrid sequences have a significant place in clinical MRI.

PARALLEL IMAGING TECHNIQUES

Parallel imaging or **sensitivity encoding** is a technique that fills K space more efficiently than conventional imaging by filling multiple lines of K space per TR (as in FSE). Unlike FSE, however, these lines are acquired by assigning them to certain coils that are coupled together to enable them to acquire data simultaneously. Therefore we need to have coils specifically designed for this purpose and software to link them electronically. Typically 2, 4, 6 or 8 coils are used and arranged around the area to be imaged. In this example let us assume a 4-coil configuration (Figure 5.52).

coil 1 acquires line 1 and every fourth line thereafter
coil 2 acquires line 2 and every fourth line thereafter
coil 3 acquires line 3 and every fourth line thereafter
coil 4 acquires line 4 and every fourth line thereafter.

Hence every TR, four lines of K space are acquired. In the first TR period:

coil 1 acquires line 1
coil 2 acquires line 2
coil 3 acquires line 3
coil 4 acquires line 4.

In TR period 2:

coil 1 acquires line 5
coil 2 acquires line 6
coil 3 acquires line 7
coil 4 acquires line 8, and so on.

The process is repeated until all the lines are filled. As four lines are acquired per TR, the scan time is decreased by a factor of 4. This is sometimes called the **reduction factor** and is similar to the turbo factor in FSE. The reduction factor equals the number of coils in the configuration.

Now let's look at the lines acquired by each coil. You can see from Figure 5.52 that each coil has acquired every fourth line and that as a result the gap between each line is four times greater than if K space had been filled normally. Using the chest of drawers analogy in Chapter 3, this means that the depth of each drawer has quadrupled and, as this dimension is inversely proportional to the size of the FOV in the phase direction, the size of the FOV in the phase direction is reduced to a quarter of its

5

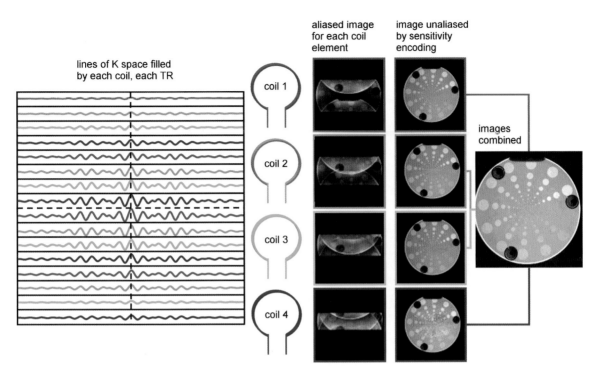

Figure 5.52 Parallel imaging.

original size as in a rectangular FOV (*see* Chapter 4). As a result, aliasing of tissue outside the FOV in the phase direction occurs and therefore each coil produces a wrapped image (*see* Chapter 7). To rectify this, the system uses the sensitivity profile of each coil to calculate where the signal is coming from relative to the coil so that it can map it correctly onto the image. This profile determines the position of the signal relative to the coil based on its amplitude. The signal coming from near to the coil has a higher amplitude than that from furthest away. As a result of this process, the image is unwrapped and combined with the unwrapped images from the other coils to form one image of the slice (*see* Figure 9.21).

Uses

Parallel imaging is an important development and can be used to either reduce scan times or improve resolution. It can be used with most pulse sequences with the appropriate software and coil configurations. Although it has obvious benefits in terms of scan time and/or resolution, it results in a slight loss of SNR. In addition, chemical shift may increase due to different resonant frequencies being mapped across each coil. Patient movement also causes misalignment between under-sampled data and reference scans.

Table 5.2   A comparison of acronyms used by manufacturers.

	GE	Philips	Siemens	Picker
Spin echo	SE	SE	SE	SE
Fast spin echo	FSE	TSE	TSE	FSE
Inversion recovery	IR	IR	IR	IR
Short Tau inversion recovery	STIR	STIR	STIR	STIR
Fluid attenuated inversion recovery	FLAIR	FLAIR	FLAIR	FLAIR
Coherent gradient echo	GRASS	FFE	FISP	FAST
Incoherent gradient echo	SPGR	T1FFE	FLASH	RF spoiled FAST
Balanced gradient echo	FIESTA	BFFE	True FISP	–
Steady state free precession	SSFP	T2 FFE	PSIF	CE FAST
Fast gradient echo	Fast GRASS/SPGR	TFE	Turbo FLASH	RAM FAST
Echo planar	EPI	EPI	EPI	EPI
Parallel imaging	ASSET	SENSE	iPAT	SMASH
Spatial pre-saturation	SAT	REST	SAT	Pre-SAT
Gradient moment rephasing	Flow comp	Flow comp	GMR	MAST
Signal averaging	NEX	NSA	AC	NSA
Anti-aliasing	No phase wrap	Foldover suppression	Oversampling	Oversampling
Rectangular FOV	Rect FOV	Rect FOV	Half Fourier imaging	Undersampling
Respiratory compensation	Resp comp	PEAR	Resp trigger	Resp gating

Abbreviations used above

AC	number of acquisitions
ASSET	array spatial and sensitivity encoding technique
CE FAST	contrast enhanced FAST
FAST	Fourier acquired steady state technique
FFE	fast field echo
FIESTA	free induction echo stimulated acquisition
FISP	free induction steady precession
FLAIR	fluid attenuated inversion recovery
FLASH	fast low angled shot
Flow comp	flow compensation
FSE	fast spin echo
GMR	gradient moment rephasing
GRASS	gradient recalled acquisition in the steady state
iPAT	integrated parallel acquisition technique
MAST	motion artefact suppression
MP RAGE	magnetization prepared rapid gradient echo
NEX	number of excitations
NSA	number of signal averages
PEAR	phase encoding artefact reduction
PSIF	mirrored FISP
RAM FAST	rapid acquisition matrix FAST
REST	regional saturation technique
SENSE	sensitivity encoding
SMASH	simultaneous acquisition of spatial harmonics
SPGR	spoiled GRASS
SSFP	steady state free precession
STIR	short tau inversion recovery
TFE	turbo field echo
TSE	turbo spin echo
Turbo FLASH	magnetization prepared sub second imaging

5

Table 5.3 Single and multi-shot methods.

	Sequence	Readout	Time
FSE	90/180	multiple SE	min/sec
GRASE	90/180	GE	min/sec
SE-EPI	90/180	GE	sec/sub sec
GE-EPI	variable flip	GE	sec/sub sec

The choice of each pulse sequence is often a quite difficult one. There are now so many that we are really spoilt for choice. However, generally speaking every pulse sequence is designed to produce a certain contrast, image quality and data acquisition. These factors should be taken into account when selecting a particular pulse sequence. Table 5.2 should help most readers apply the terms used in this and other chapters to their type of system. Table 5.3 compares the various rapid imaging techniques.

Questions

1   Explain why RF spoiled pulse sequences are not the best choice when T2* weighting is required.

2   How does balanced gradient echo differ from coherent gradient echo?

3   What parameters are used in FLAIR sequences and why?

4   What are the effects of lengthening the turbo factor in fast spin echo?

5   In which sequence is the stimulated echo only sampled?

6   When using parallel imaging how many coils should you use to halve the scan time compared with normal sequencing?

5

6

Flow phenomena

Introduction

This chapter specifically explores artefacts produced from nuclei that move during the acquisition of data. Flowing nuclei exhibit different contrast characteristics from their neighboring stationary nuclei, and originate primarily from nuclei in blood and CSF. The motion of flowing nuclei causes mismapping of signals and results in artefacts known as phase ghosting. The causes of flow artefact are collectively known as **flow phenomena**. The principal phenomena are:

- time of flight
- entry slice phenomenon
- intra-voxel dephasing.

First, however, the common mechanisms and types of flow are analyzed.

THE MECHANISM OF FLOW

There are four principal types of flow (Figure 6.1):

- **Laminar flow** is flow that is at different but consistent velocities across a vessel. The flow at the center of the lumen of the vessel is

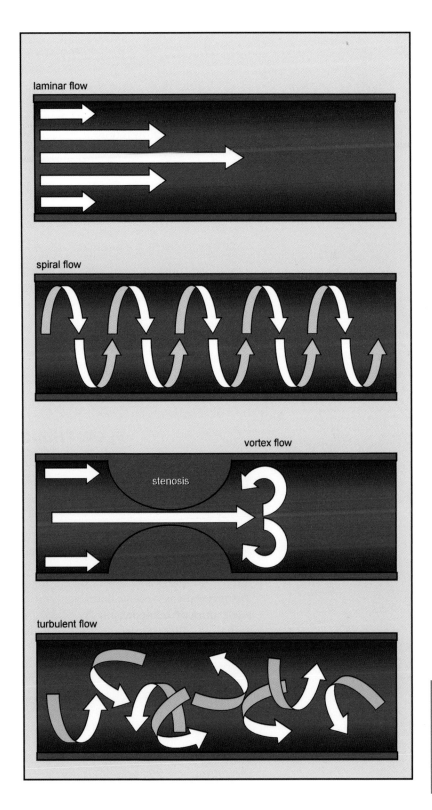

Figure 6.1 The different types of flow.

faster than at the vessel wall, where resistance slows down the flow. However, the velocity difference across the vessel is constant.

- **Spiral flow** is where the direction of flow is spiral.
- **Vortex flow** is flow that is initially laminar but then passes through a stricture or stenosis in the vessel. Flow in the center of the lumen has a high velocity, but near the walls, the flow spirals.
- **Turbulent flow** is flow at different velocities that fluctuates randomly. The velocity difference across the vessel changes erratically.

Learning point: flow mechanisms

Flow mechanisms are often termed as follows:

- First order motion laminar flow (constant velocity)
- Second order motion acceleration
- Third order motion jerk

Only first order flow can be compensated for as the system can only correct for flow that is at a constant velocity and direction during data acquisition.

FLOW PHENOMENA

Time of flight phenomenon

To produce a signal, a nucleus must receive an excitation pulse and a rephasing pulse. If a nucleus receives the excitation pulse only and is not rephased, it does not produce a signal. Similarly, if a nucleus is rephased but has not previously been excited, it does not produce a signal. Stationary nuclei always receive both excitation and rephasing pulses, but flowing nuclei present in the slice for the excitation may have exited the slice before rephasing. This is called the **time of flight phenomenon** (Figure 6.2). The effects of the time of flight phenomenon depend on the type of pulse sequence used.

Time of flight in spin echo pulse sequences. In a spin echo pulse sequence, a 90° excitation pulse and a 180° rephasing pulse are applied to each slice. Every slice is therefore selectively excited and rephased. Stationary nuclei within the slice receive both the 90° and the 180° RF pulses and produce a signal.

Nuclei flowing perpendicular to the slices may be present within the slice during the 90° pulse, but may have exited the slice before the 180° pulse can be delivered. These nuclei are excited but not rephased and do

6

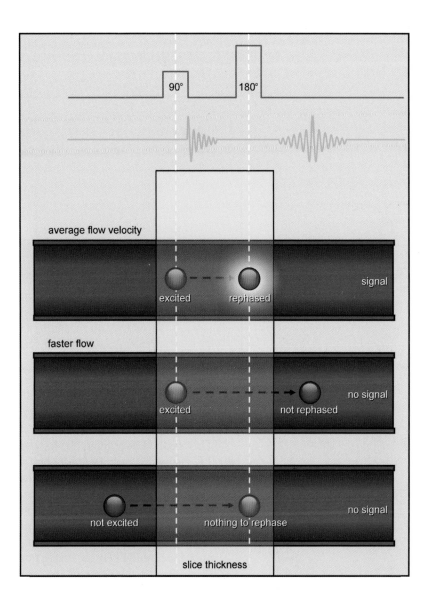

Figure 6.2 The time of flight phenomenon.

not therefore give a signal. Alternatively, nuclei not present in the slice during excitation may be present during rephasing. These nuclei have not previously been excited and do not therefore give a signal. Time of flight phenomena result in a signal void from the nuclei and so the vessel appears dark. Time of flight effects depend on the:

- *Velocity of flow.* As the velocity of flow increases, a smaller proportion of flowing nuclei are present in the slice for both the 90° and the 180° RF pulses. As the velocity of flow increases, the time of flight effect increases. This is called **high velocity signal loss**. As the velocity of flow decreases, a higher proportion of flowing nuclei are present in the slice for both the 90° and the 180° RF pulses. Therefore

6

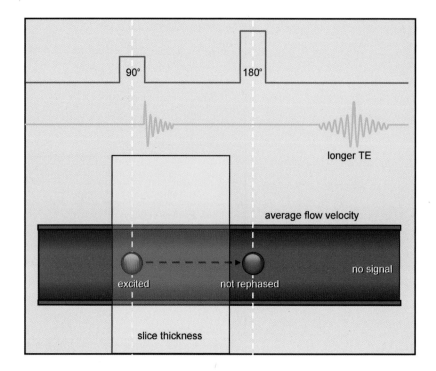

Figure 6.3   Time of flight versus TE.

as the velocity of flow decreases, the time of flight effect decreases. This is called **flow-related enhancement**.

- *TE.* As the TE increases, a higher proportion of flowing nuclei have exited the slice between the excitation pulse and the 180° rephasing pulse. Therefore, at a longer TE, more nuclei have received only one pulse and the signal void increases (Figure 6.3).
- *Slice thickness.* For a given constant velocity, nuclei take longer to travel through a thick slice compared with a thin slice. Therefore, nuclei are more likely to receive both the 90° and 180° pulse in thick slices. As the thickness of the slice decreases, the nuclei are more likely to receive only one pulse and the signal void increases.

Time of flight in gradient echo pulse sequences. In gradient echo pulse sequences, a variable excitation pulse is followed by gradient rephasing. Each slice is selectively excited by the RF pulse, but the rephasing gradient is applied to the whole body. In other words, the excitation pulse is slice selective, but the gradient rephasing is not. Therefore, a flowing nucleus that receives an excitation pulse is rephased regardless of its slice position and produces a signal. In addition, the very short TR usually associated with gradient echo sequences tends to saturate stationary nuclei which receive repeated RF pulses so that flowing nuclei appear to have a higher signal. This is explored later. In gradient echo pulse sequences therefore, flow signal enhancement is increased and these pulse sequences are often said to be flow-sensitive.

6

Summary

- Time of flight phenomena produce flow-related enhancement or high velocity signal loss
- Flow-related enhancement increases as the:
  - velocity of flow decreases
  - TE decreases
  - slice thickness increases
- High velocity signal void increases as the
  - velocity of flow increases
  - TE increases
  - slice thickness decreases

Entry slice phenomenon

Entry slice phenomenon is related to the excitation history of the nuclei. Nuclei that receive repeated RF pulses during an acquisition with a short TR are said to be **saturated** because their magnetic moments are more likely to be orientated in the spin-down direction (*see* Chapter 1). This is because the TR is not long enough for longitudinal recovery of magnetization in the tissues in which the nuclei reside. Nuclei that have not received these repeated RF pulses are said to be **fresh**, as their magnetic moments are mainly orientated in the spin-up direction. The signal that they produce is different from that of the saturated nuclei (Figure 6.4).

Stationary nuclei within a slice become saturated after repeated RF pulses, especially when the TR is short. Nuclei flowing perpendicular to the slice enter the slice fresh, as they were not present during repeated excitations. They therefore produce a different signal from the stationary nuclei. This is called the **entry slice phenomenon** or **inflow effect** as it is most prominent in the first slice of a 'stack' of slices.

The slices in the middle of the stack exhibit less entry slice phenomenon, as flowing nuclei have received more excitation pulses by the time they reach these slices. In other words, they become less fresh and more saturated and their signal intensity depends mostly on the TE, TR, flip angle and the contrast characteristics of the tissue in which they are situated.

The entry slice phenomenon only decreases if nuclei receive repeated excitations. The rate at which the nuclei receive the excitation pulses determines the magnitude of the phenomenon. Any factor that affects the rate at which a nucleus receives repeated excitations affects the magnitude of the phenomenon. The magnitude of entry slice phenomenon therefore depends on:

6

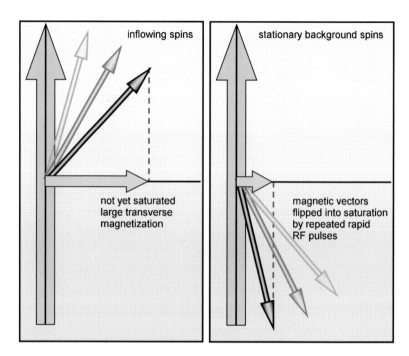

Figure 6.4 Contrast differences between saturated and fresh inflowing spins.

- *TR.* The TR is the time between each excitation pulse. A short TR results in an increase in the rate at which the RF is delivered. In other words, a short TR decreases the time between successive RF pulses. A short TR therefore reduces the magnitude of the entry slice phenomenon.
- *Slice thickness.* Flowing nuclei with a constant velocity take longer to travel through thick slices than thin slices. Nuclei traveling through thick slices are likely to receive more RF pulses than nuclei traveling through thin slices. The entry slice phenomenon therefore increases in thick slices compared with in thin slices.
- *Velocity of flow.* The velocity of flow also affects the rate at which a flowing nucleus receives RF. Fast-flowing nuclei are more likely to have traveled to the next slice when RF is delivered than slow nuclei. The entry slice phenomenon is therefore increased as the velocity of flow increases.
- *Direction of flow.* The direction of flow is probably the most important factor in determining the magnitude of the entry slice phenomenon. Flow that is in the same direction as slice selection is called **co-current** flow. Flow that is in the opposite direction to slice selection is called **counter-current** flow.
    - *Co-current flow.* Flowing nuclei travel in the same direction as slice selection. The flowing nuclei are more likely to receive repeated RF excitations as they move from one slice to the next. They therefore become saturated relatively quickly, and so the entry slice phenomenon decreases rapidly.

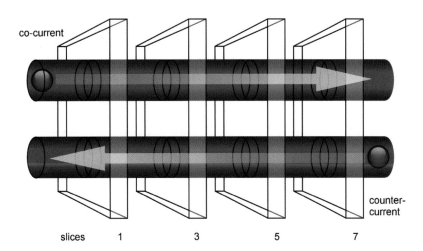

co-current

counter-current

slices   1   3   5   7

Figure 6.5 Co- and counter-current flow.

- *Counter-current flow*. Flowing nuclei travel in the opposite direction to slice excitation. Flowing nuclei stay fresh, as when they enter a slice they are less likely to have received previous excitation pulses. The entry slice phenomenon does not therefore decrease rapidly and may still be present deep within the slice stack (Figure 6.5).

Learning point: entry slice phenomenon in clinical imaging

Look at Figures 6.6 to 6.9. These are four axial slices through the abdomen prescribed and excited from the most inferior position to the most superior position, i.e. Figure 6.6 is slice 1, Figure 6.7 is slice 2, Figure 6.8 is slice 3 and Figure 6.9 is slice 4 in the stack of slices. Slice 1 was acquired first; slice 4 last, in the acquisition.

Look at the signal intensity of the aorta and IVC in these images. Although they both contain blood and should be the same signal intensity on all slices it is clear that this is not the case. In slice 1 the IVC has high signal intensity and the aorta low signal intensity. In slice 4 the contrast is opposite, i.e. the IVC is dark and the aorta is bright. In addition the IVC is darker on slice 4 than the aorta is on slice 1.

These appearances are due to entry slice phenomena. In slice 1, nuclei in the IVC are fresh because they have traveled up from the legs and have received no previous RF pulses because they are not positioned in the stack of slices. Therefore in slice 1 these nuclei receive their first RF pulse and return a high signal as their magnetic moments are mainly in the spin-up direction and are not saturated. Nuclei in the aorta, however, are saturated and return a low signal

6

because they have been excited by RF pulses as they have traveled down through the stack of slices during acquisition and their magnetic moments are primarily orientated in the spin-down direction.

In slice 4, the effect is opposite to that in slice 1. Nuclei in the aorta are now fresh as they have been traveling from the head and arms and have received no previous RF pulses. Therefore in slice 4 these nuclei receive their first RF pulse and return a high signal as their magnetic moments are mainly orientated in the spin-up direction. Nuclei in the IVC, however, are saturated by repeated RF pulses as they travel through the stack during the acquisition and their magnetic moments are primarily orientated in the spin-down direction. In slices 2 and 3, however, this inflow effect decreases as nuclei in both vessels have received RF pulses.

The IVC is darker on slice 4 than the aorta is on slice 1 because flow in the IVC is co-current to slice excitation while flow in the aorta is counter-current. Therefore nuclei in the IVC receive more RF pulses because they are traveling in the same direction as slice excitation than nuclei in the aorta that are traveling in the opposite direction to slice excitation. This effect is rarely seen in clinical imaging because flow compensation techniques such as spatial pre-saturation eliminate it. This is discussed later.

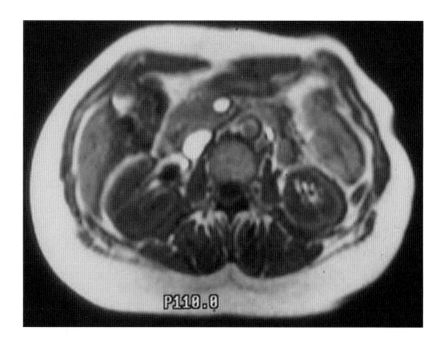

Figure 6.6   Axial T1 weighted image slice 1 (most inferior).

6

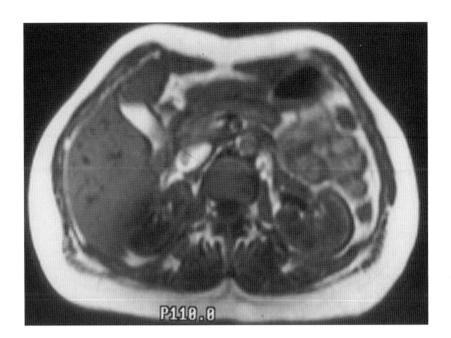

Figure 6.7 Axial T1 weighted image slice 2.

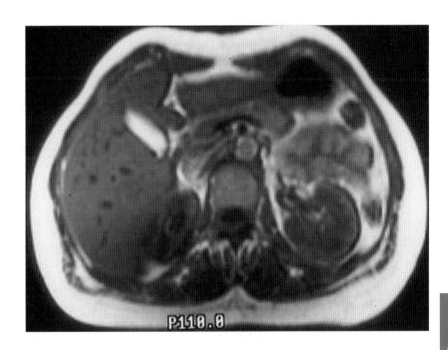

Figure 6.8 Axial T1 weighted image slice 3 .

6

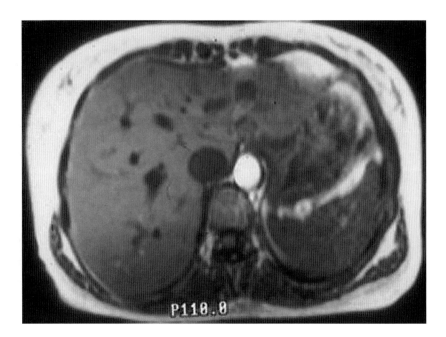

Figure 6.9 Axial T1 weighted image slice 4 (most superior).

Summary

Entry slice phenomenon increases:

- at the first slice in the stack
- when using a long TR
- in thin slices
- with fast flow
- in counter-current flow

Intra-voxel dephasing

Gradients alter the magnetic field strength, precessional frequency and phase of nuclei. Nuclei flowing along a gradient rapidly accelerate or decelerate depending on the direction of flow and gradient application. Flowing nuclei therefore either gain phase (if they have been accelerated), or lose phase (if they have been decelerated) (*see* the watch analogy in Chapter 1).

If a flowing nucleus is adjacent to a stationary nucleus in a voxel, there is a phase difference between the two nuclei. This is because the flowing nucleus has either lost or gained phase relative to the stationary nucleus due to its motion along the gradient. Therefore nuclei within the same

6

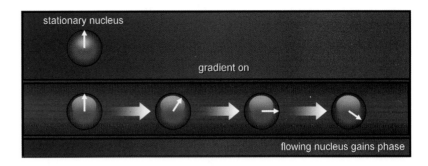

Figure 6.10 Intra-voxel dephasing.

voxel are out of phase with each other, which results in a reduction of total signal amplitude from the voxel. This is called **intra-voxel dephasing** (Figure 6.10). The magnitude of intra-voxel dephasing depends on the degree of turbulence. In turbulent flow, intra-voxel dephasing effects are irreversible. In laminar flow, the intra-voxel dephasing can be compensated for as long as the velocity and direction of flow are constant.

Summary

- Flow affects image quality
- Time of flight effects give signal void or enhancement
- Entry slice phenomenon effects give a different signal intensity to flowing nuclei
- The signal intensity of the lumen is also affected by the mechanism of flow

FLOW PHENOMENA COMPENSATION

Introduction

Flowing nuclei therefore produce a very confusing range of signal intensities. Ideally, these should be compensated for, so that their adverse effects on image quality and interpretation can be minimized. There are several methods available to help reduce flow artefacts and these are now discussed. These techniques also reduce phase mismapping in pulsed flow such as blood and CSF. This is discussed in more detail in Chapter 7. The methods for reducing flow phenomena are:

- even echo rephasing
- gradient moment nulling
- spatial pre-saturation.

6

Even echo rephasing

If two or more echoes are produced in a spin echo pulse sequence, intra-voxel dephasing may be reduced by acquiring the second and succeeding even echoes at a multiple of the first TE, for example, two echoes, first TE 40 ms and second TE 80 ms. This works on the principle that flowing nuclei that are out of phase at the first echo are in phase at the second echo as long as the nuclei are given exactly the same amount of time to rephase as they were given to dephase. In other words, if at the first TE of 40 ms they are out of phase, 40 ms later (at 80 ms) they will be in phase again. This is called **even echo rephasing** and can be used to reduce artefact in a T2 weighted image.

Gradient moment rephasing (nulling)

Gradient moment rephasing compensates for the altered phase values of the nuclei flowing along a gradient. It uses additional gradients to correct the altered phases back to their original values and follows the same principles as the balanced gradient system used in balanced gradient echo sequences (*see* Chapter 5). Flowing nuclei do not gain or lose phase due to the presence of the main gradient.

Gradient moment rephasing is performed by the slice select gradient and/or the readout gradient. The gradient alters its polarity from positive to double negative and then back to positive again. A flowing nucleus traveling along these gradients experiences different magnetic field strengths, and its phase changes accordingly. This is shown in Figure 6.11 where a flowing spin gains 90° of phase as it passes along the first positive lobe of the gradient and then loses 180° of phase as it passes through the double negative lobe of the gradient. Its net phase change at this stage is that it has lost 90° of phase. As it then passes through the last positive lobe of the gradient this is corrected so that the net phase change is zero.

Gradient moment rephasing predominantly reduces intra-voxel dephasing. As flowing nuclei have the same phase as stationary nuclei in the same voxel, their signals add constructively and therefore a bright signal results. Gradient moment rephasing gives flowing nuclei a bright signal as spins are in phase. In Figure 6.12 ghosting of the aorta is clearly seen. This is removed in Figure 6.13 where gradient moment rephasing has been applied.

Gradient moment rephasing assumes a constant velocity and direction across the gradients at all times. It is most effective on slow laminar flow and is therefore often termed **first order motion compensation**. Pulsatile flow is not strictly constant, so gradient moment rephasing is often more effective on venous, rather than arterial, flow. It is also less effective on turbulent, fast flow perpendicular to the slice.

6

no gradient

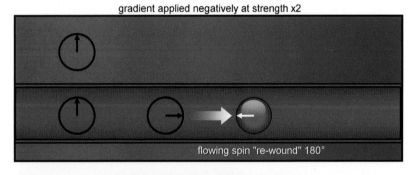

gradient applied positively at strength x1

gradient applied negatively at strength x2

Figure 6.11 Gradient moment rephasing (nulling).

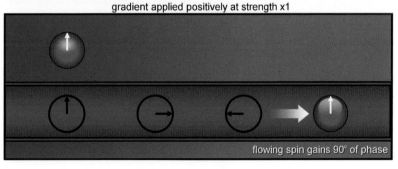

gradient applied positively at strength x1

As gradient moment rephasing uses extra gradients, it increases the minimum TE. If the system has to perform extra gradient tasks, more time must elapse before it is ready to read an echo. As a result, fewer slices may be available for a given TR or the TR and therefore the scan time may be

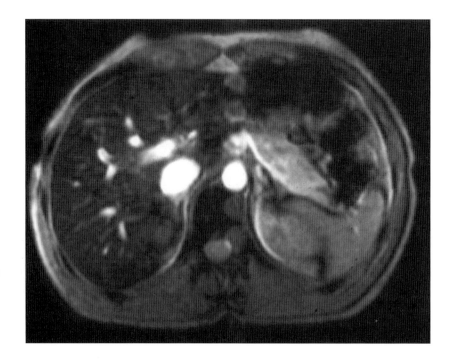

Figure 6.12 Axial T2* coherent gradient echo through the abdomen demonstrating flow artefact in the aorta, causing phase ghosting. No gradient moment rephasing was used.

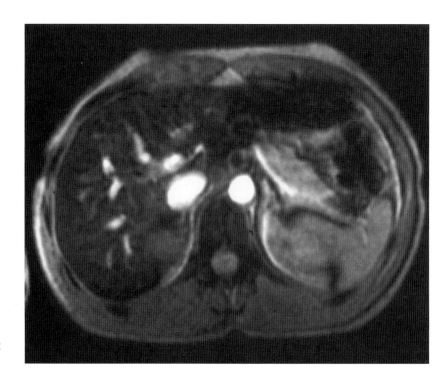

Figure 6.13 Axial T2* coherent gradient echo through the abdomen with gradient moment rephasing. The artefact has largely been eliminated.

automatically increased to scan the selected slices. As flowing nuclei are bright when gradient moment rephasing is selected, it is usually used in T2 and T2* weighted sequences where fluid (blood and CSF) is bright anyway.

Spatial pre-saturation

Spatial pre-saturation pulses nullify the signal from flowing nuclei so that the effects of entry slice and time of flight phenomena are minimized. Spatial pre-saturation delivers a 90° RF pulse to a volume of tissue outside the FOV. A flowing nucleus within the volume receives this 90° pulse. When it then enters the slice stack, it also receives an excitation pulse and is saturated. If it is fully saturated to 180°, it has no transverse component of magnetization and produces a signal void (Figure 6.14).

To be effective, pre-saturation pulses should be placed between the flow and the imaging stack so that signal from flowing nuclei entering the FOV is nullified. In sagittal and axial imaging, pre-saturation pulses are usually placed above and below the FOV so that arterial flow from above and venous flow from below are saturated. Right and left pre-saturation pulses are sometimes useful in coronal imaging (especially in the chest) to saturate flow from the subclavian vessels.

Spatial pre-saturation pulses can be brought into the FOV itself. This permits artefact producing areas (such as the aorta) to be pre-saturated so

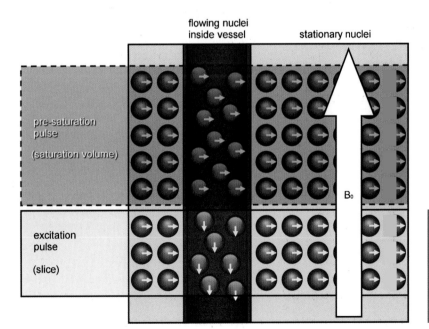

Figure 6.14 Spatial pre-saturation.

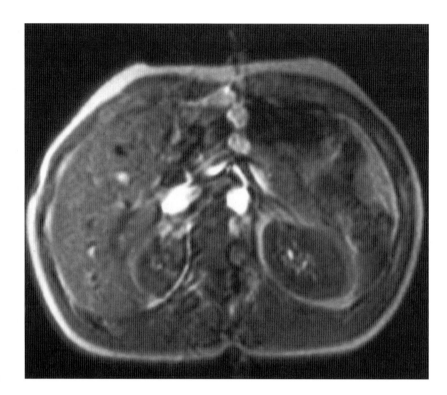

Figure 6.15 Axial T2* coherent gradient echo through the abdomen demonstrating flow artefact in the aorta, causing phase ghosting. No spatial pre-saturation was used.

that phase mismapping can be reduced (*see* Chapter 7). Pre-saturation pulses are only useful if they are applied to tissue. If they are applied to air they are not effective. They increase the amount of RF that is delivered to the patient, which may increase heating effects (*see* Chapter 10). The use of pre-saturation pulses may also decrease the number of slices available and should therefore be used appropriately.

Pre-saturation pulses are also only effective if the flowing nucleus receives the 90° pre-saturation pulse. Pulses are applied around each slice just before the excitation pulse. The TR, and the number of slices, therefore govern the interval between the delivery of each pre-saturation pulse. To optimize pre-saturation, use all the slices permitted for a given TR. As pre-saturation produces a signal void, it is usually used in T1 and proton density weighted images where fluid (blood and CSF) is dark anyway. Figures 6.15 and 6.16 show axial T1 weighted gradient echo images of the abdomen with and without pre-saturation. Ghosting of the aorta seen on Figure 6.15 is largely eliminated by using spatial pre-saturation pulses in Figure 6.16. Note also that the signal intensity of the aorta is reduced by using pre-saturation.

Pre-saturation nullifies signal and can therefore be used specifically to eliminate certain signals. The main uses of this are:

- chemical pre-saturation
- spatial inversion recovery (SPIR).

6

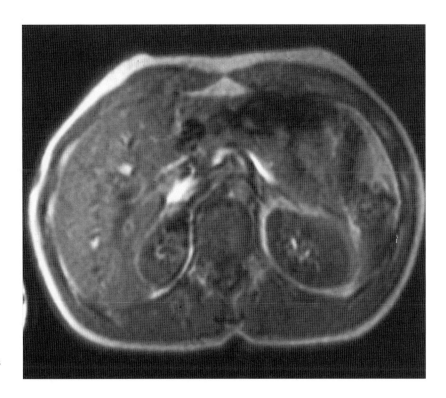

Figure 6.16 Axial T2* coherent gradient echo through the abdomen using spatial pre-saturation inferiorly and superiorly to the slice. The artefact has been largely eliminated and vessel signal has been nulled.

Chemical pre-saturation. Hydrogen exists in different chemical environments in the body, mainly in fat and water (*see* Chapter 2). The precessional frequency of fat is slightly different from that of water. As the main magnetic field strength increases, this frequency difference also increases. For example, at 1.5 T the precessional frequency between fat and water is approximately 220 Hz, so fat precesses 220 Hz lower than water. At 1.0 T this frequency difference is reduced to 147 Hz. The frequency difference between fat and water is called the **chemical shift** and can be used to specifically null the signal from either fat or water. This technique is important to differentiate pathology (which is mainly water) and normal tissue (which often contains fat). To saturate or null either fat or water, the precessional difference between the two must be sufficiently large so that they can be isolated from each other. Fat or water saturation is therefore most effectively achieved on high field systems.

Fat saturation. To saturate a fat signal, a 90° pre-saturation pulse must be applied at the precessional frequency of fat to the whole FOV (Figure 6.17). The excitation RF pulse is then applied to the slices and the magnetic moments of the fat nuclei are flipped into saturation. If they are flipped to 180°, they do not have a component of transverse magnetization and produce a signal void. The water nuclei, however, are excited, rephased and produce a signal. Figures 6.18 and 6.19 compare axial T2 weighted images of the parotid gland, with and without fat pre-saturation. Using fat saturation has increased the CNR between

6

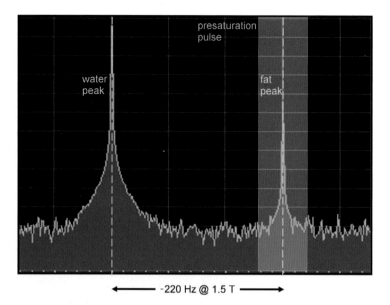

Figure 6.17   Fat saturation.

◄──────── -220 Hz @ 1.5 T ────────►

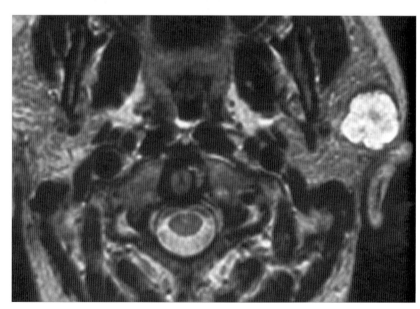

Figure 6.18   Axial FSE T2 weighted image without fat saturation.

the lesion and normal tissue as fatty components in the base of the skull have been nulled.

Water saturation. To saturate the water signal, the pre-saturation pulse must be applied at the precessional frequency of water to the whole FOV (Figure 6.20). The RF excitation pulse is then applied to the slices, and the magnetic moments of nuclei in water are flipped into saturation. If they are flipped to 180°, they do not have a transverse component of magnetization and produce a signal void. The fat nuclei, however, are

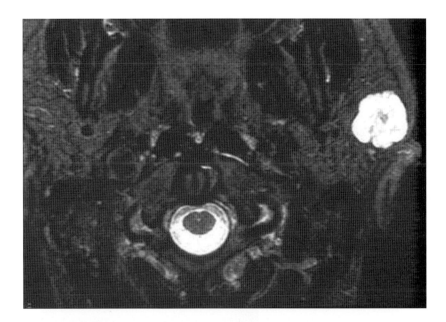

Figure 6.19   Axial T2 weighted image with fat saturation.

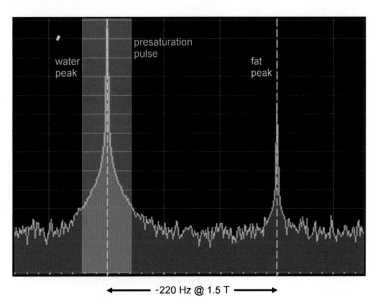

Figure 6.20   Water saturation.

excited, rephased and produce a signal. Figures 6.21 and 6.22 compare axial T1 weighted images of the liver, with and without water pre-saturation. Any fatty lesions in the liver are better demonstrated after water saturation as normal liver signal is nulled.

To be used effectively, there should be an even distribution of fat or water throughout the FOV. Pre-saturation RF is transmitted at the same frequency and evenly to the whole FOV, so that a particularly dense area of fat receives the same pre-saturation energy as an area with very little fat.

6

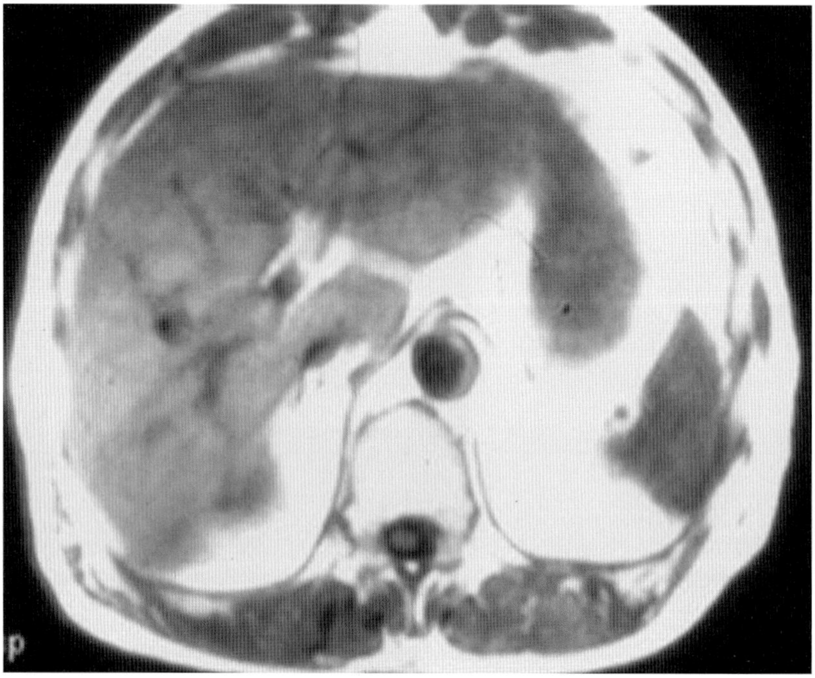

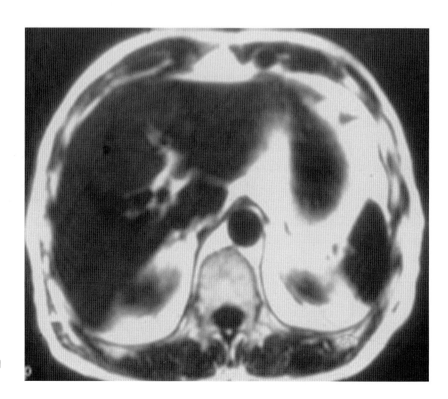

Figure 6.21 Axial T1 weighted image without water saturation.

Figure 6.22 Axial T1 weighted image with water saturation.

6

Under these circumstances fat saturation is less effective. In addition, the gradients applied for spatial encoding vary the frequency across each slice. For this reason chemical pre-saturation often appears non-uniform across the slice or imaging volume. Therefore optimal saturation occurs at the center of a slice or in the central portion of the imaging volume. Fat and water pre-saturation delivers extra RF into the patient and therefore reduces the number of slices available for a given TR.

The pre-saturation pulses are delivered to the FOV before the excitation of each slice. The interval between the pre-saturation pulses is called the **SAT TR** and is equal to the scan TR divided by the number of slices. If the SAT TR is longer than the T1 times of fat or water, the magnetic moments of fat or water may not be saturated as they have had time to recover before each pre-saturation pulse is delivered. To prevent this, always prescribe the maximum number of slices available for a given TR so that the SAT TR is reduced to a minimum.

Any tissue can be nulled in this way, as long as an RF pulse matching its precessional frequency is applied to the imaging volume before excitation. For example, silicone may be saturated to null its signal in breast imaging. This is a useful technique for ruptured implants. Spatial pre-saturation is also useful to reduce artefacts like phase mismapping and aliasing (*see* Chapter 7).

Spatial inversion recovery (SPIR). In this technique an RF pulse at the precessional frequency of fat is applied to the imaging volume but unlike chemical pre-saturation this has a magnitude of 180°. The magnetic moments of fat are therefore totally inverted into the −Z direction. After a time TI, which corresponds to the null point of fat, the 90° excitation pulse is applied. As fat has no longitudinal magnetization at this point, the excitation pulse produces no transverse magnetization in fat. Therefore the fat signal is nulled (Figures 6.23 and 6.24).

This technique therefore combines fat saturation and inverting mechanisms similar to STIR (*see* Chapter 5) to eliminate the fat signal. However, it has several advantages over both of these techniques. Chemical saturation is very dependent on homogeneity of the main magnetic field as it requires the precessional frequency of fat to be the same over the whole imaging volume. SPIR is much less susceptible to this because nulling also occurs by selecting an inversion time corresponding to the null point of fat. This depends on the T1 recovery time of fat rather than its precessional frequency and relaxation times are not affected by small changes in homogeneity. However, as STIR sequences totally rely on the T1 recovery times to null signal rather than precessional frequencies they are less likely to be affected by inhomogeneity than fat saturated methods such as SPIR or fat saturation.

Figures 6.25 and 6.26 compare a STIR image with a SPIR image and clearly show more uniform nulling of fat in the STIR sequence. However, in STIR sequences, gadolinium may be nulled along with fat, as gadolinium shortens the T1 recovery time of tissues taking up contrast to that of fat (*see* Chapter 11). Therefore STIR sequences must never be used

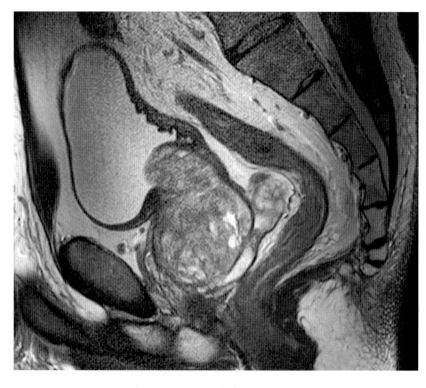

Figure 6.23 Sagittal T2 weighted FSE image of the pelvis.

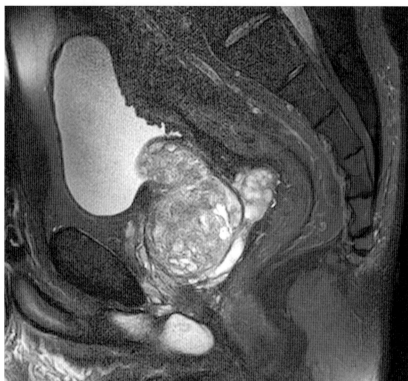

Figure 6.24 Sagittal T2 weighted FSE image of the pelvis with SPIR. Fat has been suppressed.

6

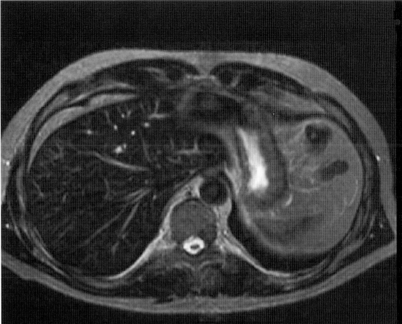

Figure 6.25 Axial STIR image. Fat is uniformly suppressed.

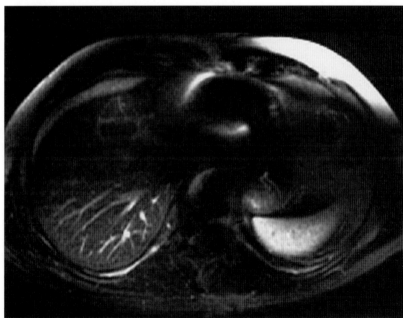

Figure 6.26 Axial SPIR image. Non-uniform suppression of fat is clearly seen due to field inhomogeneities.

after giving gadolinium. However, in SPIR sequences this does not occur because fat is selectively inverted and nulled, leaving gadolinium untouched. Therefore SPIR may be used to null the signal from fat in sequences where gadolinium has been given.

6

Learning point: fat suppression techniques

We have discussed several ways of nulling the fat signal. Unless a lipoma (a fatty tumor) is present, fat is usually considered normal tissue. In sequences where both fat and water or fat and gadolinium return a high signal it is often necessary to null the signal from fat to visualize water (which may indicate pathology) more clearly. Examples of this are in T2 weighted TSE sequences. Currently fat is nulled in the following ways:

- fat saturation
- STIR
- SPIR
- out of phase imaging (Dixon technique). This is used in gradient echo sequences to null the signal from voxels in which fat and water nuclei co-exist. This is achieved by selecting a TE when fat and water are out of phase with each other. As they are incoherent, no signal is received from the voxel (Figures 6.27 and 6.28) (*see* more on the phase difference between fat and water in Chapter 7).

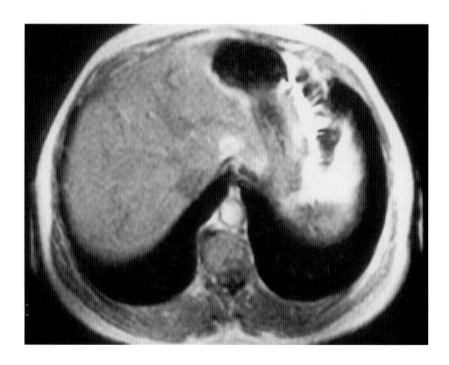

Figure 6.27 Axial gradient echo in-phase image.

6

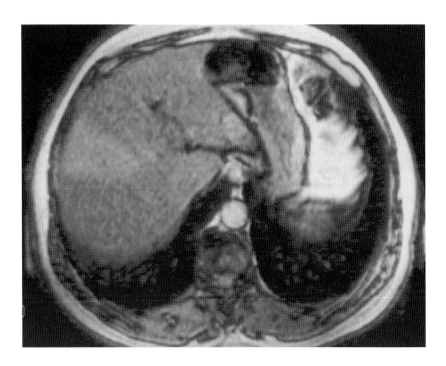

Figure 6.28 Axial gradient echo out of phase image.

Summary

Even echo rephasing:

- uses balanced echoes in which even echoes demonstrate less dephasing than odd echoes
- reduces intra-voxel dephasing
- is mainly used in T2 weighted sequences

Gradient moment rephasing:

- uses additional gradients to correct altered phase values
- reduces artefact from intra-voxel dephasing
- gives flowing nuclei a bright signal
- is mainly used in T2 or T2* weighted images
- is most effective on slow, laminar flow within the slice

Chemical pre-saturation:

- uses additional RF pulses to nullify signal from flowing nuclei
- reduces artefact due to time of flight and entry slice phenomenon
- gives flowing nuclei a signal void
- is mainly used in T1 weighted images
- is effective on fast and slow flow
- increases the RF deposition to the patient
- can be used to nullify signal from fat or water and to reduce aliasing

6

Now that flow phenomena have been discussed, it is appropriate to proceed to explore other artefacts that are commonly seen on MR images. These are described in the next chapter.

Questions

1   What factors affect time of flight flow phenomena in spin echo sequences?

2   What factors affect entry slice phenomena?

3   Is the flow in the aorta co-current or counter-current?

4   What are the consequences of using gradient moment nulling?

5   Where would you place pre-saturation volumes on a small FOV coronal left shoulder?

6   What are the advantages of using SPIR over fat saturation and STIR?

7

Artefacts and their compensation

Introduction

All MRI images have artefacts to some degree. It is therefore very important that the causes of these artefacts are understood and compensated for if possible. Some artefacts are irreversible, and may only be reduced rather than eliminated. Others can be avoided altogether. This chapter discusses the appearances, causes and remedies of the most common artefacts encountered in MRI.

Phase mismapping

Appearance

Phase mismapping or ghosting produces replications of moving anatomy across the image in the phase encoding direction. It usually originates from anatomy that moves periodically throughout the scan such as the chest wall during respiration (Figure 7.1), pulsatile movement of vessels and CSF, swallowing and eye movement. When looking at an image, the direction of phase encoding can always be determined by the direction of the phase mismapping or ghosting artefact.

7

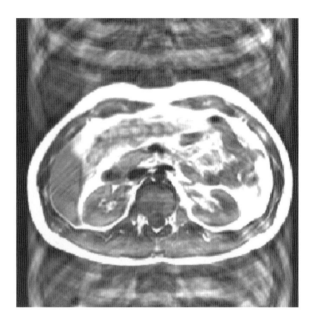

Figure 7.1 Axial image through a breathing abdomen showing phase mismapping.

Cause

Phase mismapping is produced by anatomy moving along the phase encoding gradient during the pulse sequence. It only occurs along this gradient because:

- The phase encoding gradient has a different amplitude every TR while frequency and slice select gradients have the same amplitude every TR (*see* Chapter 3). Therefore as anatomy moves during the scan it is misplaced in the phase encoding direction as the phase gradient changes. Imagine the chest wall moving during the scan as shown in Figure 7.2. The chest wall is located at a position along the phase encoding gradient during expiration, but may have moved to another position during the next phase encoding at inspiration. The chest wall is given different phase values depending on its position along the gradient e.g. 3 o'clock and 2 o'clock. Therefore moving anatomy is mismapped into the FOV along the phase encoding gradient.
- There is a time delay between phase encoding and readout (Figure 7.2). Therefore anatomy may have moved between phase encoding and when the signal is read during frequency encoding and put into K space. No mismapping occurs along the frequency axis as frequency encoding is performed as the signal is read and digitized.

Remedy

There are several ways of reducing phase mismapping. Total elimination, is, however, impossible unless of course you are imaging a cadaver! The remedies of mismapping are associated with their individual causes.

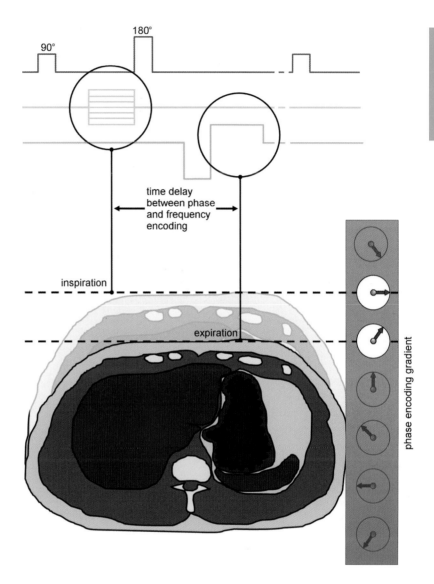

90°

180°

time delay
between phase
and frequency
encoding

inspiration

expiration

phase encoding gradient

Figure 7.2 The causes of
phase mismapping.

Swapping phase and frequency. As ghosting only occurs along the phase
axis, the direction of phase encoding can be changed, so that the artefact
does not interfere with the area of interest. For example, in a sagittal
cervical spine, frequency encoding is usually performed by the Z gradient
(head to foot) as this is the longest axis of the patient in the sagittal plane
(Figure 7.3). Phase is therefore anterior posterior and performed by the
Y gradient. Swallowing and pulsatile motion of the carotids along the
phase axis produces ghosting over the spinal cord. Swapping phase
and frequency so that the Y gradient (anterior posterior) performs frequency encoding and the Z gradient performs phase encoding, places
the artefact head to foot so that it does not obscure the spinal cord
(Figure 7.4). It should be noted, however, that this option does not reduce
or eliminate the artefact. It merely moves it so that it is less likely to
obscure important anatomy. This remedy is also useful in sagittal imaging

7

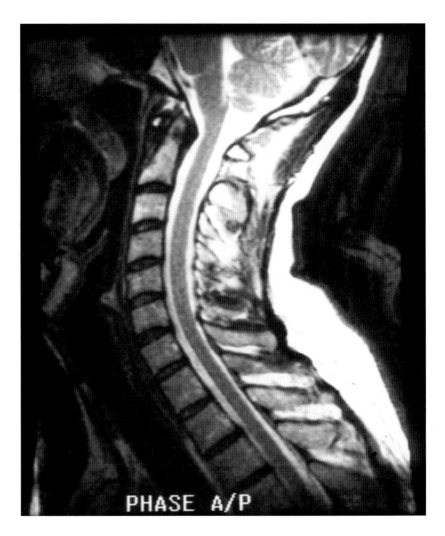

Figure 7.3 Sagittal T2 weighted image of the cervical spine with phase and therefore phase ghosting mapped anterior to posterior.

PHASE A/P

of the knee to remove artefact originating from the popliteal artery, and in axial imaging of the chest where anterior mediastinal structures are obscured by the aorta. Which way do you think phase and frequency should be located in these examples?

Using pre-saturation pulses. Pre-saturation (discussed in Chapter 6) nulls the signal from specified areas. Placing pre-saturation volumes over the area producing artefact nullifies the signal and reduces the artefact. For example, in sagittal imaging of the cervical spine, swallowing produces ghosting along the phase axis (anterior posterior) and obscures the spinal cord. Bringing a pre-saturation pulse into the FOV and placing it over the throat reduces the artefact. In addition, pre-saturation reduces artefact from flowing nuclei in blood vessels. Pre-saturation produces low signal from these nuclei and is most effective when placed between the origin of the flow and the FOV.

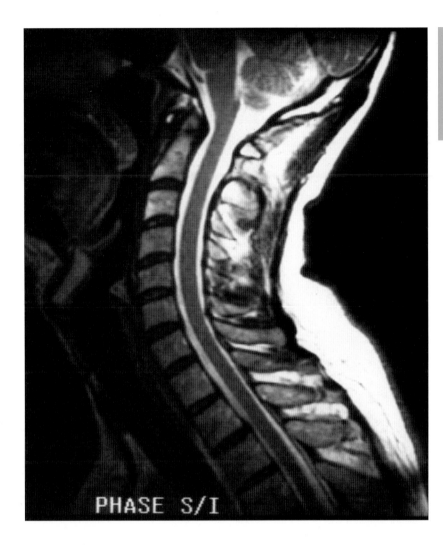

PHASE S/I

Figure 7.4 Sagittal T2 weighted image of the cervical spine with phase and therefore phase ghosting mapped superior to inferior. Note how visibility of the cervical cord has been slightly improved compared to Figure 7.3.

Using respiratory compensation techniques. When imaging the chest and abdomen, respiratory motion along the phase axis produces phase mismapping. In very fast sequences it is possible for patients to hold their breath, eliminating artefact. In longer sequences a method known as **respiratory compensation** or respiratory ordered phase encoding (ROPE) can greatly reduce ghosting from respiration. This entails placing a set of bellows around the patient's chest when imaging the chest or abdomen. These bellows are corrugated in their middle portion and expand and contract as the patient breathes (Figure 7.5). This expansion and contraction causes air to move back and forth through the bellows. The bellows are connected by hollow rubber tubing to a transducer located on the system. A transducer is a device that converts the mechanical motion of air flowing back and forth along the bellows to an electrical signal. The system therefore analyses this signal, the amplitude of which corresponds to the maximum and minimum motion of the chest wall during

7

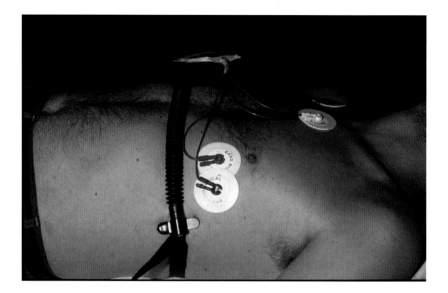

Figure 7.5 Placement of respiratory compensation bellows and cardiac gating leads.

respiration. Respiratory compensation does not affect the scan time or the image contrast. The only penalty of this method is that the number of slices available for a given TR may be slightly reduced.

Learning point: respiratory compensation and K space filling

As described in Chapter 3, the central lines of K space are filled after shallow phase encoding gradient slopes (which result in good signal and contrast), while the outer lines are filled after steep phase encoding gradient slopes that result in high spatial resolution. Anatomy that moves along a shallow phase encoding slope produces maximum ghosting as there is a higher signal to mismap in the image. Anatomy that moves along a steep phase encoding gradient slope, however, produces less ghosting as there is a smaller signal to mismap.

The system is able to read the electrical signal from the transducer and perform the shallow phase encoding gradient slopes, which fill the central lines of K space when the chest or abdominal wall movement is at a minimum. In this way most of the data that provide image signal and contrast are acquired when chest wall motion is low. The steep phase encoding slopes that fill the outer lines are reserved for when the chest wall movement is at a maximum (Figure 7.6). Therefore ghosting artefact from respiratory motion is reduced. Look at Figures 7.7 and 7.8. Phase mismapping seen in Figure 7.7 is reduced by using respiratory compensation in Figure 7.8.

7

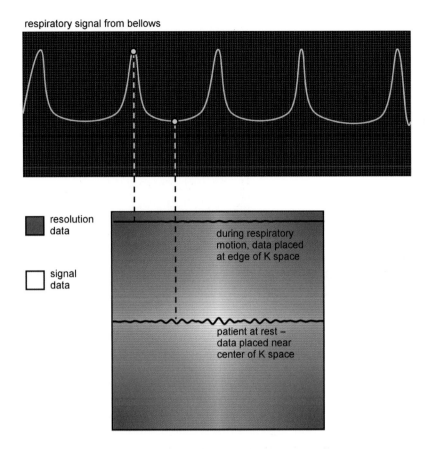

respiratory signal from bellows

resolution data

signal data

during respiratory motion, data placed at edge of K space

patient at rest – data placed near center of K space

Figure 7.6 Respiratory compensation and K space.

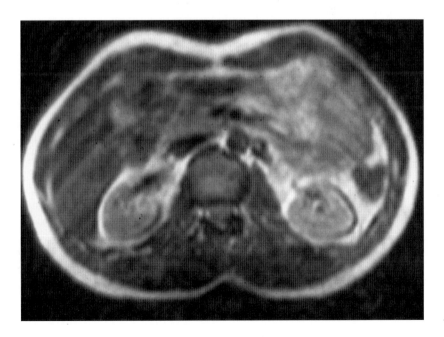

Figure 7.7 Axial T1 weighted image of the chest showing phase ghosting from respiration.

7

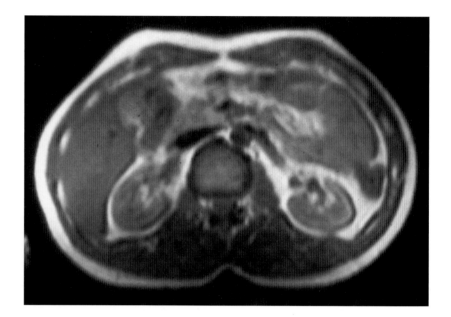

Figure 7.8 Axial T1 weighted image of the chest with respiratory compensation. Phase ghosting is reduced.

Some systems use a method known as **respiratory gating** or **triggering** that times the excitation RF with a certain phase of respiration. Each slice of the acquisition is therefore obtained at the same phase of respiration. However, this method has several drawbacks. First, the TR and therefore the contrast is determined by the rapidity of respiration and second, since respiratory rates are generally longer than the TR, the scan time is lengthened and image contrast may change.

Cardiac gating. Gating is a very general term used to describe a technique of reducing phase mismapping from the periodic motion caused by respiration, cardiac and pulsatile flow motion. Just as respiratory gating monitors respiration, cardiac gating monitors cardiac motion by co-ordinating the excitation pulse with the R wave of systole. This is achieved by using an electrical signal generated by the cardiac motion to trigger each excitation pulse. There are two forms of gating.

- Electrocardiogram (ECG, EKG) gating uses electrodes and lead wires that are attached to the patient's chest to produce an ECG (Figure 7.5). This is used to determine the timing of the application of each excitation pulse. Each slice is acquired at the same phase of the cardiac cycle and therefore phase mismapping from cardiac motion is reduced. ECG gating should be used when imaging the chest, heart and great vessels.
- Peripheral gating uses a light sensor attached to the patient's finger to detect the pulsation of blood through the capillaries. The pulsation is used to trigger the excitation pulses so that each slice is acquired at the same phase of the cardiac cycle. Peripheral gating is not as accurate as ECG gating, so is not very useful when imaging the heart itself. However, it is effective at reducing phase mismapping

7

when imaging small vessels or the spinal cord, where CSF flow may degrade the image. ECG and peripheral gating are discussed in more detail in Chapter 8.

Gradient moment nulling (discussed in Chapter 6) reduces ghosting caused by flowing nuclei moving along gradients. It produces a bright signal from these flowing nuclei and also reduces ghosting significantly. It is most effective in slow, regular flow within the imaging plane.

Other motion reducing techniques. Some types of voluntary motion, such as eye movement, can be reduced by asking the patient to focus their eyes on a particular part of the magnet/room. Other involuntary motion, such as bowel motion, is reduced by administering antispasmodic agents (Figures 7.9 and 7.10). Increasing the NEX may also help, as this increases the number of times the signal is averaged. Motion artefact is averaged out of the image as it is more random in nature than the signal itself. Voluntary motion can be reduced by making the patient as comfortable as possible, and immobilizing them with pads and straps. A nervous patient always benefits from thoughtful explanation of the procedure, and a constant reminder over the system intercom to keep still. A relative or friend in the room can also help in some circumstances. In extreme cases, sedation of the patient may be required.

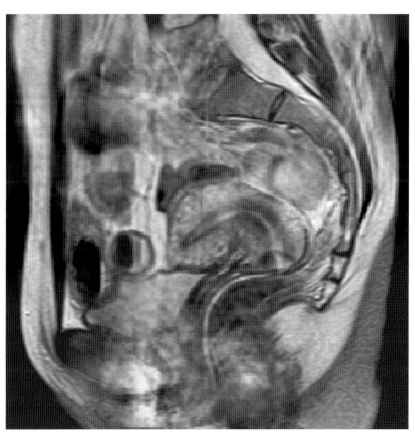

Figure 7.9 Sagittal T2 weighted images of the pelvis. Bowel motion has caused blurring of structures.

7

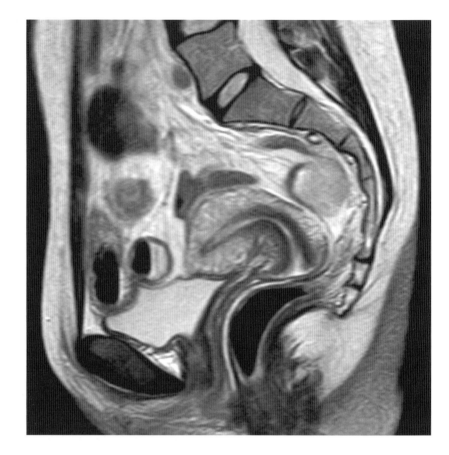

Figure 7.10 Sagittal
T2 weighted image of the
pelvis after administration of
anti-spasmodic agents. Bowel
motion has been reduced.

Aliasing or wrap around

Appearance

Wrap or aliasing produces an image where anatomy that exists outside the
FOV is folded onto the top of anatomy inside the FOV. In Figure 7.11 the
FOV in the phase direction is smaller than the anterior posterior dimensions of the head. Therefore signal outside the FOV in the phase direction
is wrapped into the image.

Cause

Aliasing is produced when anatomy that exists outside the FOV is mapped
inside the FOV. Anatomy outside the selected FOV still produces a signal
if it is in close proximity to the receiver coil. Data from this signal must
be encoded, i.e. allocated a pixel position. If the data are under-sampled,
the signal is mismapped into pixels within the FOV rather than outside.
Aliasing can occur along both the frequency and phase axis.

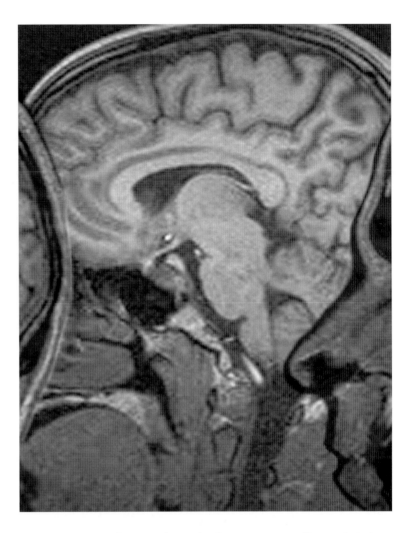

7

Figure 7.11   Sagittal image of the brain showing aliasing or wraparound.

Frequency wrap. Aliasing along the frequency encoding axis is known as **frequency wrap**. This is caused by undersampling the frequencies that are present in the echo. These frequencies originate from any signal, regardless of whether the anatomy producing it is inside or outside the selected FOV. Ideally, only the frequencies originating from inside the FOV are allocated a pixel position. This only occurs if the frequencies are sampled often enough. According to the Nyquist theorem (*see* Chapter 3), frequencies must be sampled at least twice per cycle to map them correctly. If the Nyquist theorem is not obeyed and frequencies are not sampled enough, signal from anatomy outside the FOV in the frequency encoding direction is mapped into the FOV (Figure 7.12 bottom image). Wrap around results along the frequency encoding axis.

Phase wrap. Aliasing along the phase axis of the image is known as **phase wrap**. This is caused by undersampling along the phase axis. After FFT every phase value from 0° to 360° (or 12 o'clock through to the following

7

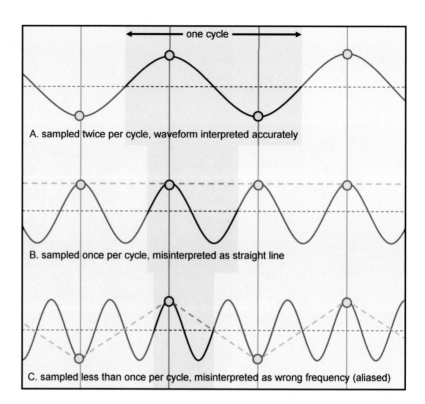

Figure 7.12 Aliasing and undersampling.

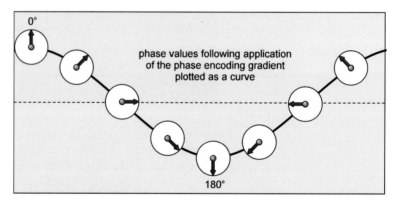

Figure 7.13 The phase curve.

12 o'clock) must be mapped into the FOV in the phase encoding direction (Figure 7.13). This phase curve is repeated on both sides of the FOV along the phase axis. Any signal is allocated a phase value according to its position along this curve. As the curve is repeated, signal originating outside the FOV in the phase direction is allocated a phase value that has already been given to signal originating from inside the FOV. There is, therefore, a duplication of phase values. This duplication causes phase wrap along the phase axis.

Look at Figure 7.14 where the FOV in the right-to-left phase axis of the image is smaller than the dimensions of the axial abdomen. The phase

axial abdomen slice, spins exhibit phase curve after phase encoding gradient application

7

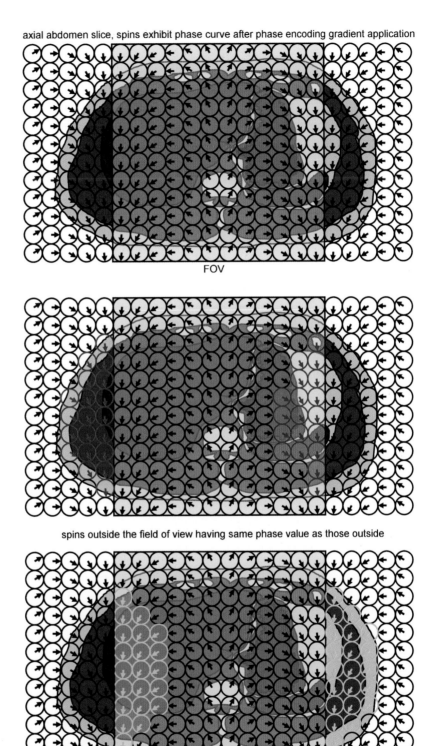

FOV

spins outside the field of view having same phase value as those outside

Figure 7.14 Phase wrap.

7

encoding gradient has been applied in this direction and produces a change of phase across the X-axis of the bore of the magnet. At this particular gradient slope, spins outside the FOV have the same phase position as spins inside the FOV (red and blue areas in the diagram). As they have the same phase value these red and blue areas are wrapped inside the image because they have a phase value exactly the same as spins within the FOV.

Remedy

Aliasing along both the frequency and phase axis can totally degrade an image and should be compensated for. Enlarging the FOV so that all anatomy producing signal is incorporated within the FOV achieves this, but also results in a loss of spatial resolution. Bringing pre-saturation bands onto areas outside the FOV that may wrap into the image can sometimes sufficiently null signal from these areas and reduce aliasing. There are, however, two anti-aliasing software methods available that compensate for wrap.

Anti-aliasing along the frequency axis. Increasing the sampling rate so that all frequencies are digitized sufficiently would eliminate aliasing in the frequency direction. However, doing so would also increase noise in the image (*see* Chapter 3). Therefore a frequency filter is used to filter out frequencies that occur outside the selected FOV. Signal originating from outside the FOV along the frequency axis is no longer mismapped as it is filtered out (Figure 7.15). Most systems automatically apply this option so that aliasing never occurs along the frequency encoding axis, which is similar to filtering out the bass and treble on a music system with a graphic equalizer.

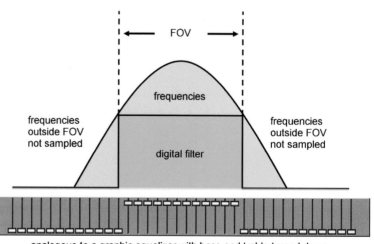

Figure 7.15 Anti-aliasing along the frequency axis.

Anti-aliasing along the phase axis. This is termed **no phase wrap** or **anti-foldover**. No phase wrap oversamples along the phase encoding axis by increasing the number of phase encodings performed. This is achieved by enlarging the FOV in the phase direction so that the phase curve extends over a wider area of anatomy. There is now no duplication of phase values as signal outside the FOV has a different phase value to that inside. Anatomy is no longer mismapped and aliasing does not occur (Figure 7.16). However, as enlarging the FOV results in a loss of spatial resolution, the number of phase encodings is increased to compensate for this. Increasing the number of phase encodings in turn increases the scan time and so some systems automatically reduce the NEX or signal averages to compensate for this. Others, however, do not, so using this option increases the scan time.

The extended portion of the FOV is usually discarded during reconstruction so that only the selected FOV is displayed. Although the SNR is not noticeably reduced, image quality may suffer slightly with no phase wrap. As a decrease in NEX reduces the number of signal averages, motion artefacts may be more apparent. Look at Figures 4.25 and 4.26 in Chapter 4 that were acquired with 1 and 4 NEX. In Figure 4.25 you may notice some ghosting along the superior sagittal sinus. This is reduced in Figure 4.26 because a higher NEX was used.

Learning point: no phase wrap, K space and the chest of drawers

The chest of drawers analogy describes this option well. The height of the chest of drawers determines the resolution of the image (i.e. if a 256 matrix has been selected then drawers +/–128 are filled with data: the top and bottom drawers). To reduce this artefact, more phase encodes must be performed, therefore more drawers must be filled. To fill more drawers and still keep the height of the chest of drawers the same, each drawer must be thinner (as discussed in Chapter 4). The depth of the drawer is inversely proportional to the FOV in the phase direction, so halving the depth of each drawer doubles the FOV in the phase direction, allowing anatomy to be included in a larger FOV and prevent aliasing. Doubling the number of phase encoding steps or drawers doubles the scan time, and some systems halve the NEX (the number of times each drawer is filled) to compensate (Figure 7.16). Hence this option eliminates aliasing (as long as anatomy is outside the larger FOV) and maintains the original resolution, FOV and scan time (Figures 7.17 and 7.18).

7

original FOV

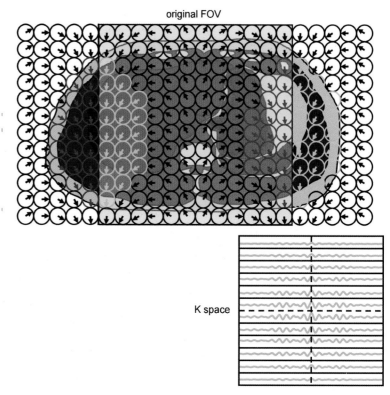

K space

phase curve extended to cover new FOV

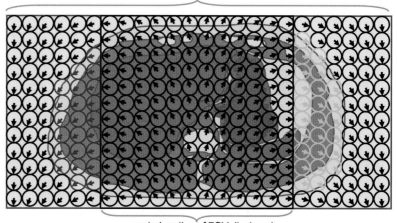

central portion of FOV displayed

K space
dimensions remain
the same,
incremental step
halved

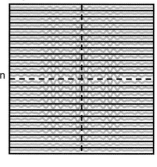

Figure 7.16   Anti-aliasing along the phase axis.

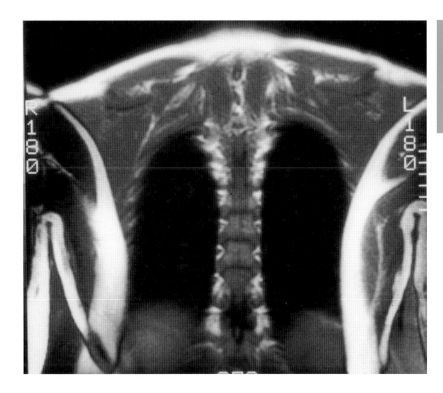

Figure 7.17 Coronal image of the chest showing phase wrap.

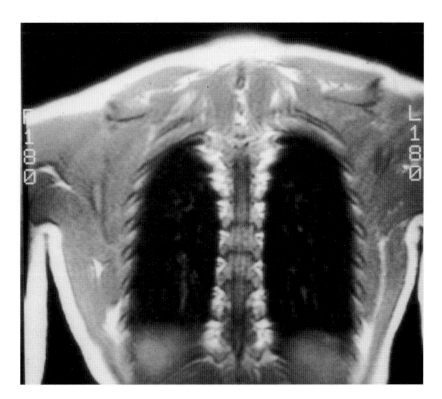

Figure 7.18 Coronal image of the chest with anti-aliasing. Wrap has been eliminated.

7

Chemical shift artefact

Appearance

Chemical shift artefact produces a dark edge at the interface between fat and water. It occurs along the frequency encoding axis only. Figure 7.19 shows a black band to the right of both kidneys. This is chemical shift artefact.

Cause

Chemical shift artefact is caused by the different chemical environments of fat and water. Although fat and water are both made up of hydrogen protons, fat consists of hydrogen arranged with carbon, while in water, hydrogen is arranged with oxygen. As a result, fat precesses at a lower frequency than water. This difference in precessional frequency is proportional to the main magnetic field strength B_0, for example, at 1.5 T the difference in precessional frequency is 220 Hz. That is, fat precesses 220 Hz less than water. At 1.0 T this difference is 147 Hz and, at lower field strengths (0.5 T or less), it is usually insignificant. However, at higher field strengths, it can lead to an artefact known as **chemical shift**. The amount of chemical shift is often expressed in arbitrary units known as parts per million (ppm) of the main magnetic field strength. Its value is always independent of the main field strength and equals 3.5 ppm. From

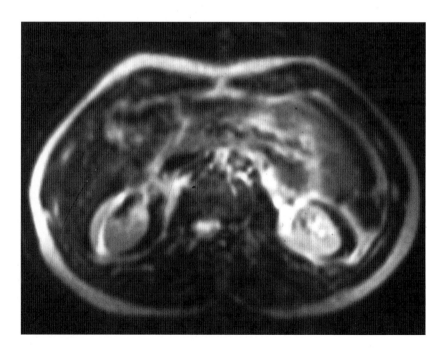

Figure 7.19 Chemical shift artefact seen has a black band to the right hand side of each kidney.

this, the chemical shift between fat and water can be calculated at different field strengths.

The receive bandwidth determines the range of frequencies that must be mapped across the FOV. The FOV is divided into pixels, the number of which is determined by the matrix size. If 256 frequency samples are selected, the receive bandwidth must be mapped across 256 pixels in the FOV. The receive bandwidth and the number of frequency samples determine the bandwidth of each pixel.

For example, if the receive bandwidth is +/−16 kHz, 32 000 Hz are mapped across the FOV. If 256 frequency samples are collected, the FOV is divided into 256 frequency pixels. Each pixel therefore has an individual frequency range of 125 Hz (32 000/256 Hz) (Figure 7.20). At a field strength of 1.5 T, the precessional frequency difference between fat and water is 220 Hz and therefore, using the above example, fat and water protons existing adjacent to one other in the patient are mapped 1.76 pixels apart (220/125) (Figure 7.20, middle diagram). This pixel shift of fat relative to water is called chemical shift artefact. The actual dimensions of this artefact depend on the size of the FOV, as this determines the size of each pixel. For example, a FOV of 24 cm and 256 frequency pixels results in pixels 0.93 mm in size. A pixel shift of 1.76 results in an actual chemical shift between fat and water of 1.63 mm (0.93 × 1.76 mm). As the FOV is enlarged this dimension increases.

Remedy

Chemical shift can be limited by scanning at lower field strengths and by keeping the FOV to a minimum. At high field strengths, the size of the receive bandwidth is one way of limiting chemical shift. As the receive bandwidth is reduced, a smaller frequency range must now be mapped across the same number of frequency pixels, for example, 256. The individual frequency range of each pixel therefore decreases, and so the 220 Hz difference in precessional frequency between fat and water is translated into a larger pixel shift (Figure 7.20 lower diagram). For example, if the receive bandwidth is reduced to +/−8 kHz, only 16 000 Hz is now mapped across 256 frequency pixels. Each pixel has a range of only 62.5 Hz (16 000/256 Hz). The 220 Hz precessional frequency difference between the two adjacent fat and water protons is now translated into a pixel shift of 3.52 pixels (220/62.5) (Figure 7.20, lower diagram).

To reduce chemical shift artefact always use the widest receive bandwidth in keeping with good SNR and the smallest FOV possible (Figure 7.21). If the bandwidth is reduced to increase the SNR, use chemical satura-tion to saturate out the signal from either fat or water (*see* Chapter 6). By doing so as either fat or water is nulled, there is nothing for one tissue to shift against, and therefore chemical shift artefact is eliminated. These measures are really only necessary at higher field strengths. At 0.5 T or less, chemical shift artefact is insignificant and usually does not need to be compensated for.

7

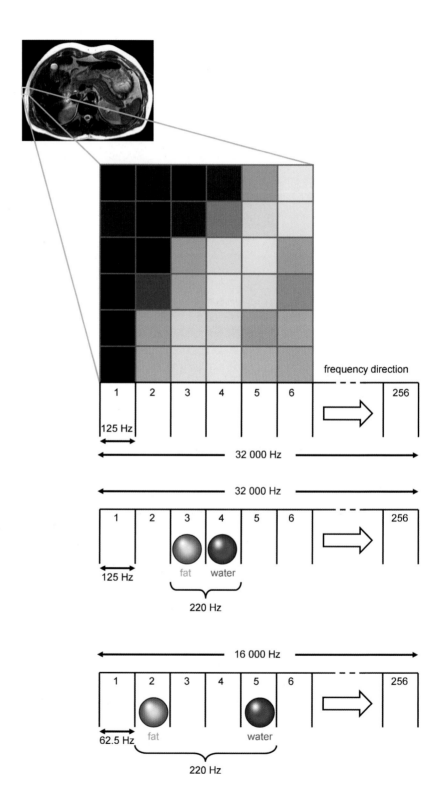

Figure 7.20 Chemical shift and pixel shift.

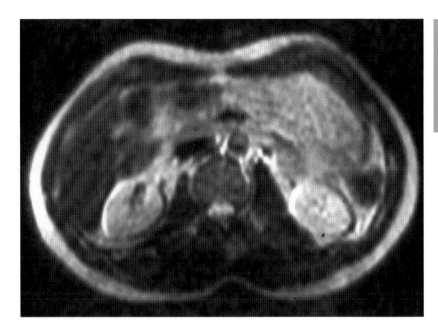

Figure 7.21   Axial image through the abdomen acquired with a wide receive bandwidth. Chemical shift artefact seen on Figure 7.19 has been reduced.

Chemical misregistration

Appearance

When fat and water are in phase, their signals add constructively, and when they are out of phase their signals cancel each other out. This cancellation effect is known as **chemical misregistration** artefact, which produces a ring of dark signal around certain organs where fat and water interfaces occur within the same voxel, for example, the kidneys (Figure 7.22). Chemical misregistration mainly occurs in the phase direction, as it is produced due to a phase difference between fat and water. It is most degrading to the image in gradient echo pulse sequences, where gradient reversal is very ineffective.

Cause

Chemical misregistration is an artefact produced as a result of the precessional frequency difference between fat and water. The artefact is caused because fat and water are in phase at certain times and out of phase at others, due to the difference in their precessional frequency. As they travel at different speeds around their precessional paths, they are at various positions on the path but periodically they are at the same position and therefore in phase.

7

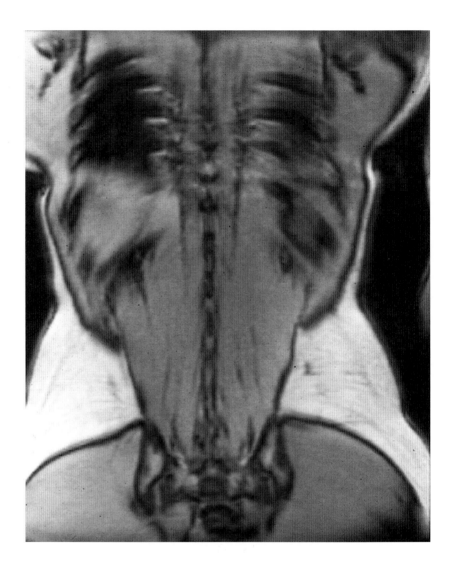

Figure 7.22 Chemical misregistration seen as a black line around the abdominal organs.

Learning point: chemical misregistration and the watch analogy

This is analogous to the hour and minute hands of a clock. Both hands travel at different speeds around the clock; the hour hand moves through 360° in 12 hours, while the minute hand moves the same distance in one hour. However, at certain times of the day, the hands are superimposed or in phase, i.e. approximately at 12 noon, 1.05 am, 2.10 am, 3.15 am, etc. (Figure 7.23).

in phase

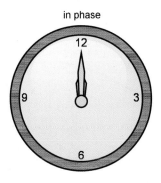

out of phase

in phase

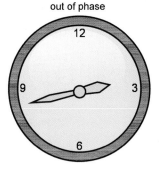

out of phase

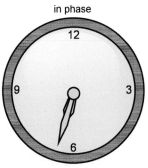

Figure 7.23 Chemical misregistration and the watch analogy.

Remedy

Select a TE that matches the periodicity of fat and water at your field strength. The periodicity of fat and water depends on the field strength (Figure 7.24). At 1.5 T, for example, selecting a TE that is a multiple of 4.2 ms reduces chemical misregistration artefact, while at 0.5 T the periodicity of fat and water is 7 ms. In addition, use spin echo sequences rather than gradient echo as 180° RF pulses are very effective at compensating for differences in phase between fat and water, while gradient echo sequences are very poor at this.

Truncation artefact

Appearance

This artefact produces a banding artefact at the interfaces of high and low signal (this artefact is called Gibbs artefact when seen in sagittal images of the cervical spine). Figure 7.25 shows this at the edges of the brain where high signal from fat in the scalp lies adjacent to low signal from the skull.

Cause

This artefact results from undersampling of data so that interfaces of high and low signal are incorrectly represented on the image. Truncation artefact occurs in the phase direction only and produces a low intensity band running through a high intensity area.

Remedy

Undersampling of data must be avoided. To do so, increase the number of phase encoding steps. For example, use a 256×256 matrix instead of 256×128.

Magnetic susceptibility artefact

Appearance

This artefact produces distortion of the image together with large signal voids. Figure 7.26 shows magnetic susceptibility artefact from a dental brace present within the image volume.

7

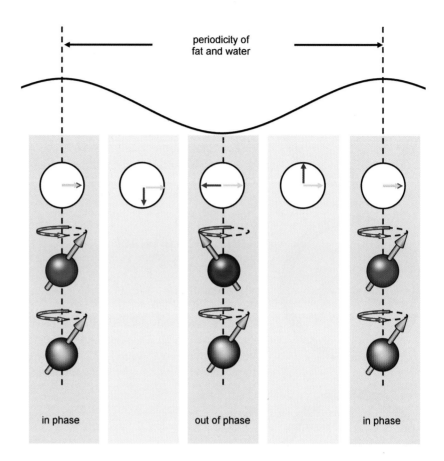

Figure 7.24 The periodicity of fat and water.

Cause

Magnetic susceptibility is the ability of a substance to become magnetized. Some tissues magnetize to a different degree than others, which results in a difference in precessional frequency and phase. This causes dephasing at the interface of these tissues and a signal loss. In practice, the main causes of this artefact are metal objects within the imaging volume, although it can also be seen from naturally occurring iron content of hemorrhage, as these magnetize to a much greater degree than the surrounding tissue. Ferromagnetic objects have a very high magnetic susceptibility and cause distortion of the image. Magnetic susceptibility artefact is more prominent in gradient echo sequences as the gradient reversal cannot compensate for the phase difference at the interface.

Remedy

This artefact can, under some circumstances, aid diagnosis. In particular, small hemorrhages are sometimes only seen because they produce a magnetic susceptibility effect. However, in general this artefact is undesirable and can ruin an image. There are several remedies available.

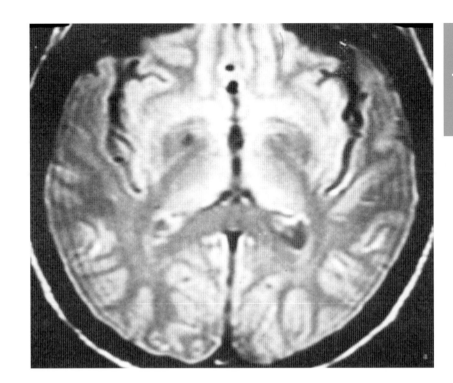

Figure 7.25 Axial image of the brain showing truncation artefact seen as faint lines adjacent to the skull–brain interface.

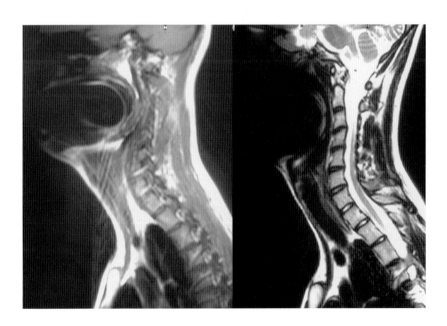

Figure 7.26 Magnetic susceptibility from a dental brace causing massive distortion of the image.

7

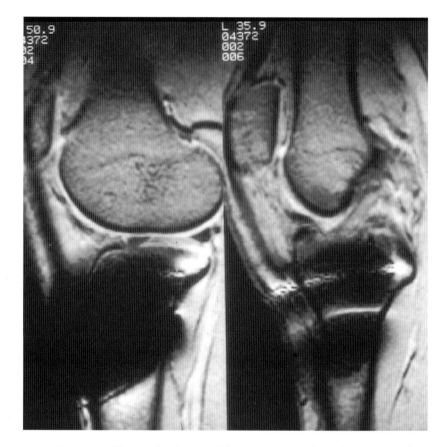

Figure 7.27 Sagittal gradient echo images of the knee with pins in the tibia. Magnetic susceptibility has produced a large distortion of the image.

- *Remove all metal objects.* Always ensure that the patient has removed all metal objects where possible before the scan. Always check whether the patient has aneurysm clips or metal implants. Most implants can be scanned but may cause local heating effects (*see* Chapter 10).
- *Use spin echo sequences instead of gradient echo.* The 180° rephasing pulse used in spin echo sequences is very effective at compensating for phase differences between fat and water while gradient echo sequences are very poor at this. In Figures 7.27 and 7.28 gradient echo and spin echo sequences respectively have been used. Metal artefact in the tibia produces magnetic susceptibility artefact on both images but this is significantly reduced in the spin echo sequence. The same effect is also produced when using SS-FSE as opposed to standard FSE. The long echo train used in single shot imaging produces increased rephasing from added 180° rephasing pulses. The artefact is therefore significantly reduced.
- *Decrease the TE.* Longer echo times allow for more dephasing between tissues with susceptibility differences, therefore using a short TE reduces this artefact. Broad receive bandwidths also reduce the TE (*see* Chapter 3), so this is also a useful remedy when faced with this artefact.

7

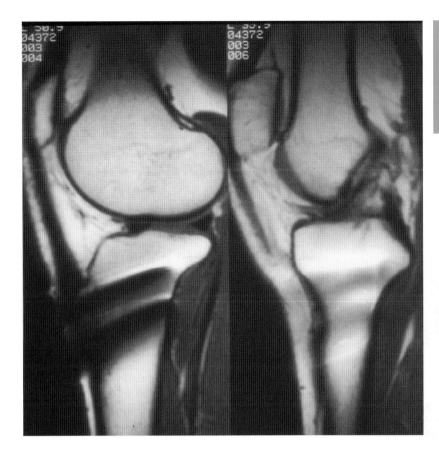

Figure 7.28   Sagittal spin echo images of the same patient as shown in Figure 7.27. The artefact is reduced.

Cross excitation and cross talk

Appearance

Adjacent slices in an acquisition have different image contrasts (Figure 7.29).

Cause

An RF excitation pulse is not exactly square. The width of the pulse should be half its amplitude, but this normally varies by up to 10%. As a result, nuclei in slices adjacent to the RF excitation pulse may become excited by it. Adjacent slices receive energy from the RF excitation pulse of their neighbors (Figure 7.30).

This energy pushes the NMV of the nuclei towards the transverse plane, so that they may become saturated when they themselves are excited. This

7

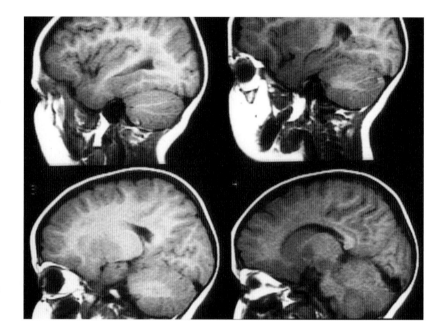

Figure 7.29 Contrast changes between slices as a result of cross excitation.

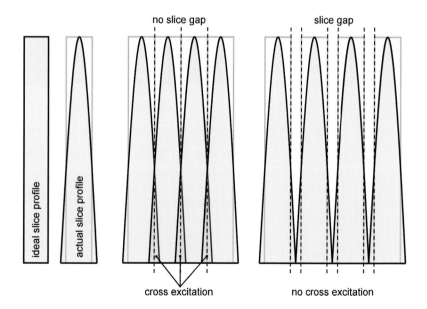

Figure 7.30 Cross excitation.

effect is called **cross excitation** and affects image contrast. The same effect is produced by energy dissipation to adjacent slices, as nuclei within the selected slice relax to B_0. These nuclei lose their energy due to spin lattice relaxation and may dissipate this energy to nuclei in neighboring slices. This is specifically called **cross talk** and should not be confused with cross excitation.

7

Remedy

Cross talk can never be eliminated as it is caused by the natural dissipation of energy by the nuclei. Cross excitation can be reduced by ensuring that there is at least a 30% gap between the slices. This is 30% of the slice thickness itself, and reduces the likelihood of RF exciting adjacent slices. For example, if the slice thickness selected is 5 mm, use a skip or gap of 2 mm (40% of 5 mm), rather than a 1 mm gap (20% of 5 mm). In addition, most systems excite alternate slices during the acquisition so that there is some time for cross excitation in adjacent slices to decay before it is their turn to be excited. For example: excitation order of slices is 1, 3, 5, 7, 2, 4, 6, 8. Slices 1 to 7 have time to decay their cross excitation, while slices 2 to 8 are being excited (approximately half the TR).

A process known as **interleaving** extends this time even further. When interleaving slices, alternate slices are excited and divided into two acquisitions. In this way, cross excitation created in adjacent slices has the time of a whole acquisition to decay before it is its turn to be excited. For example: excitation order of slices is 1, 3, 5, 7 in the first acquisition and 2, 4, 6, 8 in the second. Slices 1 to 7 have the time of a whole acquisition (several minutes) to decay, while slices 2 to 8 are being excited. When using interleaving, no gap is required between the slices.

Some systems use software to 'square off' the RF pulses so that the adjacent nuclei are less likely to become excited. This reduces cross excitation but often results in some loss of signal, as a proportion of the RF pulse is lost in the squaring off process. It is still wise to use a small gap of 10% when employing this software.

Zipper artefact

Appearance

Zipper artefact appears as a dense line on the image at a specific point (Figure 7.31).

Cause

This is caused by extraneous RF entering the room at a certain frequency, and interfering with the inherently weak signal coming from the patient. It is caused by a leak in the RF shielding of the room.

Remedy

Call the engineer to locate the leak and repair it.

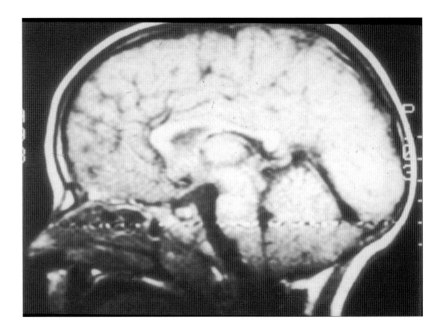

Figure 7.31   Zipper artefact seen as a horizontal line across the image.

Shading artefact

Appearance

This produces a difference in signal intensity across the imaging volume.

Cause

Shading is an artefact that produces a loss of signal intensity in one part of the image. Its main cause is the uneven excitation of nuclei within the patient due to RF pulses applied at flip angles other than 90° and 180°. Shading is also caused by abnormal loading on the coil or by coupling of the coil at one point. This may occur with a large patient who touches one side of the body coil and couples it at that point. Shading can also be caused by inhomogeneities in the main magnetic field, which can be improved by shimming (*see* Chapter 9).

Remedy

Always ensure that the coil is loaded correctly, i.e. that the correct size of coil is used for the anatomy under examination, and that the patient is not touching the coil at any point. The use of foam pads or water bags between the coil and the patient will usually suffice. In addition, also ensure that

7

appropriate pre-scan parameters have been obtained before the scan (*see* Chapter 3), as these determine the correct excitation frequency and amplitude of the applied RF pulses.

Moiré pattern

Appearance

This is shown as a black and white banding artefact on the edge of the FOV in Figure 7.32. It is always seen in gradient echo imaging typically when a large FOV is used.

Cause

This is a combination of wrap and field inhomogeneity in gradient echo sequences. In coronal imaging of the body, especially if the patient's arms are touching the bore of the magnet, pixels are wrapped on top of each

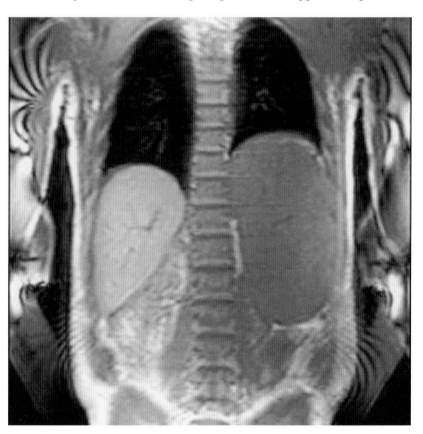

Figure 7.32 Moiré pattern, seen as zebra lines on the edge of the FOV.

7

other because anatomy exists outside the FOV but is producing signal. Inhomogeneities cause this wrap to be in and out of phase causing the banding appearance.

Remedy

Use spin echo sequences or ensure the patient keeps their arms within the FOV.

Magic angle

Appearance

This is seen in certain tendons as high signal intensity. In Figure 7.33 this is seen in the patellar tendon and may mimic pathology.

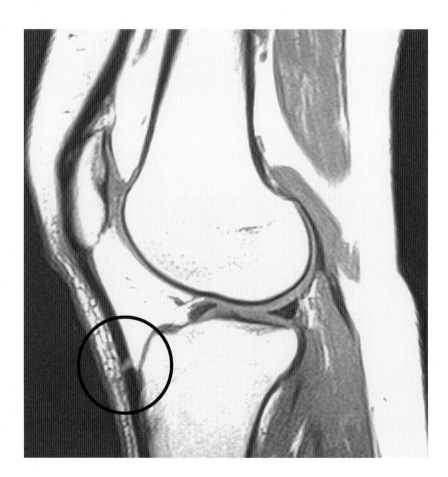

Figure 7.33 Magic angle artefact has high signal intensity seen at the lower border of the patellar tendon.

Cause

This is caused when structures that contain tightly bound fibers lie at an angle of 55° to the main field, altering its signal intensity.

Table 7.1 Artefacts and their remedies.

Artefacts	Axis	Remedy	Penalty
Truncation	phase	respiratory compensation	may lose a slice
		swap phase and frequency	may need anti-aliasing
		gating	variable TR
			variable image contrast
			increased scan time
		pre-saturation	may lose a slice
		gradient moment rephasing	increases minimum TE
Chemical shift	frequency	increase bandwidth	decrease minimum TE available
			decrease SNR
		reduce FOV	reduces SNR
			decreases resolution
		use chemical saturation	reduces SNR
			may lose slices
Chemical misregistration	phase	select a TE at periodicity of	may lose a slice if TE is
		fat and water	significantly reduced
Aliasing	frequency and phase	no frequency wrap	none
		no phase wrap	may reduce SNR
			may increase scan time
			increases motion artefact
			due to reduced NEX
		enlarge FOV	reduces resolution
Zipper	frequency	call engineer	irate engineer!
Magnetic susceptibility	frequency and phase	use spin echo	not flow sensitive
			blood product may be missed
		remove metal	none
Shading	frequency and phase	check shim	none
		load coil correctly	none
Motion	phase	use antispasmodics	costly
			invasive
		immobilize patient	none
		counseling of patient	none
		all remedies for mismapping	see previous
		sedation	possible side effects
			invasive
			costly
			requires monitoring
Cross talk	slice select	none	none
Cross excitation	slice select	interleaving	doubles the scan time
		squaring off RF pulses	reduces SNR
Moiré	frequency and phase	use SE	none
		patient not to touch bore	none
Magic angle	frequency	change TE	none
		alter position of anatomy	none

7

Remedy

Alter the angle of the structure or change the TE.

There are some other artefacts caused by major equipment malfunction. The loss of a gradient, for example, causes distortion of the image, and eddy currents induced in the gradient coils can cause phase artefacts as they create additional unwanted phase shifts. On the whole, however, artefacts produced in MR can be compensated for to some extent, and this is summarized in Table 7.1.

Questions

1   What is magnetic susceptibility and how do you reduce it?

2   You are examining a knee with a prosthesis *in situ*. What artefact would you expect to see, and how would you try to achieve the optimum image quality?

3   What is the difference between chemical shift and chemical misregistration?

4   Under what conditions would you get phase wrap?

5   What is the difference between cross talk and cross excitation? Which can be reduced and how?

6   List the different ways of reducing phase mismapping.

8

Vascular and cardiac imaging

8

Introduction

There are several methods that can be used to evaluate both the neuro-vascular and cardiovascular systems with the use of MRI. A series of magnetic resonance vascular imaging techniques are available to evaluate non-invasively both the morphology and hemodynamics of the vascular system. Such techniques include conventional MRI, acquired with imaging options to enable vascular visualization and magnetic resonance angiography (MRA) acquired to visualize moving blood.

Before MRA, the patient would be required to undergo both conventional angiographic and/or cardiac catheterization procedures to study vascular anatomy, and Doppler ultrasound to study flow velocity and direction. MRI enables direct imaging correlation between hemodynamic flow velocity and morphologic display, with little or no discomfort to the patient or to the radiographer. The current techniques used are now discussed.

Conventional MRI vascular imaging techniques

MR imaging techniques for vascular imaging include a number of imaging sequences based in spin echo and gradient echo techniques. Spin echo imaging generally uses sequences that combine RF pulse combinations of

90° and 180° pulses or, in the case of fast spin echo, 90° and several 180° pulses depending upon the turbo factor selected by the operator. IR sequences generally utilize spin echo sequences that begin with 180° inversion pulse (or several inversion pulses) followed by a 90° and 180° pulse. Gradient echo sequences can be acquired with an initializing RF pulse, of a given flip angle, followed by a gradient refocusing pulse (*see* Chapter 5).

These pulse sequences are supplemented with options such as gradient moment rephasing and pre-saturation. As previously discussed in Chapter 6, these options can be used to reduce motion artefact from flowing nuclei. However, as they give nuclei flowing in blood either signal void or signal enhancement, they also produce contrast between vessels and the surrounding tissue. These techniques can therefore be very useful to demonstrate occlusion of a vessel, if the MRA sequences are not available. Pre-saturation and gradient moment rephasing are now described in the context of vascular imaging.

Black blood imaging

To give an anatomic structure contrast relative to other tissues within the body, the structure must appear either darker or brighter than the surrounding tissues. Several techniques can be employed to produce images where vessels appear dark. These include spin echo acquisitions and the application of pre-saturation pulses. In spin echo sequences, rapidly flowing blood appears dark, enabling visualization of the vessel relative to surrounding tissues. Nuclei that receive both the 90° and 180° pulses produce an MR signal. However, flowing nuclei that receive either the 90° pulse or the 180° pulse (but not both) produce no signal.

When spin echo acquisitions produce images where blood is dark they can be referred to as **black blood images** (Figure 8.1). This technique can be further improved by the application of pre-saturation pulses (*see* Chapter 6). Short TR/TE spin echo imaging with the use of pre-saturation pulses enables visualization of the vascular system in that flowing vessels appear black. Saturation eliminates phase ghosting and provides intraluminal signal void for excellent distinction between patent and obstructed vessels.

Pre-saturation can be used to evaluate vascular patency throughout the head and body. However, since pre-saturation uses additional RF pulses, the specific absorption rate (SAR, discussed in Chapter 10) is increased, and the slice number available per TR may be reduced as a result. Additional pre-saturation pulses outside the FOV or the imaging volume transfer magnetization of flowing spins through 90° into the transverse plane (Figure 8.2). Flowing spins, which then enter the imaging field, receive an additional 90° RF pulse within the imaging volume. The magnetization of flowing spins is therefore flipped an additional 90° to 180°. Signal saturation from flowing spins occurs because no time is allowed for recovery of magnetization. Given that flowing blood in vessels should appear black, persistent signal within vessel lumen after the application of saturation pulses indicates slow flow, clot or vascular occlusion.

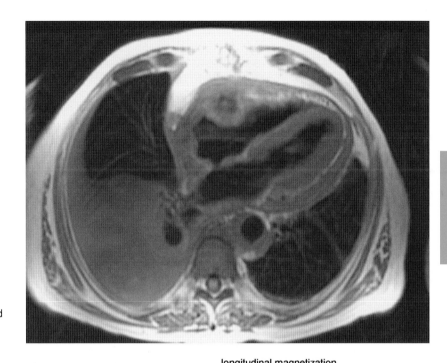

8

Figure 8.1 Axial black blood image through the heart. Blood in the chambers of the heart and great vessels has low signal intensity.

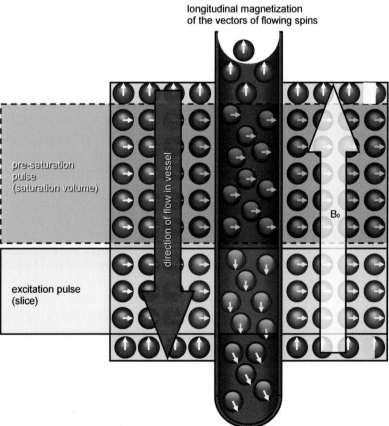

Figure 8.2 Spatial pre-saturation to produce black blood.

8

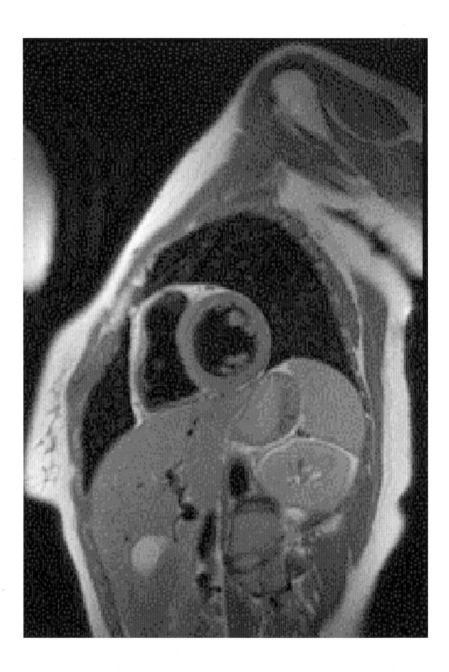

Figure 8.3 Double IR prep
short axis image of the heart.

In addition to conventional spin echo imaging, FSE sequences can also
provide images with intraluminal signal void in areas where there is flow
within vessels. To make flowing vessels even darker, FSE sequences can
be initiated with inversion pulses. These pulses can be known as driven
equilibrium, whereby the sequence begins with a 180° pulse and then
another 180° pulse for a total of 360° pulse. In this case the magnetization
is 'driven' back to equilibrium, or back to the starting point or the original
point along the Z-axis. This technique is also known as **double inversion
recovery or double IR prep** (Figure 8.3)(*see* Chapter 5).

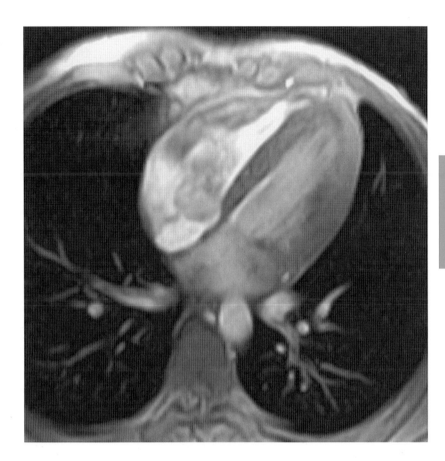

Figure 8.4 Axial bright blood image through the heart. Blood in the chambers and great vessels has high signal intensity.

Bright blood imaging

In addition to making the vessels appear black, vascular structures can also be visualized by making them bright. Several techniques can be used to enhance the signal from flowing blood, including gradient echo imaging and/or gradient moment rephasing and/or contrast enhancement. In gradient echo imaging, flowing spins are refocused by the rephasing gradient and hence patent vessels appear bright on the image. As a result, this technique can be referred to as **bright blood imaging** (Figure 8.4) and can be further improved by the application of an imaging option known as gradient moment rephasing (*see* Chapter 6).

Gradient moment rephasing is a first order velocity compensation technique used to visualize slow-moving protons with constant velocity. Protons in venous blood or CSF are put into phase with the stationary protons, so that intra-voxel dephasing is reduced. Gradient moment rephasing complements flow by making vessels containing slow-flowing spins appear bright, so enhancing the signal from blood and CSF.

Gradient moment rephasing is widely used in the chest and abdomen, brain, extremities and for the myelographic effect of CSF in T2 weighted images of the spine. There are, however, several trade-offs for using

8

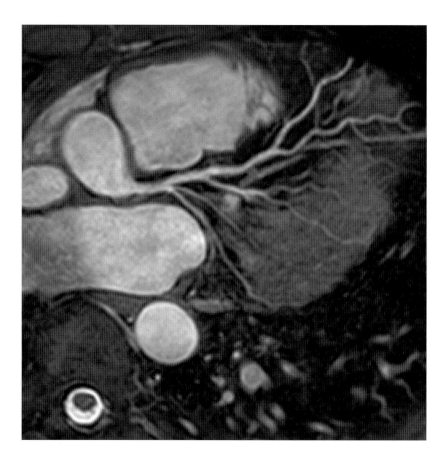

Figure 8.5 Balanced gradient echo sequence of the coronary arteries.

gradient moment rephasing. One such trade-off is that it requires a longer minimum TE due to the use of additional gradients, and results in a reduction in the number of slices available. Another trade-off is that gradient moment rephasing is not particularly effective on rapid flow in the chest or abdomen. However, it is helpful for the visualization of slow flow found in these areas.

In addition to conventional gradient echo imaging, there is a relatively new gradient echo technique that uses a balanced gradient system (*see* Balanced gradient echo in Chapter 5). The utilization of this balanced gradient technique yields a net phase shift of zero within the proton spins. Balanced gradient echo images are acquired with a very short TR and TE. In fact, the TE is generally half the TR value. For example, if the TR is 8 ms then the TE is 4 ms (depending upon the gradient capabilities of the imaging system). In this imaging acquisition the image contrast is weighted to T2/T1. Tissues with a high T2/T1 ratio (such as CSF or blood) appear bright. Balanced gradient echo imaging sequences are used for cardiac imaging (Figure 8.5) and also for MR cholangiopancreatography, MR myelography and for the evaluation of the internal auditory canals (*see* Figures 5.40 and 5.41).

Learning point: saturation techniques in vascular imaging

Pre-saturation can be used on both spin echo and gradient echo pulse sequences and in some instances it is appropriate to use both pre-saturation and gradient moment rephasing in the same sequence. Another technique to enhance the signal from flowing blood is the administration of contrast agents (*see* Chapter 11).

Magnetic resonance angiography (MRA)

A more sophisticated means of imaging the vascular system is with the use of a technique known as **magnetic resonance angiography** (**MRA**). Vascular contrast is maximized by enhancing the signal from moving spins in flowing blood and/or suppressing the signal from stationary spins residing in tissue. When stationary spins are suppressed, the appearance of vasculature is enhanced by the increased signal from fresh spins which flow into the imaging volume and receive RF excitation for the first time (sometimes known as the **inflow effect**). There are two methods available to suppress stationary spins. First, two acquisitions can be performed which treat stationary spins identically, but which differentiate moving spins and subtract them. Second, if a short TR that saturates spins within the imaging volume is used in combination with the inflow effect, a high degree of vascular contrast can be achieved. At present, there are four basic MRA techniques, which utilize different phenomena to increase the signal from flowing spins and can be used to evaluate the cardiovascular system non-invasively. These techniques include:

- digital subtraction MR angiography (DS-MRA)
- time of flight MR angiography (TOF-MRA)
- phase contrast MR angiography (PC-MRA)
- velocity encoding techniques
- contrast enhanced MRA.

Digital subtraction MRA

Digital subtraction MRA has been compared to digital subtraction angiography as contrast is selectively produced for moving spins during two acquisitions. These are then subtracted to remove the signal from the stationary spins, leaving behind an image of only the moving spins. An early subtraction angiogram has been performed while gating to the cardiac cycle. An acquisition during systole (fast flow) was subtracted from an acquisition during diastole (slow flow). In this case, the stationary spins were subtracted out, visualizing only the moving spins (and hence the vasculature) on the resultant image. Although this is an outdated technique and not widely used, it does deserve a brief mention in that it laid the groundwork for some of the techniques used today.

Time of flight MRA

Time of flight MRA (TOF-MRA) produces vascular contrast by manipulating the longitudinal magnetization of the stationary spins. TOF-MRA uses a coherent gradient echo pulse sequence in combination with gradient moment rephasing to enhance flow. In TOF-MRA, the TR is kept well below the T1 time of the stationary tissues so that T1 recovery is prevented. This beats down the stationary spins, while the inflow effect from fully magnetized flowing fresh spins produces a high vascular signal. However, if the TR is too short, the flowing spins may be suppressed, along with the stationary spins, which reduce vascular contrast.

TOF-MRA can be acquired in 2D or 3D. In 2D TOF-MRA, a flip angle of 45°–60° in conjunction with a TR of 40–50 ms is usually sufficient to maximize signal without suppressing the signal from flowing nuclei. Within this flip angle and TR range, saturation of flowing spins only occurs at flow velocities of approximately 3 cm/s or less. In addition, signal intensities in flowing spins may be increased by shortening their T1 times with the use of contrast enhancement agents (*see* Chapter 11).

To evaluate signals from arterial flow, it may be advisable to apply saturation pulses in the direction of venous flow. For example, to evaluate the carotid arteries in the neck, apply saturation pulses superior to the imaging volume to saturate the signal from inflowing venous blood (Figure 8.6).

TOF-MRA is most sensitive to flow that is perpendicular to the FOV and the slice. Any flow that is parallel to (or remains in) the FOV can be saturated along with the stationary tissue if the flow velocities are slow relative to the TR. In addition, vessels with flow within the FOV may demonstrate some saturation of flowing spins, since T1 recovery occurs over the time in which spins move downstream in the imaging volume (Figure 8.7). The result of these phenomena is a reduction in vascular signal.

Another disadvantage of TOF-MRA is high signal in some background tissues, especially those with a short T1 relaxation time such as fat. As a result, high signal intensity can be seen, for example, in the orbit, caused by the short T1 of retro-orbital fat. This can be minimized by choosing a TE so that to a certain extent the signals from fat and water are out of phase with each other, and therefore cancel each other out. The TE should, however, be kept relatively short, to minimize intra-voxel dephasing and subsequent phase ghosting and signal loss.

Another remedy for this high signal is an option known as **magnetization transfer contrast (MTC)**. In this option, off resonance RF pulses are added to the imaging sequences to suppress the signals from

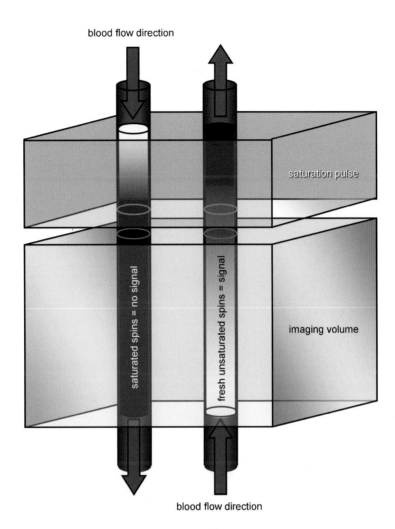

blood flow direction

saturation pulse

8

saturated spins = no signal

fresh unsaturated spins = signal

imaging volume

blood flow direction

Figure 8.6 Pre-saturation volume relative to the imaging stack.

macromolecules, like those found in gray and white matter in brain tissue (*see* Chapter 4).

Both solutions should help to minimize unwanted background signals and can be used for TOF-MRA and/or for post-contrast enhanced brain imaging by suppressing brain tissue, structures such as vasculature in MRA or lesions in enhanced brain imaging. In addition blood components with a short T1 recovery time, such as methemaglobin, also appear bright on TOF-MRA. Therefore, there can be a problem in distinguishing sub-acute hemorrhage from flowing blood on TOF-MRA images.

Another method for the improvement in vascular signal is with an increase in field strength. Signal to noise in MRI is directly proportional to field strength. For example, as field strength doubles, SNR doubles. As in clinical MRI, MRA also shows a marked improvement in SNR and contrast to noise (CNR) with an increase in field strength. With the increase in the number of ultra-high field scanners for clinical MRI and MRA,

8

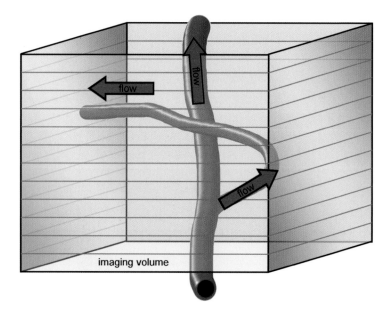

Figure 8.7 Flow within the imaging volume.

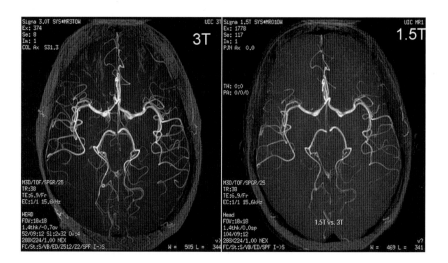

Figure 8.8 Axial TOF-MRA images at 3T (left) and 1.5T (right). Note greater SNR and CNR in the 3T image.

vascular signal (SNR and CNR) can be improved with higher field strength imagers such as 3.0 T and above (Figure 8.8).

2D vs 3D TOF-MRA. TOF-MRA can be acquired in either 2D (slice by slice) or 3D (volume) acquisition modes. In general, 3D volume imaging offers high SNR and thin contiguous slices for good resolution. However, as TOF-MRA is sensitive to flow coming into the FOV or the imaging volume, spins in vessels with slow flow can be saturated in volume imaging. For this reason, 3D TOF should be used in areas of high velocity flow (intracranial applications), and for high resolution to visualize small

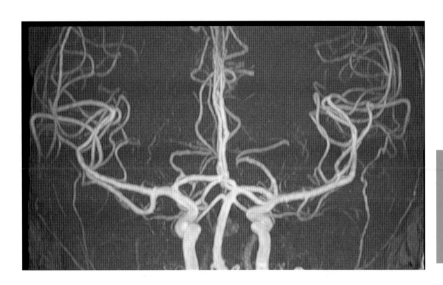

8

Figure 8.9 TOF-MRA of the Circle of Willis.

vessels (Figure 8.9). 2D TOF is optimal in areas of slower velocity flow (carotids, peripheral vascular, and the venous systems) and when a large area of coverage is required. In 3D techniques, there is a higher risk of saturating signals from spins within the volume.

Parameters and clinical suggestions for TOF-MRA

The carotid bifurcation, the peripheral circulation and cortical venous mapping can be imaged with 2D TOF-MRA. The parameters used for 2D TOF-MRA vary with manufacturer but generally the following should optimize image quality:

TR	45 ms
TE	minimum allowable
flip angles	approximately 60°

The selection of a short TR and medium flip angles allows for saturation of stationary nuclei but the moving spins coming into the slice remain fresh, and so vascular image contrast is maximized. The short TE reduces phase ghosting and susceptibility artefacts found on MR images acquired with gradient echo. Gradient moment rephasing, in conjunction with saturation pulses to suppress signals from areas of undesired flow, should be used to enhance vascular contrast relative to stationary tissue. Axial slice planes with slice thicknesses ranging from 1.5 mm (for the carotids and cortical venous structures) to 2.9 mm (for the peripheral vascular structures) should suffice.

TOF-MRA advantages

- reasonable imaging times (approximately 5 mins depending on parameters)
- sensitive to slow flow
- reduced sensitivity to intra-voxel dephasing

TOF-MRA disadvantages

- sensitive to T1 effects (short T1 tissues are bright so that hemorrhagic lesions may mimic vessels)
- saturation of in-plane flow (any flow within the FOV or volume of tissue can be saturated along with background tissue)
- enhancement is limited to either flow entering the FOV or very high velocity flow

2D TOF-MRA advantages

- large area of coverage
- sensitive to slow flow
- sensitive to T1 effects

2D TOF-MRA disadvantages

- lower resolution
- saturation of in-plane flow
- venetian blind artefact (occurs as respiration and patient motion moves tissue in and out of the slice that is being suppressed)

3D TOF-MRA advantages

- high resolution for small vessels
- sensitive to T1 effects

3D TOF-MRA disadvantages

- saturation of in-plane flow
- small area of coverage

Overcoming the disadvantages of TOF-MRA. There are a number of ways to overcome the limitations of TOF-MRA for both 2D and 3D acquisitions. These are listed above and there are several imaging options and protocol modifications that compensate for these pitfalls.

To overcome the susceptibility artefacts that are present on any gradient echo sequence, including MRA, short TEs and small voxel volumes should be used. In general, longer TEs permit more dephasing and therefore a TE of less than 4 ms minimizes this artefact. The larger the voxel, the more intra-voxel dephasing and therefore small FOVs, thin slices and fine matrices will reduce this effect.

Poor background suppression can be corrected by either using TEs that acquire data when fat and water are out of phase or by implementing magnetization transfer techniques. Out of phase images minimize the signal from tissues, such as fat, that have a short T1 relaxation time (*see* Chapter 7). MTC suppresses signal from macromolecules in fat and gray and white matter. As a result of improved background suppression, smaller peripheral vessels may be visualized (*see* Chapter 4).

Suppression of in-plane vascular signal, especially in 3D acquisitions, can be overcome by the utilization of ramped RF pulses and via the administration of contrast media. Ramped RF pulses set flip angles across a 3D acquisition so that the flip angle increases across the volume of the slab. As a result, signal from spins that have flowed across the volume of tissue still produce signal at the end of the imaging volume. The administration of intravenous contrast agents also enhances signal from blood that might have otherwise been suppressed.

Motion artefacts can arise from a number of sources including respiration and pulsatile blood flow. Respiratory motion artefacts, known as Venetian blind artefacts, can be minimized by reducing respiration via breath-hold techniques. Pulsation artefacts can be reduced by timing the acquisition to the cardiac cycle. This technique is known as gating and will be discussed later in the chapter.

To overcome the limited coverage provided by 3D TOF-MRA, one can either acquire images in another plane or combine a number of 3D acquisitions in a technique known as MOTSA. MOTSA is **multiple overlapping thin section angiography**. It combines a number of high-resolution 3D acquisitions to produce an image that has good resolution and a large area of coverage.

MRA image reformation

The manner in which the data from MRA images are reformatted plays a large part in determining the way in which vascular anatomy is perceived in the images. One method for reformatting TOF-MRA image data uses a technique known as **maximum intensity projection (MIP)**. In this technique, a projection ray is passed through the volume of data so that these data are projected onto a two-dimensional plane. There is a mathematical correlation between each pixel in the projection image and the pixels along each line of the volume data. A projection pixel is assigned the

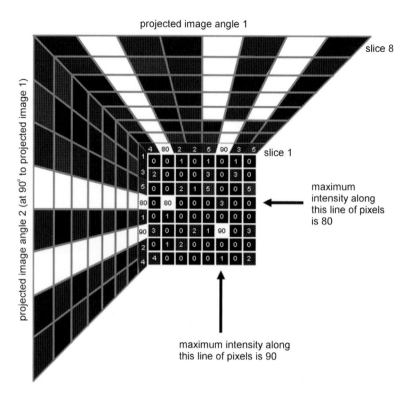

Figure 8.10   MIP reformatting.

maximum intensity found along the projection ray passing through the volume data. Subsequent intensities detected by the ray are assigned lesser signal intensities.

This process is repeated at different projection angles and the resultant images are then combined to give a three-dimensional perception of vascular structures. This technique is known as MIP with a ray trace algorithm or depth queuing. With the use of a ray trace algorithm, the image is viewed so that the vascular anatomy nearest to the observer appears brighter than that which is furthest away. As a result, the viewer has a perception of the depth of the image data (Figures 8.10 and 8.11).

Another method of reformatting MRA images is with a Shaded Surface Display (SSD). This technique reformats image data such that the display appears as though a light is shone onto structures (as opposed to MIP which appears as a light shining *through* structures). This results in a 3D appearance of the vasculature.

To visualize contrast enhanced MRA images without obstruction of background tissues, subtraction techniques can be used. This technique takes the image acquired without contrast, and 'subtracts' the image from that acquired during contrast enhancement. The resultant image demonstrates vascular signal free from background signal (Figure 8.12).

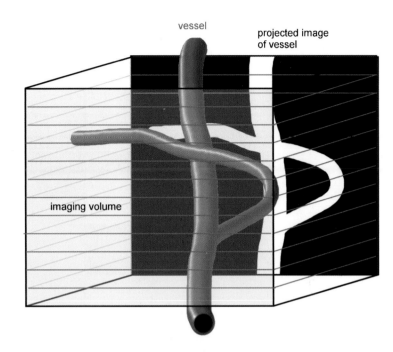

vessel

projected image
of vessel

imaging volume

8

Figure 8.11 MIP reformatting.

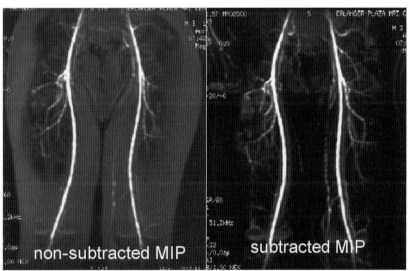

non-subtracted MIP   subtracted MIP

Figure 8.12 These images
were acquired un-subtracted
(left) and subtracted (right).

Phase contrast MRA

Phase contrast MRA uses the velocity differences, and hence the phase
shifts in moving spins, to provide image contrast in flowing vessels. The
variation in phase originates from physiological conditions such as sys-
tolic and diastolic velocity changes. Phase shifts can also be generated in
the pulse sequence by phase encoding the velocity of flow with the use of a
bipolar (two lobes that are equal in strength, one negative one positive)

8

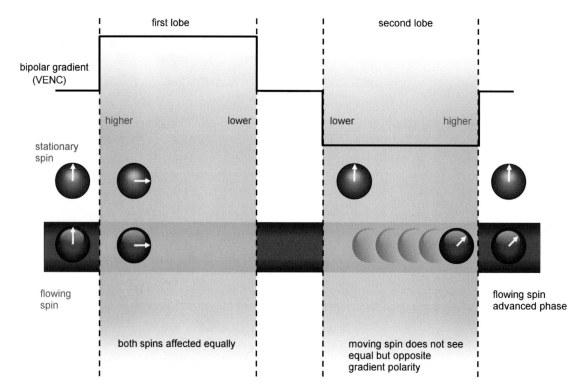

Figure 8.13   Bipolar gradients in PC-MRA.

gradient. In this method, phase shift is introduced selectively for moving spins with the use of magnetic field gradients. This technique is known as **phase contrast magnetic resonance angiography (PC-MRA)**. PC-MRA is sensitive to flow within, and that coming perpendicularly into the FOV and the slice (Figure 8.13).

Immediately after the RF, excitation pulse spins are in phase. In PC-MRA a gradient of a given strength is applied to both stationary and flowing spins. During initial application of the first bipolar gradient there is a shift of phases of stationary and flowing spins but both are affected equally. After the second part of the application of the bipolar gradient, the stationary spins return to their initial phase, but those of moving spins acquire some phase.

The bipolar gradient is then applied with opposite polarity or direction but at the same strength or amplitude so that the same variants occur, but in the opposite direction. PC-MRA then subtracts the two acquisitions so that the signals from stationary spins are subtracted out leaving only the signals from flowing spins. The combination of PC-MRA acquisitions results in what are known as magnitude and phase images. The un-subtracted combinations of flow sensitized image data are known as **magnitude images,** while the subtracted combinations are called **phase images.**

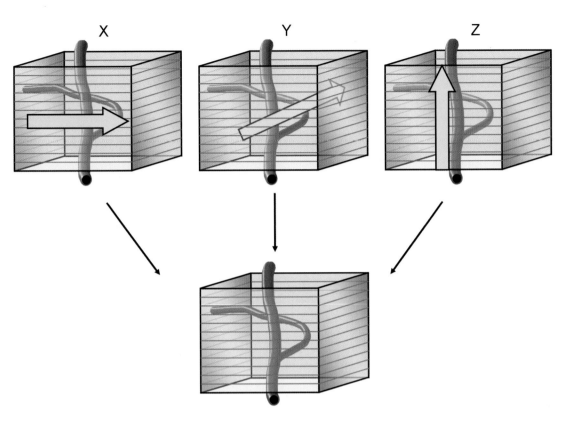

Figure 8.14 Flow encoding axes.

Flow encoding axes

Sensitization to flow is obtained along the direction of the applied bipolar gradient. If the bipolar gradient pulses are applied along the Z-axis, phase shifts are induced in flow that occurs along this axis, so sensitizing the PC-MRA to flow that runs from head to foot. Since flow can occur in other directions, bipolar gradients are applied in all three dimensions and in doing so, sensitize flow in all three directions X, Y and Z (Figures 8.14 and 8.15). These are known as **flow encoding axes**. However, an increase in the number of flow encoding axes also increases the imaging time.

Velocity encoding (VENC)

PC-MRA can also be sensitized to flow velocity. Velocity encoding technique (VENC) compensates for projected flow velocity within vessels by controlling the amplitude or strength, of the bipolar gradient. If the VENC selected is lower than the velocity within the vessel, aliasing can occur. This results in low signal intensity in the center of the vessel, but better delineation of the vessel wall itself. It occurs because high velocity laminar flow is found in the center of the vessel, the signal from which is aliased or

8

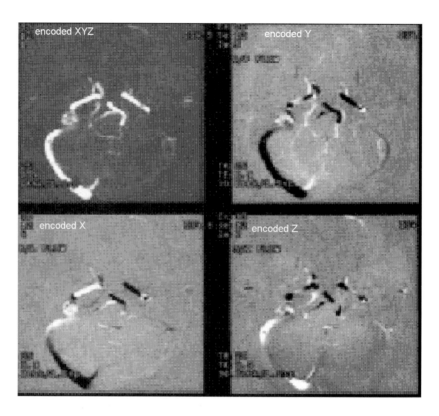

Figure 8.15 These images were acquired with PC-MRA encoded with various flow encoding axes. The top right hand and all bottom images are known as phase images and were encoded in only one direction. The top left hand image is known as a magnitude image and was encoded in all three orthogonal axes.

mismapped out of the vessel lumen. However, there is better delineation of the vessel wall above background noise levels. Conversely, with high VENC settings, intraluminal signal is improved, but vessel wall delineation is compromised (Figures 8.16 and 8.17).

2D and 3D PC-MRA

PC-MRA can be acquired with the use of either 2D or 3D acquisition strategies. Two-dimensional techniques provide acceptable imaging times (1 to 3 min) and flow direction information. If a 2D PC-MRA acquisition has been flow encoded from superior to inferior, flow from the head appears white, while flow from the feet appears black. 2D acquisitions, however, sometimes cannot be reformatted and viewed in other imaging planes. As in clinical imaging, 3D offers SNR and spatial resolution superior to 2D imaging strategies, and the ability to reformat in a number of imaging planes retrospectively. The trade-off, however, is that in 3D PC-MRA, imaging time increases with the TR, NEX, the number of phase encoding steps, the number of slices and the number of flow encoding axes selected. For this reason, scan times can approach 15 min or more.

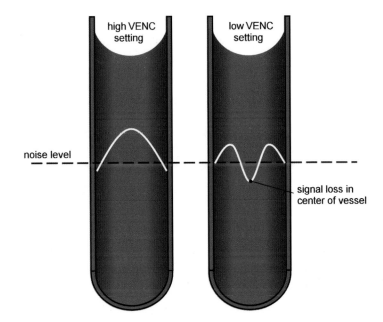

high VENC
setting

low VENC
setting

noise level

signal loss in
center of vessel

8

Figure 8.16 VENC settings.

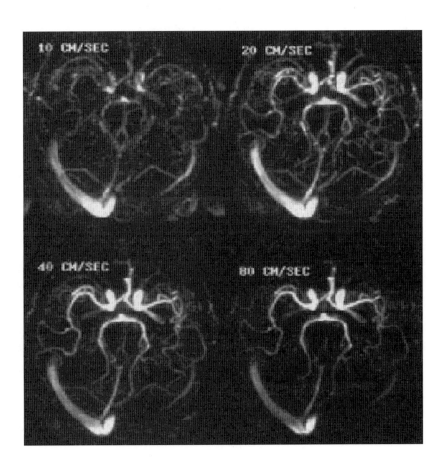

Figure 8.17 These images
were acquired with PC-MRA
and were acquired with various
velocity encoding settings
(VENC) 10, 20, 40 and 80 cm/s.

Parameters and clinical suggestions for PC-MRA

PC-MRA can be used effectively in the evaluation of arteriovenous malformations, aneurysms, venous occlusions, congenital abnormalities and traumatic intracranial vascular injuries. 3D volume acquisitions can be used to evaluate intracranial vasculature (Figure 8.18). Suggested parameters are:

28 slices volume, 1 mm slice thickness
flip angle   20° (60 slice volume flip angle reduced to 15°)
TR   less than or equal to 25 ms
VENC   40–60 cm/s
flow encoding in all directions.

2D techniques offer more acceptable imaging times of approximately 1 to 3 min. For intracranial applications of 2D PC-MRA suggested parameters are:

TR   18–20 ms
flip angle   20°
slices thickness   20–60 mm
VENCs   20–30 cm/s for venous flow
                    40–60 cm/s for higher velocity with some aliasing
                    60–80 cm/s to determine velocity and flow direction

For carotids 2D PC-MRA parameters include:

flip angles   20°–30°
TR   20 ms
VENCs   40–60 cm/s for better morphology with aliasing
                    60–80 cm/s for quantitative velocity and directional information

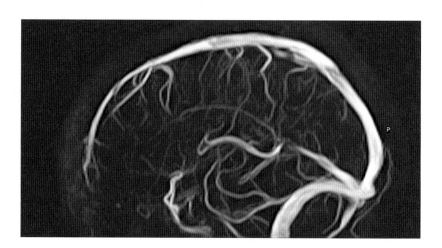

Figure 8.18   Sagittal PC-MRA image of the sagittal sinus.

Advantages of PC-MRA

- sensitivity to a variety of vascular velocities
- sensitivity to flow within the FOV
- reduced intra-voxel dephasing
- increased background suppression
- magnitude and phase images

Disadvantages of PC-MRA

8

- long imaging times with 3D
- more sensitive to turbulence

Velocity encoding techniques

Velocity encoding techniques are designed to evaluate flow velocity and direction providing information similar to Doppler ultrasound. The projection plane is located at right angles to the excitation plane. The location of vascular plugs on the projection plane shows flow direction, and length of the projection defines the velocity of flow.

Contrast enhanced MRA

Sometimes it is advantageous to acquire images in the plane that best covers the anatomy. For example, to cover adequately the ascending and descending aortic arch the sagittal plane is optimal, while the coronal plane is better for the renal arteries and aorta. The problem with this strategy is that it is prone to in-plane flow. To overcome this, a combination of 3D imaging with contrast enhancement with rapid dynamic imaging may be used. To overcome small coverage, images can be acquired in the desired plane for adequate coverage.

Therefore, another more invasive technique is to introduce a bolus injection of contrast medium followed by a 3D T1 gradient echo sequence. This technique uses a 3D gradient echo sequence followed by a bolus injection of gadolinium and a dynamic imaging sequence. This sequence is generally timed to the arterial phase and then repeated several times to acquire images during intermediate and venous phases of the vascular system. Technical considerations for enhanced MRA include:

- injection bolus (hand injection vs power injector)
- scan timing (estimating, test injection, or bolus tracking)
- image parameters (adequate coverage, SNR and fat suppression) (Figure 8.19).

8

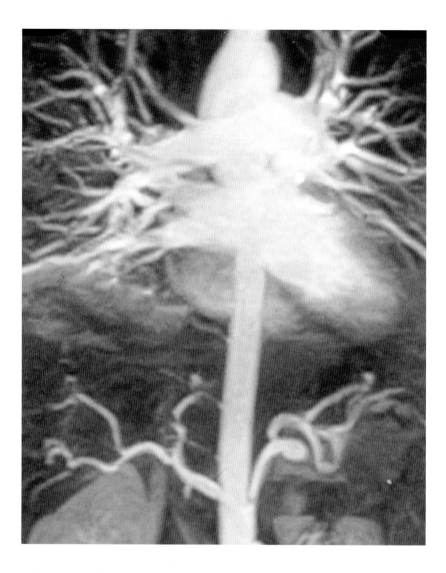

Figure 8.19   CE-MRA of the aorta and vessels.

Magnetic resonance angiography summary

The information provided by PC and TOF-MRA differs from that of conventional contrast angiography as MRA produces a flow sensitive image, rather than a morphological image. Consequently, clinical situations that require hemodynamic information are more suited to MRA than those requiring fine anatomic detail. Using MRA, laminar flow can be clearly imaged. However, as turbulent flow contains dispersion velocities that result in dephasing within a voxel, a loss of signal intensity results. In many respects, information provided by MRA is a combination of the flow information obtained in a Doppler ultrasound examination, and the morphological information contained in conventional contrast angiography. This is especially true when PC and TOF-MRA are used in combination with velocity encoding techniques.

Perfusion and diffusion imaging

It appears that perfusion and diffusion imaging represents the next step, after MRI and MRA, in non-invasive tissue characterization. Diffusion is the translational motion of water molecules in any direction, but distinct from those rotations responsible for T1 recovery and T2 decay. Diffusion imaging uses balanced gradients to preserve signal intensity in stationary spins, but also to reduce the signal intensity of diffusing water protons. In water diffusion is usually isotropic, but in tissue that restricts diffusion it occurs anisotropically (*see* Chapter 12).

Perfusion is micro-circulation or the delivery of blood to tissues. Perfusion imaging is the measurement of blood volume in these areas. This measurement, however, is complicated because fewer than 5% of tissue protons are intravascular. To measure perfusion either stationary spins can be suppressed, or signal intensity in perfusing spins increased. This can be achieved either by employing motion-sensitive gradients, or introducing enhancement agents (*see* Chapter 12). Figure 8.20 shows a perfusion study of the heart to assess myocardial perfusion in a patient, post-myocardial infarction.

Vascular imaging techniques have now been described in general. To image the heart and great vessels specifically, the motion of these organs during cardiac activity must be compensated for, if good quality images are to be obtained. This is achieved using a technique known as cardiac gating.

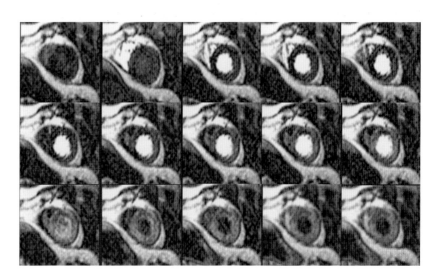

Figure 8.20 Perfusion study of the myocardium.

8

Cardiac gating

Cardiac gating is a method that reduces the phase mismapping produced as a result of heart motion and pulsatile blood flow. It uses the electrical signal of the heart, or the mechanical flow of the vascular bed, to trigger each pulse sequence (Figure 8.30). Two methods are used:

- *Electrocardiogram* (ECG, EKG) gating uses electrodes and lead wires placed on to the patient's chest to detect the electrical activity of the heart.
- *Peripheral gating* uses a photo-sensor placed on the patient's finger to detect a pulse in the capillary bed.

The ECG

The ECG is acquired by measuring the voltage difference between two electrodes attached to the patient's chest. Most systems color code the electrodes so that they can be placed correctly. The red and the white electrodes are usually placed across the heart, as these measure the voltage difference between two points. The green electrode is the ground, and should be placed as near to (but not touching) either the red or the white electrode. The ECG consists of:

- a P wave that represents atrial systole (contraction)
- a QRS complex that represents ventricular systole
- a T wave that represents ventricular diastole (relaxation).

The peak of the R wave is used to trigger each pulse sequence because, electrically, it has the greatest amplitude (Figure 8.21). This technique is known as prospective gating. Prospective means that the scan is timed to, and triggered from, the beats of the heart during the acquisition. Prospective gating is the technique that occurs during image acquisition, as opposed to retrospective gating. Retrospective gating (performed during many cardiac ciné acquisitions) acquires image data and times to the cardiac cycle during reconstruction (after the scan acquisition – retrospectively).

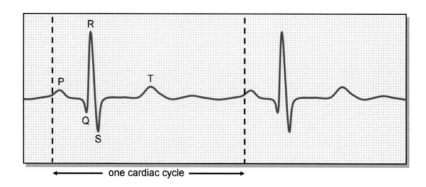

Figure 8.21 The ECG.

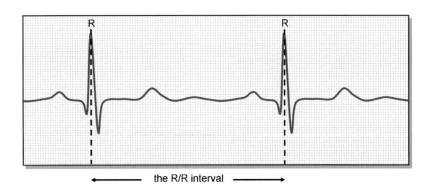

Figure 8.22 The R to R interval.

The effective TR

As cardiac gating uses each R wave to trigger the pulse sequence, the TR depends entirely on the time interval between each R wave. This is called the **R to R interval** and is controlled by the patient's heart rate (Figure 8.22). If a patient has a fast rate, the RR interval is shorter than if the patient has a slow heart rate. The TR, and therefore the image weighting and number of slices, depends totally on the heart rate. The TR is now termed 'effective' as the heart rate is not perfectly constant and varies from one heartbeat to another.

For example, if the heart rate is 60 beats per minute then:

R to R interval = 60 000 ms ÷ 60 = 1000 ms.

(There are 60 seconds per minute and 1000 milliseconds per second or 1 heartbeat every second.)

If the patient's heart rate is 120 beats per minute then:

R to R interval = 500 ms.

This seems to be very restrictive in terms of weighting and slice number. To a certain extent this is true, in that there is no control of the R to R interval itself. In some patients the effective TR is 500 ms, and in others the TR is over 1000 ms, which reduces the T1 weighting considerably. This has to be tolerated when using gating techniques, as a penalty for producing images with reduced cardiac motion artefact.

Obtaining T2 weighted images can be more troublesome, but most systems use a method whereby every second or third R wave can be used as a trigger. In this way, the effective TR is lengthened so that saturation (and therefore T1 weighting) does not prevail, and proton density (short TE), and T2 (long TE) images can be obtained.

For example, if the R to R interval is 1000 ms:

1 R to R selected effective TR = 1000 ms
2 R to R selected effective TR = 2000 ms
3 R to R selected effective TR = 3000 ms.

To achieve T1 weighting, use each R wave to trigger each pulse sequence. This gives an effective TR of 600 to 1000 ms, depending on the patient's heart rate. For proton density and T2 weighting, use every second or third R wave to trigger, as this gives an effective TR of 2000 to 3000 ms, depending on the patient's heart rate.

Slice acquisition

The slices are acquired during the effective TR in the same way as in conventional imaging. Phase encoding data from each slice are acquired during the R to R interval. During the next interval data from another phase encoding step are acquired (Figure 8.23). This is repeated until the acquisition of data (or all the phase encoding steps) for each slice is complete. Data from each slice are always acquired when the heart is at the same phase of cardiac activity. In other words, slice 1 is always acquired when the heart is at a certain position in its cycle, and so are slices 2, 3, etc. In this way, the motion artefact of each slice is reduced.

This of course, only applies if the patient's heart rate remains constant throughout the scan. If the rate changes at all, data are obtained at different times during the cardiac cycle, and the images contain a great deal of artefact. Most patients' heart rates do not remain constant, but fluctuate due to anxiety or the gradient noise during the sequence. To compensate for this, certain safeguards are built into the effective TR so that gating is more efficient. These safeguards occur in the form of waiting periods around each R wave. These waiting periods are termed in many different ways, but basically there is a waiting period just before each R wave, and one just after. Many imaging systems automatically build these waiting periods into the pulse sequences. Others provide these as user-selectable parameters.

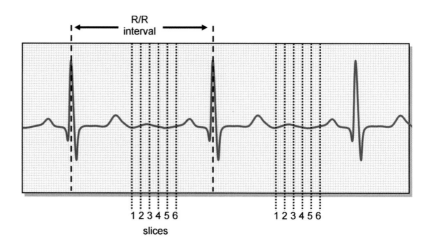

Figure 8.23 Slice acquisition during the R to R interval.

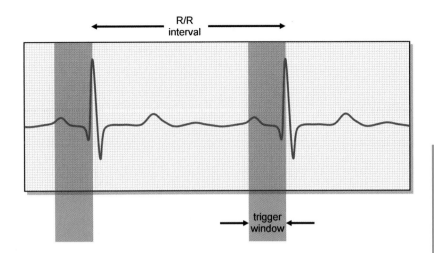

Figure 8.24 The trigger window.

8

The trigger window

The waiting period before each R wave is often called the **trigger window**. This is a time delay, usually expressed as a percentage of the total R to R interval, where the system stops scanning and waits for the next R wave (Figure 8.24).

This delay allows for the fact that the patient's heart rate may increase during the scan, moving the R wave nearer to the beginning of the window. If the system has stopped scanning and is waiting for the next R wave, it triggers the pulse sequence, regardless of whether the R wave is occurring sooner than expected. If the heart rate speeds up even more, so that the R wave occurs while the system is still acquiring data, the R wave is missed and the effective TR suddenly lengthens (Figure 8.25).

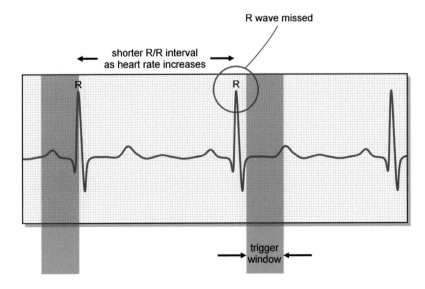

Figure 8.25 A missed R wave as the heart rate increases.

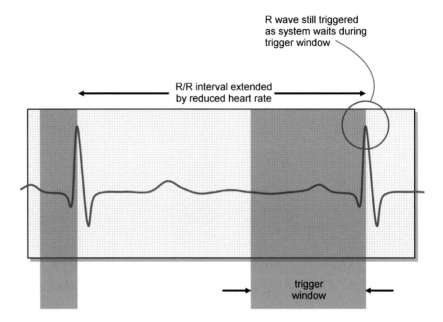

Figure 8.26 The R wave is not missed as the heart rate decreases.

If the heart rate slows down, the R wave moves further away from the beginning of the window, but the system is still waiting to trigger the scan and does so when it detects the next R wave. The effective TR is lengthened but the R wave is not missed (Figure 8.26).

The trigger window is usually expressed as a percentage of the R to R interval. Clearly, the correct window must be selected so that any increase in the heart rate is compensated for. Selecting a very large window, however, reduces the amount of time available to acquire slices, and so a balance is required. In practice, most patients' heart rates vary by about 10% during the scan, so selecting a window of about 10 to 20%

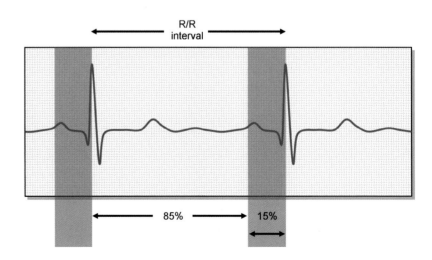

Figure 8.27 What would the trigger window be if the RR interval was 1000 ms?

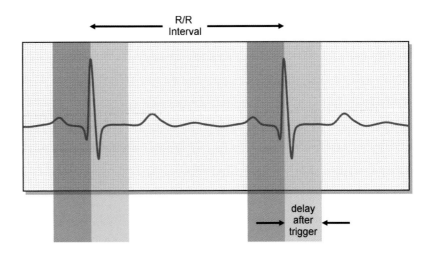

Figure 8.28 The delay after trigger.

compensates adequately for any variations in the heart rate and still allows a reasonable number of slices to be acquired (Figure 8.27).

The trigger delay

The waiting period after each R wave is often termed the delay after trigger or **trigger delay**. There is always a slight hardware delay between the system detecting the R wave and transmitting RF to excite the first slice. This is usually in the order of a few milliseconds. This period can often be extended, however, to delay the acquisition of the slices until the heart is in diastole and is therefore relatively still (Figure 8.28).

The available imaging time

The available imaging time is the time available to acquire slices. It is defined as the effective TR minus the trigger window and the delay after trigger.

Available imaging time
= R to R interval − (trigger window + trigger delay)

If the R to R interval is 1000 ms, the trigger window 10% and the trigger delay 100 ms the time available to acquire the data is:

1000 − 100 − 100 = 800 ms

The available imaging time is not the effective TR. The effective TR is the time between the excitation of slice 1 in the first R to R interval, to its excitation in the second R to R interval. The available imaging time is purely the time allowed to collect data, and governs the number of slices that can be obtained (Figure 8.29).

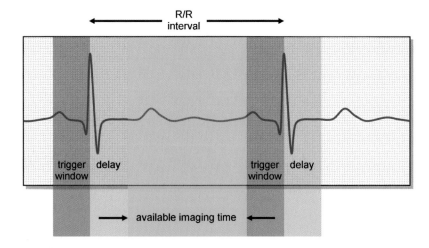

Figure 8.29   The available imaging time.

Peripheral gating

Peripheral gating works in exactly the same way as ECG gating. A photo-sensor attached to the patient's finger detects the increase in blood volume in the capillary bed during systole. This, in turn, affects the amount of light reflected back to the sensor and a wave form is obtained. The peaks of the waves are now termed the R waves, but these represent the peripheral pulse that occurs approximately 250 ms after the R wave of the ECG. The trigger window, trigger delay and available imaging time still apply.

Parameters used in gating

T1 weighting

  short TE
  1 R to R interval

PD/T2 weighting

  short TE (PD)/long TE (T2)
  2 or 3 R to R intervals

Safety aspects of gating

The electrodes used in gating are attached to cables that are conductors and are therefore capable of carrying relatively high currents. The cables lie within the high intensity region of the gradient field during the scan. As

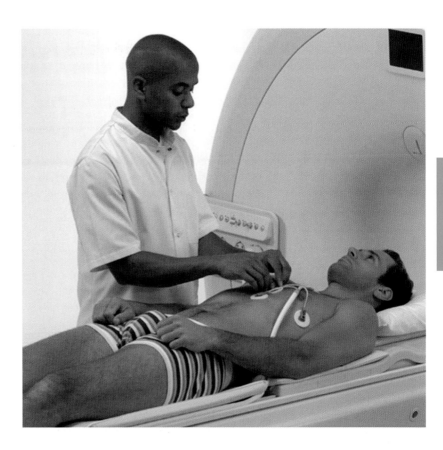

Figure 8.30   Placement of gating leads.

a result, currents may be induced in the cables, which can potentially store and transfer heat to the patient. It is therefore possible to burn or blister the patient, if strict safety rules are not adhered to.

Always check the cables and electrodes for damage. If they are frayed or splitting, do not use them under any circumstances. When positioning the cables, avoid looping or crossing them over. The point of crossover creates extra heat that could burn through the insulating material of the cable. When positioning the patient within the bore of the magnet, make sure that the cables do not touch either the patient or the bore of the magnet. Running the cables down the center of the patient avoids contact with the bore, and placing pads between the cables and the patient prevents possible injury (Figure 8.30).

The uses of gating

Gating is useful when imaging any area that contains pulsatile flow, or the heart itself. This includes the chest and great vessels, the abdomen, the spinal cord (CSF pulsations) and the brain. Virtually any area where pulsatile motion degrades the image lends itself to gating of some sort. The decision to use ECG or peripheral gating is often difficult. ECG gating is more time consuming because of the electrode placement, and because arrhythmias can alter the ECG to such an extent that the system cannot detect an adequate R wave. These difficulties are usually not present with peripheral gating, but this is not adequate when imaging the heart itself. Generally, peripheral gating is adequate for the brain, spine and vessels away from the heart. ECG gating should be used for the heart itself.

Gating is a rather lengthy process as the time of the scan is determined (among other things) by the patient's heart rate. A patient with bradycardia is not welcomed in an MRI suite! For this reason, many sites reserve gating only for chest imaging. ECG gating reduces motion artefact so that anatomy can be demonstrated well. It requires electrode and lead placement on the patient.

Usually there is no control over the TR, weighting or slice number when using gating. Gating is relatively time consuming, especially if the heart rate is slow.

Pseudo-gating

This is a very simple method of gating that involves selecting a TR that matches the R to R interval. ECG and peripheral gating is not employed but, instead, the patient's heart rate is measured before the examination by taking the pulse. The R to R interval is then calculated (60 000/heart rate in ms) and the TR corresponding to this is selected. As long as the heart rate does not significantly change during the examination, data from each slice are acquired at exactly the same time during the cardiac cycle as in conventional gating. This technique may be useful when conventional gating fails due to a poor ECG signal or low peripheral pulse. However, to be most effective, the heart rate must remain unaltered during the examination.

Gating is essential when studying the anatomy of the heart and great vessels. However, a study of heart function requires multiple images acquired at multiple phases of the cardiac cycle. This can be achieved using multi-phase imaging or cine.

Multi-phase cardiac imaging

In multi-phase cardiac imaging, a spin echo pulse sequence is used with slices acquired at precise phases of the cardiac cycle. This technique can be performed with either single-slice or multi-slice acquisition techniques. In multi-slice acquisition, the first slice location is acquired in each of four phases of the cardiac cycle. This is then repeated at the other slice locations. All the images acquired at each slice location can be placed in a 'loop' so that they may be viewed rapidly one after the other. In this way, cardiac motion can be visualized and cardiac function evaluated. One drawback is that the imaging time increases with the number of slice locations and/or phases imaged.

Ciné

Most cardiac ciné acquisitions are generally acquired with a gradient echo sequence with retrospective gating techniques. Unlike the prospective gating acquisitions described above, retrospective gating uses a method of collecting data continuously throughout the cardiac cycle. With this type of acquisition, data from each slice location can be acquired at different phases during the cardiac cycle. These data can then be reconstructed and displayed in a loop (or a movie), so that each location slice demonstrates cardiac motion and hence, cardiac function. Since ciné is usually performed with a gradient echo sequence, flowing blood appears bright. ECG or peripheral gating must be used, but data collection is continuous (and separated later, retrospectively) not triggered (prospective). The ECG is purely used to determine the phase of the cardiac cycle, so that after the acquisition the system can sort the data and reconstruct the images across the whole of the cardiac cycle.

Parameters used in ciné

We need to obtain good contrast between the vessel to be imaged with ciné and the surrounding tissue. T2* weighted coherent gradient echo sequences are used, so that blood or CSF appears bright. Gradient echo sequences are flow sensitive, because gradient reversal is not slice selective (as in spin echo). Therefore, a flowing nucleus produces signal after gradient rephasing, regardless of its slice location during excitation (*see* Chapter 6). Using a pulse sequence that employs coherent transverse magnetization in conjunction with the steady state maximizes T2* weighting. A short TR (in the order of 40 ms) in conjunction with flip angles of 30°–45° should be selected to maintain the steady state.

Using a short TR ensures that the stationary spins within the slice become saturated or beaten down by rapid successive RF pulses, while the flowing spins enter the slices relatively fresh. This saturates the background stationary tissue and enhances the brightness of the flowing nuclei. The TE should be relatively long to enhance T2* weighting (about 20 ms) and the use of gradient moment rephasing maximizes contrast even further. Some systems also permit ciné acquisitions with incoherent gradient echo sequences. These can be used to give T1 weighted ciné images. To optimize vascular contrast, however, use:

coherent gradient echo sequences
TR   less than 50 ms
flip angles   30°–45° (to maintain the steady state and satu
                   rate stationary nuclei)
TE   15–25 ms (to maximize T2)
gradient moment rephasing (to enhance bright blood)

Data collection

The data are collected from each slice at a certain interval across the cardiac cycle. The R to R interval and the effective TR for each slice determine how many times these data can be collected during each cardiac cycle. Data are collected at data points during the cycle. In addition, the number of phases of the cardiac cycle required to make up the ciné loop can be selected. For example, if 16 phases are selected each slice must demonstrate 16 different positions of the heart in one cardiac cycle (compared with 4 phases in multi-phase imaging). This is analogous to frames per second, but in ciné it refers to the number of phases per cardiac cycle.

To do this accurately, the collection of data must correlate as much as possible to each cardiac phase (Figure 8.31). Each data point must coincide with each cardiac phase. If the system cannot match the data points and the phases, it takes some data from one point and some from another,

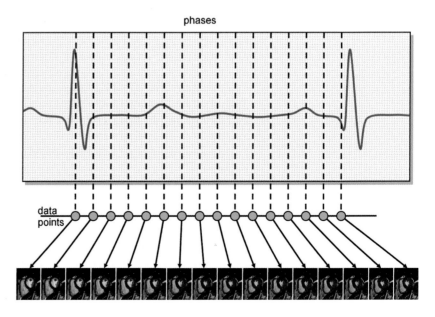

Figure 8.31 Data acquisition in ciné imaging.

phases

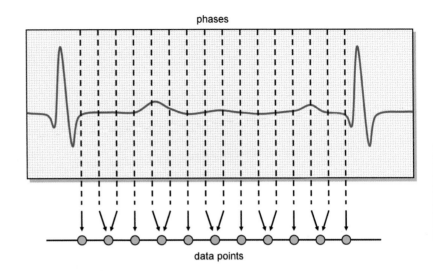

data points

Figure 8.32 Mismatching of the data points

8

to form the image at a certain phase position. Under these circumstances, ciné does not work efficiently (Figure 8.32).

In practice it is therefore important to calculate how many data points the system can collect for a given R to R interval, and ensure that the number of phases selected does not exceed this. The number of data points can be calculated by dividing the R to R interval by the effective TR. In ciné, the effective TR for each slice is the TR selected multiplied by the number of slices prescribed.

For example, if a TR of 40 ms is selected and two slices are prescribed, the effective TR is 80 ms. The effective TR in ciné is therefore very different from that used in gating, and the two should not be confused. In gating, the TR is not selectable as it is determined by the R to R interval. Although gating is used in ciné, the data are collected across the whole of the cardiac cycle and a TR is selectable. The ECG trace is purely used by the system to measure the cardiac cycle, not to trigger the pulse sequence.

The effective TR of each slice in ciné imaging is the time between the collection of data for each slice. The number of data points collected is therefore determined by this, and by the R to R interval of each cardiac cycle. If the effective TR is 80 ms and the R to R interval is 800 ms, 10 data points can be collected during each cardiac cycle. To ciné efficiently, the number of cardiac phases reconstructed should not exceed 10 in this example.

The uses of ciné

Ciné is useful for dynamic imaging of vessels and CSF. For example, ciné can evaluate aortic dissection and cardiac function (Figure 8.33). In the brain, it may be useful to demonstrate dynamically the flow of CSF in patients with hydrocephalus.

8

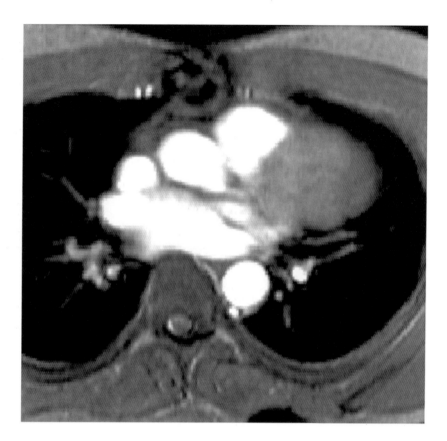

Figure 8.33   Ciné of the heart. An atrial fibroma is noted as a gray mass (adjacent to bright flow.

SPAMM

In addition to the classic cardiac imaging techniques there are new advances currently used in research. One of these techniques is known as **spatial modulation of magnetization (SPAMM)**. SPAMM modulates the magnetization thus creating a saturation effect on the image. This effect can be seen on the image appearing as cross-hatching of stripes. SPAMM is used in association with a multi-slice multi-phase acquisition and acquires data along the short axis of the left ventricle. In normal hearts, the stripes move along with the cardiac muscle. However, in cases of infarction, the infarcted area does not contract along with the normal muscle, and can therefore be easily identified in relation to the stripes (Figure 8.34).

Cardiac and vascular imaging can be a useful tool in the evaluation of a whole host of clinical situations. However, there are many logistical drawbacks. Motion artefact is a constant problem and patient co-operation is essential. In addition, radiographer education is a fundamental necessity if

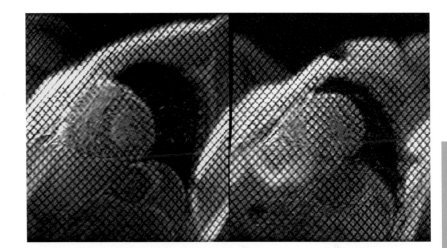

Figure 8.34 These images were acquired with SPAMM tagging, normal (left) and hypertrophic cardiomyopathy (right).

8

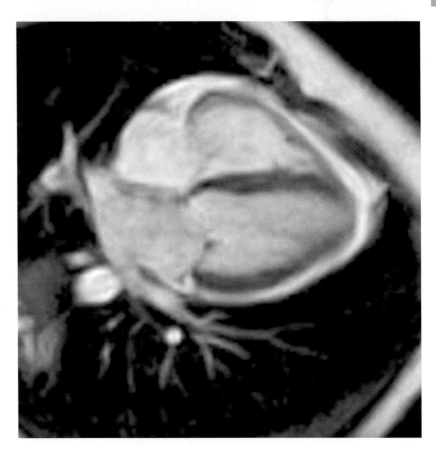

Figure 8.35 Four-chamber view of the heart.

consistently diagnostic cardiac and vascular images are to be obtained. The quality and applications of cardiac MRI have increased with the use of EPI sequences and software options that allow rapid filling of K space (Figure 8.35) (*see* Chapters 3 and 5).

Questions

1   What sequences are appropriate for bright blood imaging?

2   In what ways can tissues with a short T1 relaxation time be suppressed in TOF-MRA?

3   Why do we use a trigger window in gating?

4   What is the available imaging time using these parameters: RR 800 ms trigger window 10% delay after trigger 4 m?

5   Indicate when you would use ECG, peripheral gating, or nothing when examining the following areas:
brain
knee
liver
mediastinum.

9

Instrumentation and equipment

9

Introduction

Several processes must be completed to produce magnetic resonance images. These processes include nuclear alignment, radio frequency excitation, spatial encoding and image formation. The hardware required to complete such processes includes:

- a magnet
- a radio frequency source
- an image processor
- a computer system.

The magnet aligns the nuclei into low-energy (parallel) and high-energy (anti-parallel) states (*see* Chapter 1). To maintain magnetic evenness or homogeneity, a shim system is necessary. A radio frequency (RF) source perturbs or excites nuclei. The RF system requires a transmitter and a receiver. Magnetic field gradients determine spatial locations of RF signals (*see* Chapter 3). The MR signal is changed to an understandable format from a FID into a spectrum by a series of mathematical equations known as Fourier transform. This process occurs via the array processor. The host computer oversees the process and allows a means for operator interface with the system (Figure 9.1). This chapter discusses magnetic resonance instrumentation in more detail. First, however, magnetism and magnetic properties in general are described, as this helps one to understand different magnet types.

9

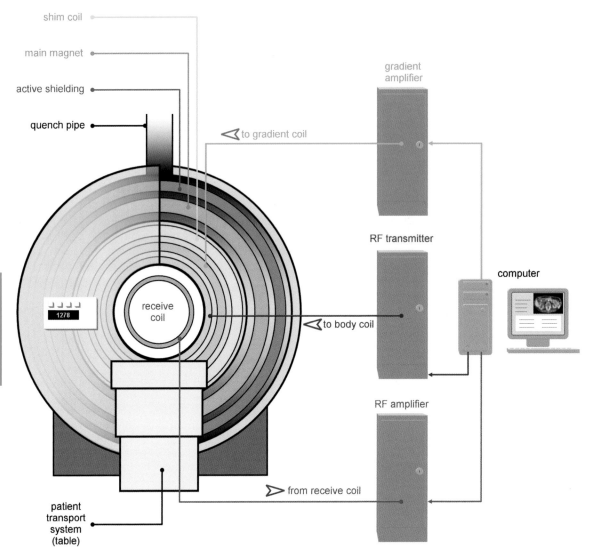

Figure 9.1   MR instrumentation.

Magnetism

Like the mass and electrical charge of a particular substance, **magnetism** is a fundamental property of matter. All substances possess some form of magnetism.

The degree of magnetism exhibited by a substance is due to a property known as the atomic magnetic dipole (or moment). These dipoles are generated in an atom by the movement of electrons. In the classical model of the atom, electrons exhibit two principal kinds of movement – an orbital

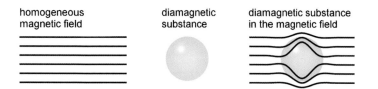

| homogeneous magnetic field | diamagnetic substance | diamagnetic substance in the magnetic field |

Figure 9.2   Diagmagnetism.

motion around the nucleus and a spinning motion around their own axes. The laws of electromagnetic induction indicate that whenever a charged particle such as an electron exhibits motion, a corresponding magnetic field is induced (*see* Chapter 1). The net magnetic moment of an atom is a combination of the magnetic moments of all the electons present.

Electrons present in the energy shells of atoms can be described as 'spin-up' or 'spin-down' depending on the direction in which they spin. Typically there are equal numbers of each type in a fully filled electron shell. The opposing polarities of these electrons will cancel out leaving no net magnetic moment. In certain atoms having partially filled shells there will be unpaired electrons, the presence of which will create a net magnetic effect in the atom.

The magnetic behavior of an atom is therefore dictated by the configuration of the orbiting electrons. Changes in the electron configuration between elements lead to them being classified as belonging to one of four main categories. In increasing order of magnetic strength these categories are:

- diamagnetism
- paramagnetism
- ferromagnetism.

Diamagnetism

With no external magnetic field present, diamagnetic substances such as silver and copper show no net magnetic moment. This is due to the fact that the electron currents caused by their motions add to zero. However, when an external magnetic field is applied, diamagnetic substances show a small magnetic moment that opposes the applied field. Substances of this type are therefore not attracted to, but are slightly repelled by, the magnetic field. For this reason, diamagnetic substances have negative magnetic susceptibilities and show a slight decrease in magnetic field strength within the sample (Figure 9.2). Examples of diamagnetic substances include inert gases, copper, sodium chloride and sulfur.

Paramagnetism

As the result of unpaired electrons within the atom, paramagnetic substances have a small magnetic moment. With no external magnetic field, these magnetic moments occur in a random pattern and thus cancel each

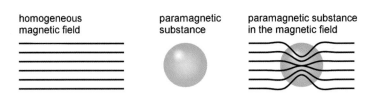

Figure 9.3   Paramagnetism.

other out. However, in the presence of an external magnetic field, paramagnetic substances align with the direction of the field and so the magnetic moments add together (Figure 9.3). Therefore paramagnetic substances affect external magnetic fields in a positive way, by attraction to the field resulting in a local increase in the magnetic field. One example of a paramagnetic substance is oxygen. Another is gadolinium chelates used as MR contrast agents.

Diamagnetic effects appear in all substances. However, in materials that possess both diamagnetic and paramagnetic properties, the positive paramagnetic effect is greater than the negative diamagnetic effect, and so the substance appears paramagnetic. The apparent magnetization of an atom can be shown by the following equation:

$$B_0 = H_0 (1 + x)$$

where

B_0 is the magnetic field
H_0 is magnetic intensity.

A substance is diamagnetic when $x < 0$. A substance is paramagnetic when $x > 0$.

Ferromagnetism

Ferromagnetic substances differ a great deal from diamagnetic and paramagnetic substances. When a ferromagnetic substance such as iron comes in contact with a magnetic field, the results are strong attraction and alignment. Objects made of substances of this type can become dangerous projectiles when inadvertently brought near a strong magnetic field. They retain their magnetization even when the external magnetic field has been removed. Therefore, ferromagnetic substances remain magnetic, are permanently magnetized and subsequently become **permanent magnets**. The magnetic field in permanent magnets can be hundreds or even thousands of times greater than the applied external magnetic field (Figure 9.4).

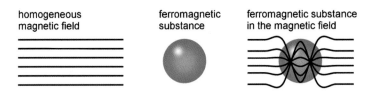

Figure 9.4   Ferromagnetism.

Learning point: paramagnetism and contrast agents

Superparamagnetic materials have positive magnetic susceptibilities that are greater than paramagnetic materials and less than those of ferromagnetic materials. Such substances include iron oxide particles which can be used as T2 or T2* agents for MRI. At present there is one intravenous superparamagnetic iron oxide contrast agent (for liver imaging) and one oral agent that are USA Food and Drug Administration (FDA) approved for use in MRI. These agents, when used with T2 or T2* imaging, make tissue appear dark (*see* Chapter 11).

Permanent magnets are bipolar as they have two poles, north and south. The magnetic field exerted by a permanent magnet produces magnetic field lines or lines of force running from the magnetic south to the north poles of the magnet. The magnetic field of the Earth also illustrates this phenomenon, which can be demonstrated with the use of a compass. The magnetic needle of the compass aligns with the lines of force of the Earth and points toward the North Pole.

In MRI a number of magnetic fields are used to create images:

- the main magnetic or static field – this is known as the primary field B_0
- the radio frequency field or RF field which is used to excite spins and produce resonance – this is known as the secondary magnetic field B_1.

The magnetic field strength is measured in one of three units:

- gauss (G)
- kilogauss (kG)
- tesla (T).

Gauss is used to measure low field strengths. For example, the strength of the Earth's magnetic field is approximately 0.6 G (depending upon one's location relative to the equator). Tesla, on the other hand, is the unit used to measure higher magnetic field strengths. The three units of measurement can be compared by the use of the equation:

$$1\,T = 10\,kG = 10\,000\,G$$

Most clinical MR systems operate from as low as 0.2 T to as high as 4 T. Most clinical imagers are 1.5 T. Until July 2004, the FDA limited clinical imaging in the USA to 2 T. This has since been increased to a limit of 4 T for infants up to one month old and up to 8 T for any age above this. This has spurred an increase in high field systems (mainly 3 T at present).

Even higher field strength systems are used for research purposes. However, the strength of the magnetic field is not perfectly even across the entire field. The evenness within the magnetic field is termed **homogeneity**. Inhomogeneity within a particular magnetic field is expressed in an arbitrary unit known as parts per million (ppm). An inhomogeneity of 1 ppm in a 1 tesla magnet yields a range in field strength from 10 000.00 to 10 000.01 G.

Now the various magnetic properties of matter have been described, the different types of magnet available are explored. These are:

- permanent magnets
- electromagnets (solenoid and resistive)
- superconducting magnets.

Permanent magnets

Since ferromagnetic substances retain their magnetism after being exposed to a magnetic field, these substances are used in the production of a permanent magnet. Examples of substances used are iron, cobalt and nickel. The most common material used to produce a permanent magnet is an alloy of aluminum, nickel and cobalt known as **alnico**. There are also some ceramic bricks possessing ferromagnetic properties that can be magnetized and used to produce permanent magnets.

The main advantage of permanent magnets is that they require no power supply or cryogenic cooling and are therefore relatively low in operating costs. In addition, the magnetic field created by a permanent magnet has lines of flux running vertically from the south to the north pole (bottom to the top) of the magnet, keeping the magnetic field virtually confined within the boundaries of the system and hence the scan room (Figure 9.5). As a result, these systems have almost no fringe field. This means that they have little or no safety considerations with respect to projectiles in the MR scan room (*see* Chapter 10). Such systems can also be designed with open configurations. Despite the low field strengths and associated lower SNR, open systems have become popular for claustrophobic and obese patients, kinematic musculoskeletal studies and interventional procedures, all of which are difficult in a closed solenoid configuration.

Electromagnets

The laws of electromagnetism state that moving electrical charges induce magnetic fields around themselves. Therefore, if a current (or a moving charge) is passed through a long straight wire, a magnetic field is created around that wire (Figure 9.6). The strength of the resultant magnetic field

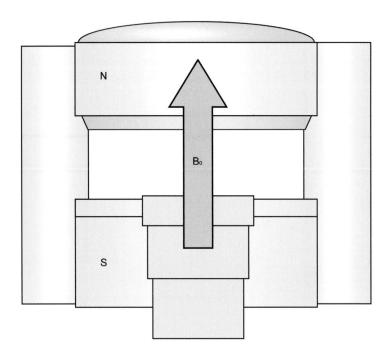

Figure 9.5 A permanent magnet.

9

is proportional to the amount of current moving through the wire. The magnetic field strength created by introducing current through a wire is calculated from the following equation:

$$B_0 = KI$$

where

 I is the current
 K is the proportionality constant (quantity of charge on each body)
 B_0 is the magnetic field strength.

Therefore the current passing along the wire is proportional to the magnetic field induced around it. The direction of the magnetic field induced can be expressed by the right-hand thumb rule. This rule states that if the fingers of the right hand are curled around a wire and the thumb points in the direction of the current, the fingers point in the direction of the magnetic field (Figure 9.6). In the case of a coil, the fingers represent the windings *and* the direction of the current and the thumb represents the net magnetic field direction.

 If current is passed through two parallel straight wires in opposing directions, the two magnetic fields tend to cancel each other out in the region between the two wires. Conversely, if the current passing along the parallel wires is flowing in the same direction, contributions to the resultant magnetic field are additive. This property is exploited for the generation of large magnetic fields.

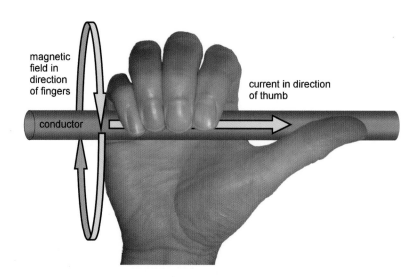

magnetic field in direction of fingers

current in direction of thumb

conductor

Figure 9.6   The right-hand thumb rule.

Solenoid electromagnets

Instead of using several parallel wires, one wire can be wrapped around to form many loops like a spring. The loops of wire form a coil and act as though they are parallel straight wires. This is called a **solenoid electromagnet** and, as the loops of wire appear to be evenly spaced, the magnetic field is considerably uniform, as it generates similar field strengths from one end to the other.

A factor that governs the efficiency of the passage of current is the inherent resistance of the coil. The degree of resistance along a wire is determined by **Ohm's law**. Ohm's law states:

V = IR

where V is equal to the applied voltage (which for our purposes is constant)

I is the current
R is the resistance within the wire.

Therefore, the solenoid electromagnet is often said to be a **resistive magnet**.

Resistive magnets

The magnetic field strength in a resistive magnet depends on the current that passes through its coils of wire. The direction of the main magnetic field in a resistive magnet follows the right-hand thumb rule, and produces lines of flux running horizontally from the head to the foot of the magnet (Figure 9.7). As a resistive system primarily consists of loops carrying current, it is lighter in weight than the permanent magnet and, although its capital costs are low, the operational costs of the resistive magnet are quite high due to the large quantities of power required to maintain the magnetic field.

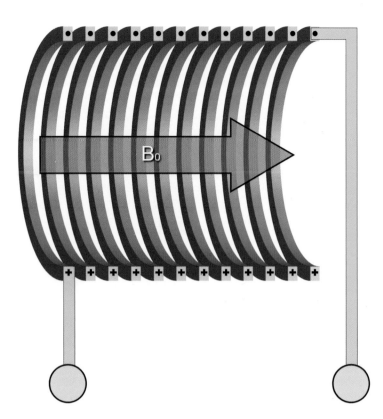

Figure 9.7 A simple electromagnet.

The maximum field strength in a system of this type is less than 0.3 T, due to its excessive power requirements. The resistive system is relatively safe as the field can be turned off instantly with the flick of a switch. However, due to the orientation of the wires and hence magnetic field lines (lines of flux), there is considerable stray magnetic field.

Superconducting electromagnets

As resistance decreases, the current dissipation also decreases. Therefore if the resistance is reduced, the energy required to maintain the magnetic field is decreased. Resistance depends on the material of which the loops of wire are made, the length of the wire in the loop, and the cross-sectional area of the wire itself. In addition, resistance depends on the temperature of the wires, which can be controlled so that resistance is minimized. In particular, some materials called superconductors exhibit zero resistance below a certain very low temperature. This is called the critical temperature. These wires are used to make the wires of superconducting magnets. A widely used material is an alloy of niobium and titanium, which becomes superconductive below approximately 4 K (kelvin).

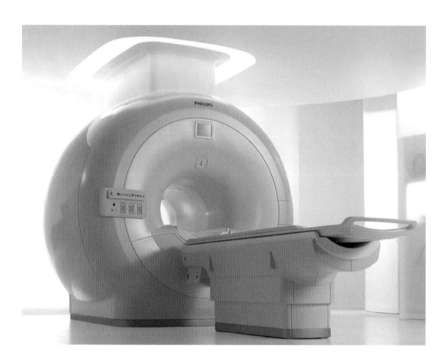

Figure 9.8   A superconducting system.

9

Initially, current is passed through the loops of wire to create the magnetic field or bring the field up to strength (ramping). Then the wires are supercooled with substances known as **cryogens** (usually liquid helium) to eliminate resistance. This is called a **cryogen bath** – it surrounds the coils of wire and is housed in the system between insulated vacuums.

When used to produce MR images, the superconducting magnet produces relatively high magnetic field strengths with virtually no power requirements (after the magnetic field has been ramped up). With resistance virtually eliminated, there is no longer a mechanism to dissipate current, so no additional power input is required to maintain the high magnetic field strength. Although the superconducting magnet has a relatively low operating cost, a system of this type is expensive to buy. However, the superconducting system offers extremely high field strengths of 0.5 to 4 T for clinical imaging, and anything up to 9 T for spectroscopic and high-resolution studies. The direction of the main magnetic field runs horizontally – like that of the resistive system – from the head to the feet of the patient. Figure 9.8 shows a typical superconducting system.

Hybrid magnets

In an attempt to get the best of both worlds, some manufacturers have combined superconducting with permanent systems to create high field 'open' magnets. The example shown in Figure 9.9 uses a permanent system supplemented with superconducting coils to increase field strength.

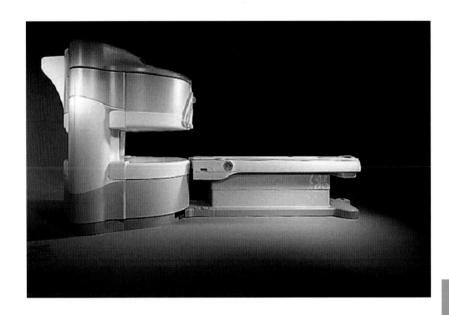

Figure 9.9 A hybrid magnet.

9

Niche magnets

Since shortly after the inception of MR imaging, system manufacturers have tried to invent variations in system designs for specialty imaging concerns. For example, several imaging companies have developed ultra-low imaging systems orthopedic applications (Figure 9.10). Some of these operate at field strengths as low as 0.01 T. As the field strength of these systems is very low, there are SNR problems. To create diagnostic images with low SNR, trade-offs are made in imaging parameters that generally result in an increase in scan time.

Summary

Permanent magnets:

- remain magnetized permanently
- flux lines run vertically
- require no power supply
- low operational costs
- small fringe fields
- heavy
- low field strengths (SNR lower/usually longer scan times)

Resistive magnets:

- field can be switched off immediately
- flux lines horizontal

- high operational cost as power supply required
- large fringe fields
- poor homogeneity at higher field strengths

Superconducting magnets:

- flux lines horizontal
- lower power requirements (cheap to run)
- expensive to buy
- large fringe fields
- high field strength (higher SNR/usually shorter scan times)

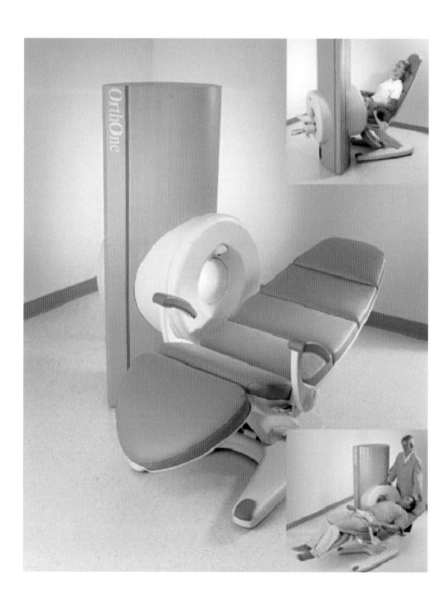

Figure 9.10   An example of a niche magnet for imaging extremities.

Image reproduced courtesy of ONI Medical Systems, Inc, MA, USA.

Fringe fields

The static magnetic field has no respect for the confines of conventional walls, floors or ceilings. The stray magnetic field outside the bore of the magnet is known as the **fringe field**. To some extent, all magnets have a fringe field. The field associated with a permanent magnet is relatively low, but in solenoid electromagnets, the fringe field is significant. These fringe fields must therefore be taken into account when siting a magnet, so that they do not extend into areas where potentially contraindicated patients, monitoring devices and other mechanical and magnetically activated devices are present.

Shielding

Magnetic shielding can significantly reduce the area covered by the fringe field. There are two methods of magnetic shielding – 'passive' and 'active' shielding.

Passive shielding is accomplished by surrounding the magnet (or lining the magnet room) with steel plates. This is an undesirable method for two main reasons. First, if the shielding is located in the magnet gantry it increases the size and weight of the machine. Passive shielding can weigh up to 40 tonnes, necessitating a ground floor magnet room with specially prepared foundations. Second, it is expensive.

The modern method of reducing the fringe field is to use **active shielding**. Active shielding uses additional superconducting coils located at each end of the main magnet inside the cryostat. These have an opposite effect to the main solenoid and can reduce the footprint of the 5 G fringe field to within a few feet of the gantry. Because of the reduced fringe field and the fact that no heavy steel cladding is required, the size and weight of the scanner is reduced to an unimposing and manageable package that can be sited in many more locations inside the hospital building. Actively shielded systems can also be sited in trailers to provide mobile services.

Shim coils

Due to the tolerances of manufacture, an MRI superconducting magnet has field homogeneity of approximately 1000 ppm on delivery from the factory. Imaging requires homogeneity of approximately 4 ppm across the imaging volume to provide good geometric sharpness and to allow even spectral fat saturation. Spectroscopic procedures require better than 1 ppm.

To achieve this, a process known as **shimming** is used. The term shimming comes from the discipline of carpentry where it refers to the use of wooden wedges (or shims) to level a surface. In the context of MRI,

9

shimming makes the field even and is achieved by the use of metal discs/plates (**passive shimming**) and an additional solenoid magnet (**active shimming**).

In the first instance, the cryostat is surrounded by a non-magnetic structure designed to hold the shims. This construction can vary in design. One type features a fiberglass tube with a number of circular hollows cut at regular intervals around its circumference and along its whole length. Each of these hollows can hold a number of circular metal discs. Another common design has moveable trays that can hold the shim plates.

Passive shimming is performed by scanning a phantom and adjusting the position of the shims until optimum field homogeneity is achieved. Passive shimming is performed at the time of installation and also counteracts any inhomogeneity due to the physical location of the magnet (due to nearby metal structures in the building or room construction).

Active shimming is performed by an electromagnetic coil and can be used to shim the system for each patient or even each sequence within a protocol. This ensures that the magnetic field is as homogeneous as possible irrespective of patient size.

Gradient coils

MRI pulse sequences use gradient magnetic fields in the process of spatial encoding of signal and in the formation of gradient echoes (*see* Chapter 3). By definition a gradient is simply a slope, in this case a very linear slope in magnetic field strength across the imaging volume in a particular direction. Gradients are created by the use of electromagnetic coils. To understand how the strength of a magnetic field can be altered, we need to consider the factors that change the strength of an electromagnet. They are the:

- number of loops in the coil
- current passing through the loops
- diameter of the loops
- spacing of the loops.

By changing the first three factors, the field strength would alter in a uniform way and therefore no gradient would be created. If a coil were made with the loops closely spaced at one end and becoming further apart at the other, or if a coil had more windings at one end than the other it could (theoretically) be used as a gradient coil. In practice, however, coils tend to be more symmetrical in design and rely on a three-terminal arrangement to achieve the gradient field.

To understand this concept, it is first necessary to visualize a simple electromagnet coil as shown in Figure 9.7. This coil has twelve windings uniformly spaced and is attached to an electrical terminal at each end.

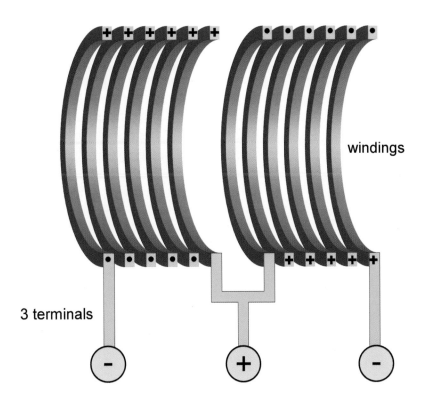

windings

3 terminals

Figure 9.11 A three terminal electromagnet.

9

Current therefore flows in one direction through the coil and the resulting direction of the magnetic field can be demonstrated with the right-hand rule, in this case left to right. Note that the direction of flow is represented by a dot and a cross indicating flow towards and away from the observer respectively (think of an arrow with a dot as its point and a cross as its tail feathers).

If this design is altered slightly to include a third terminal in the center of the coil (Figure 9.11), the polarity of the terminals can be arranged so that current flows in opposite directions at each end of the coil. This generates two magnetic fields of equal but opposite direction.

Consider a combination of these two coils as shown in Figure 9.12. The first coil represents the main magnet, and the second represents the Z gradient coil. To the left the secondary coil is producing a magnetic field in the opposite direction to B_0 and will therefore reduce the field strength at this end of the bore. To the right the secondary coil is creating a magnetic field in the same direction as B_0 and will therefore add to the field at this end of the bore. The result is a magnetic field gradient in the Z direction along the magnet bore.

By varying the magnetic field strength, gradients provide position-dependent variation of signal frequency and are therefore used for slice selection, frequency encoding, phase encoding, rewinding and spoiling (Figure 9.13). Gradient coils are powered by gradient amplifiers. Faults in the gradient coils or gradient amplifiers can result in geometric distortions in the MR image.

9

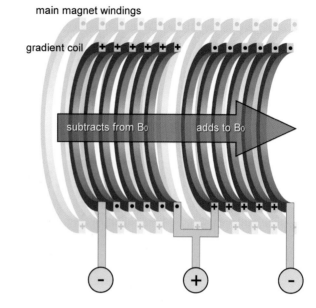

main magnet windings

gradient coil

subtracts from B₀   adds to B₀

Figure 9.12 A gradient coil.

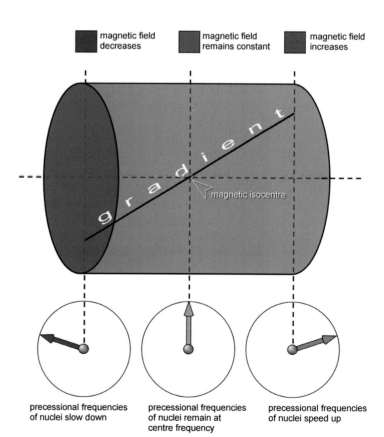

magnetic field
decreases

magnetic field
remains constant

magnetic field
increases

gradient

magnetic isocentre

precessional frequencies
of nuclei slow down

precessional frequencies
of nuclei remain at
centre frequency

precessional frequencies
of nuclei speed up

Figure 9.13 How gradients
change field strength, frequency
and phase.

Gradient strength can be expressed in units of G/cm or mT/m where:

1 G/cm = 10 mT/m

This means that the magnetic field changes by 1 gauss over each centimeter or 10 milli-tesla over each meter. Stronger gradients (15 or 40 mT/m) permit high-speed or high-resolution imaging.

High-speed gradient systems

One of the greatest factors that affects the timing of a pulse sequence is gradient switching. During the sequence each of the three gradients (X, Y and Z) are switched on and off many times for spatial encoding and for signal refocusing. Each time a gradient is switched on, power is applied to the gradient until it reaches maximum amplitude. The gradient is then left on for a period of time and then reversed for the same period of time. The application of each gradient therefore represents 'dead time' and, as gradients are applied many times during the sequences, each millisecond of wasted time is multiplied for each acquisition.

The sum of wasted seconds represents a considerable time loss, resulting in longer TRs and TEs, shorter turbo factors, fewer imaging slices and longer scan times. Significant time savings are therefore achievable by modifying the gradient system. To investigate this, we need to evaluate the main components of a balanced gradient system which include:

- gradient amplitude measured in milli-tesla per meter (mT/m) or gauss per centimeter (G/cm)
- gradient rise time measured in microseconds (ms)
- slew rate measured in milli-tesla per meter per second (mT/m/s)
- duty cycle, the percentage of time that the gradient is permitted to work.

Gradient amplitude is the strength of the gradient. Gradient amplitudes vary but typical gradient strengths are between 10 and 60 mT/m, depending on the power of the gradient set purchased. This means that when the gradient has reached maximum amplitude, its strength changes the magnetic field 10 mT over each meter or 1 gauss over each centimeter (10 mT/m = 1 G/cm). Gradient amplitudes directly affect image resolution, as high gradient amplitudes are required for a small FOV and thin slices (Figure 9.14).

Gradient rise time is the time that it takes for gradients to reach their maximum strength or amplitude (Figure 9.14). If the rise time is reduced, time is saved within the pulse sequence, which is then translated into shorter overall imaging times. High gradient amplitudes allow for shorter rise times. As shown in Figure 9.15, the application of enough power to create high gradient amplitudes shortens rise times but yields a power overshoot. In addition, high gradient amplitudes permit high amplitude balancing lobes, allowing for time savings within pulse

9

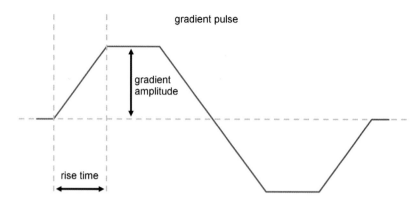

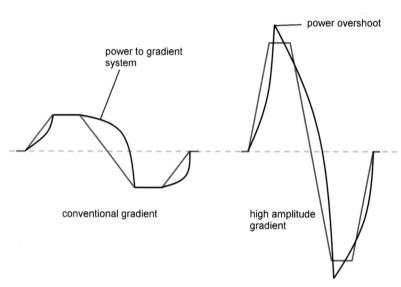

Figure 9.14 Gradient amplitude vs. rise time.

Figure 9.15 Comparison of the power supply to conventional and high speed gradient systems.

sequences (this technique will be described in more detail later in this chapter). Therefore for ultra-fast and/or ultra-high-resolution images, higher gradient amplitudes of 20 mT/m or greater are required.

Slew rate is described as the strength of the gradient over distance. Typical gradient slew rates are in the order of 70 mT/m/s. High-speed gradients are generally 120 mT/m/s. Some investigational slew rates approach 240 mT/m/s but at present this exceeds the FDA guidelines for gradient strength.

Duty cycle is a percentage of time during the TR period that the gradient is permitted to be at maximum amplitude, or to 'work', during an imaging sequence. This work time is known as the duty cycle. The duty cycle increases with slew rate but, as the duty cycle increases, the number of attainable slices is reduced. In spin echo imaging the typical duty cycle is 10% while in EPI it is closer to 50% of the TR period.

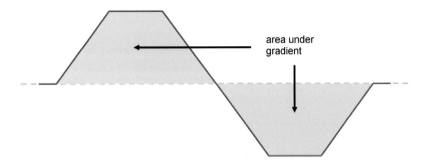

Figure 9.16 Balanced gradients.

As gradients become stronger with higher rise times, and as the noise heard during image acquisition is due to gradient noise, scanner noise is also increased. Therefore in addition to stronger gradients, manufacturers have modified gradient systems in an attempt to reduce gradient noise. These are known as quiet systems.

Balanced gradient systems

In a balanced gradient system, each gradient pulse is balanced by an equal but opposite gradient pulse. For example, a positive gradient pulse is followed by a negative pulse to undo the changes caused by the positive lobe. Therefore, in a balanced gradient system, the area under the positive lobe of the gradient equals the area under the negative lobe (Figure 9.16).

During readout, the amplitude of the positive lobe is limited by the desired resolution chosen by the FOV. The time that the gradient is left on (sampling time) is determined by the readout/receive bandwidth (*see* Chapter 3). If this time is doubled by the application of positive and negative lobes of the same amplitude and sampling, time is wasted within the pulse sequence. This wasted time results in fewer slices or, in the case of fast spin echo or EPI, shorter turbo factors and/or fewer slices. However, since it is the area under the lobes that must be equal, the negative lobe can have higher amplitude and shorter sampling time and still complete the same area. This asymmetric gradient paradigm permits time savings in the sequence and hence more slices and/or longer turbo factors can be used (Figure 9.17).

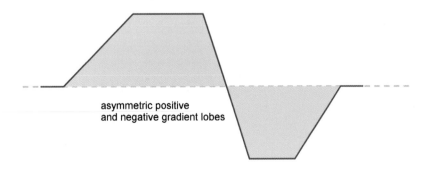

Figure 9.17 Asymmetric gradients.

9

Safety and power considerations

There are safety and power considerations associated with the application of high-speed gradients. Rapid gradient switching can cause peripheral nerve stimulation. Such stimulation results in mild cutaneous sensations, muscle contractions and stimulation of the retinal phosphenes. For this reason, many ultra-fast gradient systems operate just below the stimulation threshold. The FDA limits gradient strength to 6 T/s for all gradients but permits 20 T/s for axial gradients.

High-speed gradient switching has high power requirements in the order of 1000 kW. This necessitates high-quality gradient amplifiers. Resonant gradient systems that oscillate at a particular frequency provide a suitable alternative. Such systems produce a sinusoidal readout gradient, which reduces gradient demands, but is often incompatible with other imaging techniques that benefit from gradient switching (*see* Chapter 5).

Sampling sequelae

MR signals are sampled during readout when the frequency encoding gradient is applied. Signals are sampled only after the gradient has reached maximum amplitude. This type of sampling is known as conventional sampling. Unfortunately time is wasted within the pulse sequence waiting for the frequency encoding gradient to change.

Time within the sequence is reduced if sampling is performed while the frequency encoding gradient is changing. This is accomplished with a technique known as **ramp sampling**, in which data points are collected when the rise time is almost complete. Sampling occurs while the gradient is still reaching maximum amplitude, while the gradient is at maximum amplitude and as it begins to decline (Figure 9.18). However, this technique requires reconstruction programs to reduce artefact, and resolution may be lost. Resonant gradient systems that oscillate at a particular frequency produce a sinusoidal readout gradient that permits sinusoidal sampling. This technique provides an efficient sampling mechanism but is not compatible with all imaging sequences (Figure 9.19).

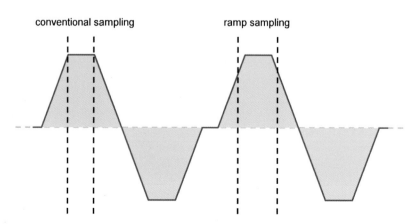

conventional sampling   ramp sampling

Figure 9.18 Conventional vs. ramped sampling.

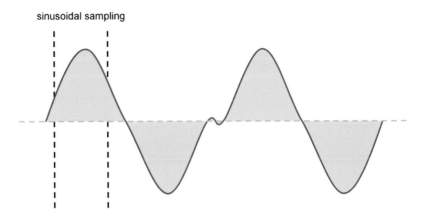

sinusoidal sampling

Figure 9.19 Sinusoidal sampling.

All the previously described time savings within pulse sequences can be translated into practical applications for MR system users. Such savings result in shorter imaging times, more slices and higher resolution matrices than in conventional imaging.

Radio frequency coils

As discussed in Chapter 1, the energy required to produce resonance of nuclear spins is expressed as a frequency and can be calculated by the Larmor equation. At field strengths used in MRI, energy within the radio frequency (RF) band of the electromagnetic spectrum is necessary to perturb or excite the spins. As shown by the Larmor equation, the magnetic field strength is proportional to the radio frequency, the energy of which is significantly lower than that of X-rays. To produce an image, RF must first be transmitted at the resonant frequency of hydrogen so that resonance can occur. The transverse component of magnetization created by resonance must then be detected by a receiver coil.

RF transmitters

Energy is transmitted at the resonant frequency of hydrogen in the form of a short intense burst of radio frequency known as a **radio frequency** pulse. This is achieved by a radio transmitter that sends frequency with enough energy to force phase coherence and flip some of the spins from a low- to a high-energy state. This RF pulse transfers the NMV from a position parallel to B_0, to an orientation at right-angles to B_0. Such a pulse is therefore called a 90° RF pulse.

The 90° RF pulse is created by an oscillating secondary magnetic field (B_1) formed as a result of passing current through a loop of wire called an **RF transmitter coil**. To accomplish excitation, the secondary B_1 field must be situated at right angles to the main magnetic field B_0. The main magnetic field of a permanent magnet is usually vertical, while a solenoid type of magnet has horizontal flux lines. Therefore the secondary field of the RF coil should occur in the horizontal axis in permanent magnets, and in the transverse or vertical axes in solenoid magnets.

As shown by the laws of electromagnetism, this field is created perpendicular to the transmitter coils themselves. In practice when using solenoid electromagnets, for example, the RF transmitter coil should be oriented above, below, or at the sides of the patient. For this reason, RF transmitter coils used in electromagnets are usually cylindrical. The main RF transmitter coils in most systems are:

- a body coil, usually located within the bore of the magnet itself
- a head coil, which is coupled to a receiver coil.

The body coil is the main RF transmitter and transmits RF for most examinations that are acquired without a transmit receive coil. Typical transmit receive coils are head, extremity and some breast coils.

Receiver coils

As previously discussed, passing current through a wire produces a magnetic field. Conversely, if a loop of wire is exposed to an oscillating field, a current is induced in the loop. This induced current and the resulting voltage constitute the MR signal. Receiver coils must be placed properly to adequately detect the MR signal. At first, receiver coils were primarily used to detect signal. Now coil elements can detect and, to a certain extent, also encode MR signal. These coil elements are required for parallel imaging techniques (*see* Chapter 5).

The configuration of the RF transmitter and receiver probes or coils directly affects the quality of the MR signal. Several types of coil are currently used in MR imaging. These are:

- volume or birdcage coils
- surface coils
- Helmholtz pair (coils specifically designed for permanent magnets)
- phased array
- encoding coil elements.

Volume coils. A volume coil can both transmit RF and receive the MR signal and is often called a transceiver. It encompasses the entire anatomy and can be used for head, extremity or total body imaging. Head and body coils of a type known as the birdcage configuration are used to image relatively large areas and yield uniform SNR over the entire imaging volume. However, even though volume coils are responsible for uniform excitation over a large area, because of their large size they generally produce images with lower SNR than other types of coils. The signal quality produced by volume coils has been significantly increased by the advent of a process known as quadrature excitation and detection. This enables signal to be transmitted and received by two pairs of coils orientated at right angles to each other, either physically or electronically. In most cases quadrature coils are used to transmit RF and to receive the MR signal.

Surface coils. Coils of this type are used to improve the SNR when imaging structures near the surface of the patient (such as the lumbar spine). Generally, the nearer the coil is situated to the structure under examination, the greater the SNR. This is because the coil is closer to the signal-emitting anatomy, and only noise in the vicinity of the coil is received, rather than the entire body. Surface coils are usually small and especially shaped so that they can be easily placed near the anatomy to be imaged with little or no discomfort to the patient. However, signal (and noise) is received only from the sensitive volume of the coil that corresponds to the area located around the coil. The size of this area extends to the circumference of the coil and at a depth into the patient equal to the radius of the coil.

For example, if a coil with a diameter of 10 cm is used, then the length of tissue that can be imaged is also 10 cm, to a depth of 5 cm. There is therefore a falloff of signal as the distance from the coil is increased in any direction. However, with the advent of intra-cavity coils such as endorectal, endovascular, endovaginal, urethral and esophageal coils, surface or local coils – as they are often now called – can be used to receive signal deep within the patient. As the SNR is enhanced when using local coils, greater spatial resolution of small structures can often be achieved. When using local coils, a body coil is generally used to transmit RF and the local coil is used to receive the MR signal unless the local coil is also a transmitter.

Phased array coils consist of multiple coils and receivers whose individual signals are combined to create one image with improved SNR and increased coverage. The smaller the RF coil, the better the SNR. Unfortunately, the smaller the coil the smaller the area of coverage. In an attempt to get both good SNR and large coverage, manufacturers have combined multiple small coils with multiple receivers. This is known as phase array coil technology. Phased array coils are now widely used. Therefore the advantages of small surface coils (increased SNR and resolution) can be combined with a large FOV for increased anatomy coverage. Usually up to four coils and receivers are grouped together in a line to increase longitudinal coverage (known as linear array for spine imaging), or two coils on top and two below for body imaging (known as volume array). During data acquisition, each individual coil receives signal from its own small usable FOV. The signal output from each coil is separately received and processed, but then combined to form one single larger FOV. As each coil has its own receiver, the amount of noise received is limited to its small FOV, and all the data can be acquired in a single sequence rather than four individual ones. Several types of phased array coils are now available. These include:

- spine phased array (Figure 9.20)
- pelvic phased array
- breast coil phased array
- cardiac array
- temperomandibular joint-phased array.

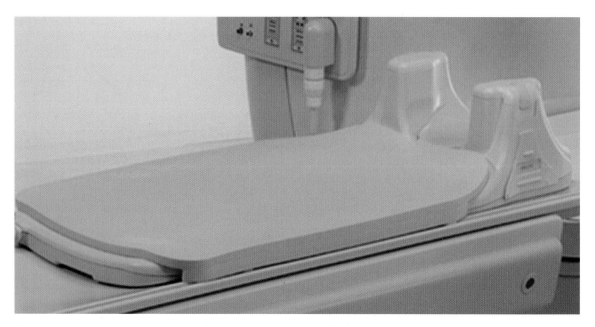

Figure 9.20   Spinal phased array coil.

9

Encoding coil elements allow for coil elements to detect and – to a certain extent – encode signal. They are used in parallel imaging techniques and discussed in detail in Chapter 5. These techniques use coils to detect a sensitivity map of the signal near the coil (Figures 9.21 and 9.22). Some manufacturers have coil systems with as many as 32 coil elements to produce images in much shorter scan times than conventional imaging.

Summary

Large coil:

- large area of uniform signal reception
- increased likelihood of aliasing with small FOV
- positioning of patient not too critical
- lower SNR and resolution
- used in examinations of torso where signal coverage is necessary (chest, abdomen)

Small coil:

- small area of signal reception
- less likely to produce aliasing artefact
- positioning of coil and patient critical
- high SNR and resolution
- used in examinations of small body parts (wrist, spine, knee)

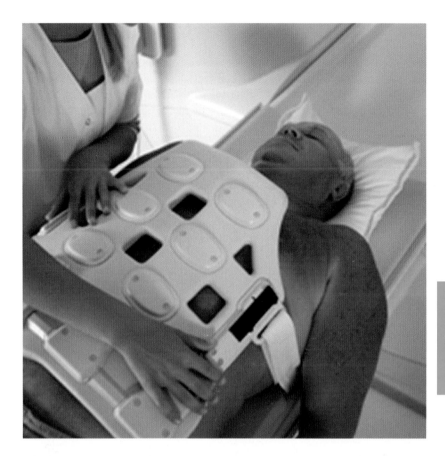

Figure 9.21 Parallel imaging coils.

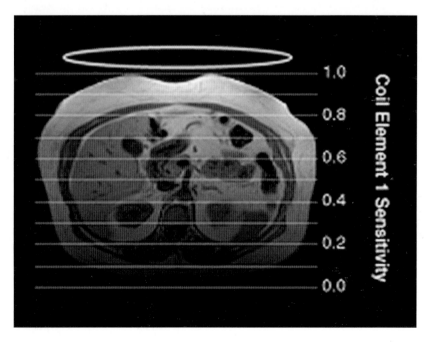

Figure 9.22 Sensitivity encoding in parallel imaging.

Coil safety

There are a few basic rules to ensure the safe operation of RF coils. Coils are connected to the system by cables, which must consist of a conductive material so that the RF power can be delivered to the coil and the signal can be sent to the image processor. They therefore have the capacity to transmit the heat that occurs during normal operation. However, under certain circumstances, this heat may burn the patient or the insulating material of the cable. To prevent such an occurrence, always make sure the cables are not looped and do not touch the patient or the bore of the magnet.

Coil cables should be inspected regularly and should not under any circumstances be used if the insulation is damaged. To receive optimum signal from the patient, the coils must be correctly tuned. Each manufacturer achieves this in a different way.

Now that the individual components of the magnet system have been discussed, the larger hardware elements are now described.

The pulse control unit

Gradient coils are switched on and off very rapidly and at precise times during the pulse sequence. They spatially localize signal along the three axes of the magnet and are also used to rewind or spoil transverse magnetization and to rephase magnetization. The same three gradients perform all these tasks and accurate pulsing of the gradient coils is essential. Gradient amplifiers supply the power to the gradient coils and a pulse control unit co-ordinates the functions of the gradient amplifiers and the coils so that they can be switched on and off at the appropriate times.

The pulse control unit is also responsible for co-ordinating the transmission and amplification of the RF. RF at the resonant frequency is transmitted by the RF transceiver to the RF amplifier and then through an RF monitor, which ensures that safe levels of RF are delivered to the patient.

The received RF signal from the coil is amplified and then passes to the array processor for fast Fourier transform. These data are then transmitted to the image processor so that each pixel can be allocated a grayscale color in the image.

Patient transportation system

All systems use a hydraulically or mechanically driven couch to lift the patient up to the level of the bore and to slide them into the magnet. This is usually achieved by pedals or buttons that move the couch up or down, and in or out of the bore. The table should be comfortable for the patient and allow for the attachment of coils and immobilization devices. There should also be a mechanism for evacuating the patient rapidly from the bore in an emergency. Some systems enable the couch to be undocked from the magnet, so that patients can be transported out of the room in an emergency without moving them on to another trolley first. All couches must, of course, be magnetically safe and contain no metal parts. The patient transport system has become more sophisticated to allow automated rapid movement of the patient between scanning positions during contrast enhanced MRA.

Operator interface

MRI computer systems vary with manufacturer. Most, however, consist of:

- a minicomputer with expansion capabilities
- an array processor for Fourier transformation
- an image processor that takes data from the array processor to form an image
- hard disc drives for storage of raw data and pulse sequence parameters
- a power distribution mechanism to distribute and filter the alternating and direct current.

The operator's link to the system is a boot terminal, usually in the vicinity of the minicomputer. System initialization and software modifications can be accessed with the use of this terminal. However, scanning and viewing capabilities are accessed at an operator's console, usually located directly outside the scan room.

In addition to data acquisition and viewing the recently acquired images, the operator console provides access to a whole host of image manipulation techniques. These include:

- viewing several images at the same time
- viewing images in a cine loop
- reformatting 3D volume images.

MR images are permanently stored from the image console onto single emulsion film similar to that used in computed tomography. However, filming MR images can be somewhat tricky, in that the brightness and contrast settings vary with each image. These brightness and contrast settings are referred to as window and level settings. Images with high intrinsic signal may require different window and level settings so that important anatomic and pathologic findings may be visualized adequately on the MR image.

For permanent storage, data may be archived either on to magnetic tape (rarely used), DAT tape, optical disc or CD (generally the method of choice today). This archive function can also be accessed through the operator's console. Images are stored so that cases can be retrieved for further manipulation and imaging in the future. They may also be used for comparison when repeat examinations are performed on the same patient.

Now that each component of the equipment has been described, it is appropriate to discuss the safe operation of this equipment. This is the subject of the next chapter.

Questions

1   Name the three types of magnetism.

2   In which direction is the Z-axis in a permanent magnetic?

3   What rule determines the direction of current flow through a coil?

4   What is the maximum field strength allowed for clinical imaging of adults in the USA?

5   What is the purpose of shimming?

6   What is the purpose of shielding?

7   What are the advantages of phased array coils?

10

MRI safety

Introduction

As yet, virtually no long-term adverse biological effects of extended exposure to MRI have been described. However, on examination of the separate components of the magnetic resonance imaging process, several reversible effects of magnetic, gradient and radio frequency fields can be observed. Much of the research into MR safety has been carried out in the USA, where most of the literature on safety originates. In February 1982, the Food and Drug Administration (FDA) issued guidelines to hospitals' Investigational Review Boards (IRBs) in *Guidelines for evaluating electromagnetic exposure risks for trials of clinical NMR*. This was later followed up with an evaluation of potential risks and hazards. To discuss the long-term biological effects of MRI, all the components of the imaging process must be considered. These elements include:

- the main magnetic field (also known as the primary or static magnetic field B_0)
- time varying magnetic fields (magnetic field gradients)
- radio frequency fields (created by the RF coils, known as secondary or B_1 fields).

All patients and personnel **must** be screened, as if they were having the procedure themselves, before entering the scan room. The international MR safety committee IMRSER also recommends that this screening is performed by 'trained professionals' and that each individual should be screened more than once (once by completing a screening form and at least once by a verbal interview). The International Society for Magnetic Resonance in Medicine (ISMRM) and the Institute for Magnetic Resonance Safety, Education, and Research (IMRSER) have issued a screening form that should be used as a guideline for screening all persons who enter the MR suite. This screening form can be easily accessed on-line on www.mrisafety.com. It is recommended that the form be used as it appears, and not modified.

The main magnetic field

The main magnetic field is responsible for the alignment of nuclei. In solenoid electromagnets, the field is usually horizontal, while in permanent magnets the field is generally vertical (Figure 10.1). This is a static or unchanging field. The FDA limit for static magnetic field strength used to be 2 T for clinical imaging. As of July 2004, these limits have been increased to 4 T for babies and infants up to one month of age and 8 T for children and adults. Higher field strengths are permitted for research.

Biological effects of the static magnetic field

The primary concern with the static magnetic field is the possibility of potential biological effects. In nature, the magnetic field associated with the Earth has a significant effect on lower life forms. The orientation of magneto-static bacteria and the migratory patterns of birds are influenced by the 0.6 G magnetic field that surrounds the Earth. In MR, small electrical

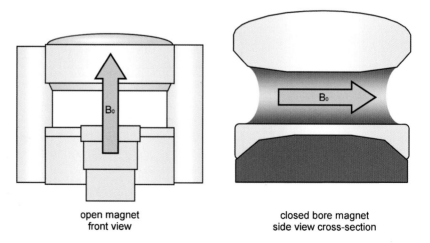

Figure 10.1 Static field directions in a permanent and superconducting system.

open magnet
front view

closed bore magnet
side view cross-section

potentials have been observed in large blood vessels that flow perpendicular to the static magnetic field. However, even at 10 T, no adverse effects have been noted on the ECGs of squirrel monkeys. Most studies show no effects on cell growth and morphology at field strengths below 2 T. Data accumulated by the National Institute for Occupational Safety, the World Health Organization and the US State Department, show no evidence of leukemia or other carcinogenesis. However, the *New England Journal of Medicine* reported an increase in leukemia in men exposed to electrical and magnetic fields in Washington State, from 1950 to 1979. In these cases the electromagnetic fields were produced by alternating currents, which resulted in changing magnetic fields. Although similar effects were detected in New York in 1987, no evidence of adverse effects has been noted in people working with linear accelerators who are exposed to static magnetic fields. The few reports of potential carcinogenesis seem controversial, since many of the study methods have been criticized.

Fringe fields

This stray magnetic field outside the bore of the magnet is known as the **fringe field** (Figure 10.2). This is considered to be a secondary concern, but can be a fatal effect of the main magnetic field. Hazards of fringe fields are associated with the siting of MR systems. The static magnetic field has no respect for the confines of conventional walls, floors or ceilings.

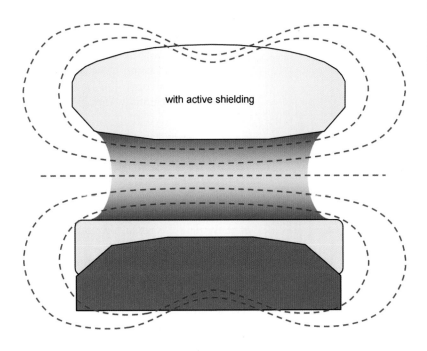

with active shielding

Figure 10.2 The fringe field.

10

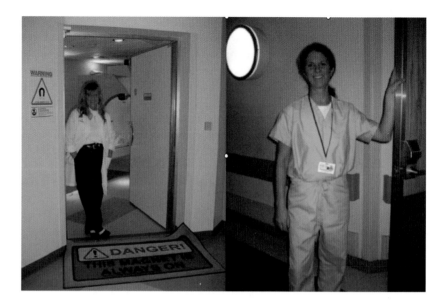

Figure 10.3 The hot and warm zones. 'Hot zone' is within the scan room. Signs displayed prominently on the wall and on floor mats indicate magnet is always on. 'Warm zone' is the area before the scan room protected by a locked door.

Protecting the general public from the fringe field. It is recommended that the general public (those persons who have not been properly screened for the effects of magnetic fields) limit exposure of magnetic field strength of 5 G and below. For this reason, many imaging facilities are situated so that public areas are below this strength, and areas above are either inaccessible or clearly marked.

Since the inception of MR imaging, there have been devastating and fatal accidents in the MR environment. For this reason, the international MR safety committee issued recommendations for a 'warm zone' near the entrance of the MR scan room. This 'warm zone' is the area near the entrance of the scan room, generally at the imager's console. The 'hot zone' is the scan room itself (Figure 10.3). In this recommendation, this warm zone has a controlled (locked) entrance such that the general public may not inadvertently wander into this area and then accidentally into the scan room.

Static fields below 2.0 T

Although no biological effects have been observed in human subjects at field strengths below 2 T, reversible effects have been noted on ECGs at these field strengths. An increase in the amplitude of the T wave can be noted on an ECG due to the **magneto-hemodynamic effect**. This is produced when conductive fluid such as blood moves across a magnetic field. It is proportional to the strength of the magnetic field. Despite this effect, no serious cardiovascular effects have been observed in patients undergoing MR.

This hemodynamic effect is considered reversible as the ECG tracing returns to normal when the patient is removed from the magnet. However, the magneto-hemodynamic effect can present problems when cardiac gating at high field. It results in the system triggering from the T wave rather than the R wave and image quality suffers as a result of insufficient cardiac gating (*see* Chapter 8). For this reason, many manufacturers have modified the ECG systems that are used for gating to reduce this effect. For this reason it is recommended that the ECG leads are not used for patient monitoring. Specific monitoring equipment should be used for pulse oximetry, for example.

Static fields above 2.0 T

Some reversible biological effects have been observed on human subjects exposed to 2.0 T and above. These effects include fatigue, headaches, hypotension and irritability. Another potential problem at these higher field strengths is the effect of magnetic interaction energy and cell orientation. Certain molecules (such as DNA) and cellular sub-units (such as sickled red cells) have magnetic properties that vary with direction. This effect is biologically important at a field strength of 2.0 T, because of the twisting force or torque that is exerted on these molecules.

Ultra-high field imaging

Most MR imaging has been acquired at field strengths of up to and including 1.5 T. There has been an increase in the distribution of ultra-high field (3.0 T and above) imaging systems. Many of these systems have been distributed for improved SNR. As field strength increases, signal to noise increases. SNR is linearly proportional to field strength. As field strength doubles, SNR doubles.

There are several safety considerations associated with field strengths higher than 1.5 T. These safety considerations include:

- an increase in the RF power (SAR) at higher field strengths
- the lack of research and testing (of implants and devices) at higher field strengths
- the relative lack of clinical experience (on humans and/or animals) at these field strengths.

For this reason, it may be advisable to avoid imaging (in any situations such as pregnancy and/or implants that are possibly contraindicated) at these ultra-high field strengths until such time that more research has been done or more clinical experience has been gained.

10

Pregnant patients

As yet, there are no known biological effects of MRI on fetuses. However, a number of mechanisms could potentially cause adverse effects as a result of the interaction of electromagnetic fields with developing fetuses. Cells undergoing division, which occurs during the first trimester of pregnancy, are more susceptible to these effects.

The FDA requires labeling of MR systems to indicate the safety of MR when used to image a fetus or infant. The current recommendation by the FDA states:

> *'If the information to be gained by MR would have required more invasive testing, MRI is acceptable.'*

In the light of the high-risk potential for pregnant patients in general, many facilities prefer to delay any examination of pregnant patients until the first trimester and then have a written consent form signed by the patient before the examination. In addition, the American College of Obstetricians and Gynecologists recommends that pregnant patients should be reviewed on a case-by-case basis. The Society of Magnetic Resonance Imaging Safety committee suggests that:

> *'Pregnant patients or those who suspect they are pregnant should be identified before undergoing MRI to assess the relative risks vs the benefits of the examination.'*

Due to the exquisite intrinsic soft tissue contrast and high resolution of MR images combined with the low risk, MR has become more common, in many cases, for the evaluation of the fetus and/or for the pregnant mother. MR can be used in cases where other non-ionizing forms of diagnostic testing are inadequate (such as ultrasound), and there is suspicion of abnormality of the fetus or the mother. Single shot FSE sequences can be acquired for the evaluation of the fetus, the placenta, uterus, fallopian tubes (for torsion), the uterus, cervix and other female pelvic structures. In some cases, fetal MRI has diagnosed lesions within the fetus, which has allowed for surgery to be performed *in utero* (before the baby was born) and has allowed for the baby to be born healthy.

In the United Kingdom, the National Radiological Protection Board (NRPB) guidelines specify that:

> *'It might be prudent to exclude pregnant women during the first three months of pregnancy.'*

However, many fetuses have undergone MRI since 1983 without any abnormalities at birth or after four years of childhood. Most imaging, however, uses field strengths up to and including 1.5 T. There has been an increase in the distribution of ultra-high field imaging systems (3 T and above). For many safety reasons – including the risk in pregnancy – there has been little or no research on humans or animals at these field strengths. For this reason, it may be advisable to avoid imaging at ultra-high field until more research has been done or more clinical experience gained.

Gadolinium enhancement is at present best avoided when examining a pregnant patient. Studies performed in pregnant baboons have shown that gadolinium does cross the placenta and enter the amniotic fluid. In this case, the gadolinium within the fluid is ingested by the fetus and passed via the urinary tract and ingested again. Since there are no research data about the safety of gadolinium chelates and their ability to stay intact (gadolinium molecules with chelates) it is prudent to avoid the administration of gadolinium chelates during pregnancy. Although fetal imaging has become more commonplace, it is still recommended to avoid gadolinium in pregnant patients.

Pregnant employees

MR facilities have established individual guidelines for pregnant employees in the magnetic resonance environment. The safety committee of the ISMRM determined that pregnant employees can safely enter the scan room, but should leave while the RF and gradient fields are employed (during the time the scanner is running). Some facilities, however, recommend that the employee stays out of the magnetic field entirely during the first trimester of pregnancy.

A survey showed no increased incidence of spontaneous abortions among MR radiographers and nurses (the natural incidence of spontaneous abortions is about 30%). Following this survey, the unit that carried out the study changed their in-house policy from one in which radiographers were kept out of the magnetic field during pregnancy, to a policy which allows pregnant radiographers and technologists to set up the patient, but not to remain during image acquisition.

It has been suggested that informed workers make their own decisions. In the US, this recommendation was influenced by a legal decision on the rights of pregnant workers in hazardous environments. Each person must make their own decision to either stay in the unit or, if possible, move back into a nearby radiology department. However, to leave an environment that is probably safe and move into one that is known to be hazardous may be inadvisable! These suggestions may change as the use of ultra-high field systems increases.

Projectiles

Ferromagnetic metal objects can become airborne as projectiles in the presence of a strong static magnetic field. Small objects, such as paper clips and hairpins, have a terminal velocity of 40 mph when pulled into a 1.5 T magnet, and pose a serious risk to the patient and anyone else present in the scan room. The force with which projectiles are pulled toward a magnetic field is inversely proportional to the strength of the magnetic

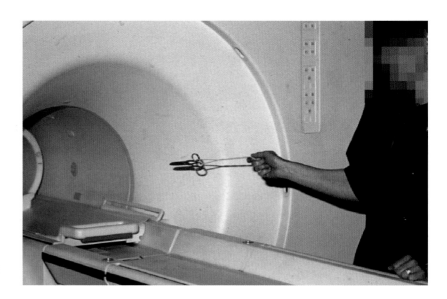

Figure 10.4 The pulling power of stainless steel scissors.

field, the mass of the object and the distance from the magnet. Even surgical tools such as hemostats, scissors and clamps, although made of a material known as 'surgical stainless steel', are strongly attracted to the main magnetic field (Figure 10.4).

Oxygen tanks are also highly magnetic and should never be brought into the scan room. However, there are non-ferrous oxygen tanks available, which are safe. Sandbags must also be inspected since some are not filled with sand but with steel shot, which is highly magnetic.

It is recommended that all objects are tested with a hand-held bar magnet before being taken into the MR scan room. In addition, it is advised that all nursing, housekeeping, fire department, emergency and MR personnel are educated about the potential risks and hazards of the static magnetic field. Signs should be attached at all entrances to the magnetic field (including the fringe field) to deter entry into the scan room with ferromagnetic objects. Metal detectors are available, but can in some cases offer a false sense of security. For this reason, most imaging facilities keep the general public well behind the 5 G line.

Medical emergencies

As in any medical facility, the MR suite should be equipped with emergency medical supplies on a crash cart. Many of these supplies can be incredibly dangerous in an MR environment. For this reason, in any critical situation, it is recommended that the patient is rapidly removed from the magnetic field before resuscitation begins.

Implants and prostheses

Metallic implants pose serious damaging effects, which include torque, heating and artefacts on MR images. Before imaging patients with MR, any surgical procedure that the patient has undergone before the MR examination must be identified. For a complete list of MR compatible implants and prosthesis refer to *Magnetic Resonance Bioeffects, Safety and Patient Management* by Shellock and Kanal. For a more up to date list of implants and devices, visit the MRI safety web page at www.mrisafety.com.

It is also important to understand that if an implanted device has been tested and deemed safe for a given field strength, it may only be imaged at that field strength or below. For example, if a device has been tested at 1.5 T then it can be used at 1.5 T and below, but not at 2 T or 3 T. As field strengths continue to increase (up to 3.0 T and beyond) the implanted devices may not have been tested at these field strengths.

Torque and heating

Some metallic implants have shown considerable torque when placed in the presence of a magnetic field. The force or torque exerted on small and large metallic implants can cause serious effects, as unanchored implants can potentially move unpredictably within the body. The type of metal used in such implants is one factor that determines the force exerted on them in magnetic fields. While non-ferrous metallic implants may show little or no deflection to the field, they could cause significant heating, due to their inability to dissipate the heat caused by radio frequency absorption. However, heating experiments have not shown excessive temperature increases in implants.

Artefacts from metallic implants

Although artefacts cannot be considered as a biological effect of the MR process, misinterpretation of MR images can yield devastating consequences. The size of the metallic implant, and type of metal (more or less ferromagnetic), the pulse sequence (spin echo or gradient echo) and some of the imaging parameters used (field strength, TE and voxel size – FOV, matrix, thickness) determine the size of the artefact shown on the MR image. Note that the artefact on the image in Figure 10.5 on the right is markedly larger than the artefact on the image on the left, even though the aneurysm clip is the same size in both patients. In this case, the artefact is larger because the susceptibility of the clip on the right is more ferrous than the clip on the left (*see* Chapter 7).

In some cases, if a metal artefact is seen and no metal is present within the patient, this could indicate the presence of blood products suggestive of a hemorrhagic lesion. The ferromagnetic properties of iron in the blood

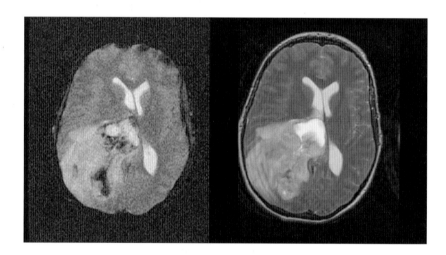

Figure 10.5   Axial images of the brain in a patient with an intracranial vascular clip acquired with spin echo (left) and gradient echo (right) sequences. Susceptibility artefact is much greater in the gradient echo image.

Figure 10.6   Axial, T2* (left) and T2 (right) images of the brain were acquired from a patient with a lesion. Note that the lesion has hemorrhagic components that are apparent on the gradient echo acquisition (left) and not apparent on the fast spin echo acquisition (right) (even though the FSE image is higher quality image).

10

may create fluctuations in local magnetic fields near the lesion. These fluctuations create 'metal artefacts' or 'susceptibility artefacts' in the area of the hemorrhage. On the FSE acquisition, the 180° pulses compensate for the local inhomogeneities caused by the ferromagnetic (iron) materials in the blood, while the gradient echo sequence does not employ a 180° refocusing pulse, and hence does not compensate for the susceptibility effects on the image (Figure 10.6).

Intracranial vascular clips

Some intracranial aneurysm clips are absolute contraindications in MR imaging. Clip motion may damage the vessel, resulting in hemorrhage, ischemia or death. Intracranial clips made of titanium have been used, and have proved safe for MR. Unfortunately there have been several cases where a clip was either 'MR compatible' or thought to be and the clip moved during an MR scan, resulting in death. The ISMRM therefore recommends that imaging of patients with aneurysm clips is not performed unless the clip has been tested for magnetic safety before insertion. IMRSER recommend that MR imaging in patients with intracranial clips is unsafe unless the clip is *'known to be safe'*.

Intravascular coils, filters and stents

Fifteen intravascular devices have been tested and five of these proved to be ferromagnetic. Although they have shown deflection in the magnetic field, these devices usually become imbedded in the vessel wall after several weeks, and are unlikely to become dislodged. Therefore it is considered safe to perform MR imaging on most patients with intravascular devices, provided a reasonable period of time has elapsed after implantation.

Extra-cranial vascular clips

Five carotid artery vascular clamps have been tested, and each showed deflection in the magnetic field. However, the deflection was mild when compared with the pulsatile vascular motion within the carotids. Extra-cranial clips tend to be surrounded by fibrous tissue or scar after surgery. Many facilities recommend that MR is delayed until 4–6 weeks after surgery but, in an emergency situation, imaging can probably be performed sooner and all studies should be evaluated on a case-by-case basis. Only the Poppen–Blaylock carotid artery clamp is believed to be contraindicated for MR, due to its large attractive response to the magnetic field.

Vascular access ports

Only two of 33 implanted vascular access ports tested showed measurable deflection in the magnetic field. These deflections are thought to be insignificant to the applications of such ports. Therefore, it is probably safe to image patients with implanted vascular access ports.

Heart valves

Twenty five of the 29 heart valve prostheses have been evaluated for magnetic susceptibility, and these showed negligible deflection to the magnetic field. The deflection is minimal compared with normal pulsatile cardiac motion. Therefore, although patients with most valvular implants are considered safe for MR, careful screening for valve type is advised because there are valves whose integrity could be compromised.

Dental devices and materials

Sixteen dental implants have been tested and twelve of these have shown measurable deflection to the magnetic field. However, most are thought to

10

be safe for MR imaging. Although most devices are not significantly affected by the magnetic field, susceptibility artefacts can adversely affect image quality in MR especially in gradient echo imaging. Some dental devices are magnetically activated, and therefore can pose potential risks for MR imaging.

Penile implants

Only one of the nine penile implants tested showed measurable deflection to the magnetic field. This, the Dacomed Omniphase™, is unlikely to cause severe damage to the patient, but may become uncomfortable, so an alternative imaging procedure may be considered. Most of today's penile implants are made of plastic.

Otologic implants

All three cochlear implants tested were attracted to the magnetic field and were magnetically or electronically activated. They are therefore definitely contraindicated for MRI. Some patients with otologic implants have been issued a card warning them to avoid MR imaging.

Ocular implants

Of twelve ocular implants tested, two were deflected by a 1.5 T static magnetic field. The Fatio eyelid spring could cause discomfort and the retinal tack could injure the eye since it is made from a ferromagnetic form of stainless steel.

Intra-ocular ferrous foreign bodies

Intra-ocular ferrous foreign bodies are a cause of major concern in MR safety. It is not uncommon for patients who have worked with sheet metal to have metal fragments or slivers located in and around the eye. Since the magnetic field exerts a force on ferromagnetic objects, a metal fragment in the eye could move or be displaced and cause injury to the eye or surrounding tissue. Small intra-ocular fragments could be missed on a standard radiograph. However, a study demonstrated that metal fragments as small as $0.1 \times 0.1 \times 0.1$ mm can be detected on standard radiographs. In addition, metal fragments from $0.1 \times 0.1 \times 0.1$ mm to $0.3 \times 0.1 \times 0.1$ mm were examined in the eyes of laboratory animals in a 2.0 T magnet. Only the $0.3 \times 0.1 \times 0.1$ mm fragments moved, but they did not cause any discernible clinical damage. Therefore, although computed tomography is more accurate in detecting the presence of small foreign bodies, plain film radiography should be adequate in screening for intra-ocular ferrous foreign bodies that have sufficient size to cause ocular damage.

The ISMRM screening form asks the patient: '*Have you ever been hit in the eye by metal?*' This is worded to imply that even if they once had metal in their eye and thought it had been removed they should still be screened with plain X-rays. It is also recommended that two views are obtained for evaluation of the orbits. Such views include a 20° posterior-anterior (Water's view) and a lateral or two Water's views with the eyes looking up and down.

Bullets, pellets and shrapnel

Although most ammunition has proved to be non-ferrous, ammunition made in some countries or produced by the military has shown traces of ferromagnetic alloys. It is advisable to take extreme caution in imaging patient with bullets or shrapnel, and to be aware of the location of such metal within the body.

Orthopedic implants, materials and devices

Each of fifteen orthopedic implants tested showed no deflection within the main magnetic field. However, a large metallic implant such as a hip prosthesis can become heated by currents induced in the metal by the magnetic and radio frequency fields. It appears, however, that such heating is relatively low. Most orthopedic implants have been imaged with MR without incident.

Surgical clips and pins

Abdominal surgical clips are generally safe for MR because they become anchored by fibrous tissue, but they produce artefacts in proportion to their size and can distort the image. It is recommended that, if possible, the MR procedure is delayed until 4–6 weeks post-operative, although this may not be necessary. As always, patients should be evaluated on a case-by-case basis.

Halo vests and other similar externally applied devices

Halo vests pose several risk factors which include deflection and subsequent dislodging of the halo, heating due to RF absorption, electrical current induction within the halo rings, electrical arcing and severe artefactual consequences which could render the imaging acquisition useless. Non-ferrous and non-conductive halo vests that are MR compatible are commercially available. Therefore, in the light of the potential risks and hazards associated with halo vests, it is advisable to identify the halo vest before proceeding with MR imaging.

Electrically, magnetically or mechanically activated or electrically conductive implanted devices

Certain implanted devices are contraindicated or require precautions for MR imaging because they are either magnetically, electrically or mechanically activated. Each device should be evaluated on a case-by-case basis. These implants include:

10

- cardiac pacemakers
- cochlear implants
- tissue expanders
- ocular prostheses
- dental implants
- neurostimulators
- bone growth stimulators
- implantable cardiac defibrillators
- implantable drug infusion pumps.

The function of such implants is impaired by the magnetic field, so patients with such devices should not be examined with MR. Also, devices which depend on magnetization to affix themselves to the patient (such as magnetic sphincters, magnetic stoma plugs and magnetic prosthetic devices) could be demagnetized and may be contraindicated for MR.

Pacemakers

Cardiac pacemakers used to be an absolute contraindication for MRI. Even field strengths as low as 5 G may be sufficient to cause deflection, programming changes and closure of the reed switch that converts a pacemaker to an asynchronous mode. In addition, patients who have had their pacemaker removed may have pacer wires left within the body. These could act as an antenna and (by induced currents) cause cardiac fibrillation. For this reason, there used to be limits for scanning such patients with implanted pacer wires.

Today, it could be acceptable to scan some patients with implanted pacer wires (patients whose pacemaker has been removed) as long as the wires are cut close to the skin and not looped outside the chest. In addition, modern pacemakers are being developed that are MR compatible. Therefore, this – as any implanted device – should be evaluated on a case-by-case basis. For specific questions about imaging of such patients, post questions on www.mrisafety.com. Warning signs should be posted at the 5 G line to prevent the exposure of anyone with a pacemaker or other electronic implants.

Some facilities have imaged non-dependent, pacemaker patients without incident. To err on the side of caution, however, most imaging facilities still do not image pacemaker patients.

Gradient magnetic fields

All MR imaging systems are equipped with a set of resistive wire windings known as gradient coils. Gradients provide position-dependent variation in magnetic field strength and are pulsed on and off during and between RF excitation pulses. The purpose of these gradients is to encode spatial information contained in the emitted RF signal. Gradient fields are switched on and off during image acquisition. In doing so, they create a time-varying magnetic field (TVMF).

Time-varying magnetic fields

Many studies have looked at the biological effects of TVMF, since they exist around power transformers and high-voltage lines. The health consequences are not related to the strength of the gradient field, but rather to changes in the magnetic field that cause induced currents. In MR, there is concern with nerves, blood vessels and muscles that act as conductors in the body. Faraday's law of induction states that changing magnetic fields induce electrical currents in any conducting medium. Induced currents are proportional to the material's conductivity and the rate of change of the magnetic field. In MR, this effect is determined by factors such as pulse duration, wave shape, repetition pattern, and the distribution of the current in the body. The induced current is greater in peripheral tissues as the amplitude of the gradient is higher away from the magnetic isocentre.

Biological effects that vary with current amplitude include reversible alterations in vision, irreversible effects of cardiac fibrillation, alterations in the biochemistry of cells and fracture union. Effects occasionally experienced during MRI examinations using echo planar techniques include mild cutaneous sensations and involuntary muscle contractions. Visual effects may occur when retinal phosphates are stimulated by induction from TVMF. This results in light flashes or 'stars in one's eyes'. The FDA limit for TVMF is expressed in the same units as Faraday's laws of induction. In the Faraday equation:

$$\Delta B / \Delta T = \Delta V$$

where:

ΔB = change in magnetic field (caused by switching gradients)
ΔT = change in time
ΔV = change in voltage.

The FDA limit for gradient fields used to be 6 T/s for all gradients. In this case, therefore, ΔB is 6 T and ΔT is 1 s. In addition, the FDA used to limit axial gradient fields to 20 T/s and gradient rise times to 120 ms. EPI sequences pose the greatest concern for TVMF effects as strong gradients are switched rapidly during image acquisition. As of July 2004, these limits have been increased so that gradient strengths are limited to those below those that are sufficient to produce severe discomfort or painful nerve stimulation.

Acoustic noise

As current is passed through the gradient coils during image acquisition, a significant amount of acoustic noise is created. Although noise levels on most commercial systems are considered to be within recommended safety guidelines, noise can cause some reversible and irreversible effects. These effects include communication interference, patient annoyance, transient hearing loss and – in patients who are susceptible to hearing impairment – permanent hearing loss.

Earplugs are an acceptable and inexpensive way of preventing hearing loss and should be used regularly. It is recommended that all patients are provided with hearing protection in the form of ear plugs or headphones. A more expensive alternative is 'anti-noise' or destructive noise apparatus, which reduces noise and permits better communication between the operator and the patient. Manufacturers are also improving 'quiet' gradient systems where there is a significant reduction in gradient noise during image acquisition (*see* Chapter 9).

Radio frequency fields

Exposure to radio frequency occurs during MR examinations as the hydrogen nuclei are subjected to an oscillating magnetic field. The source of this electromagnetic radiation is the radio frequency coils that surround the patient inside the magnet bore. As the RF pulse is doubled (from 90° pulses to 180° pulses) four times the power is used. For this reason, fast spin echo sequences give the greatest concern for RF effects as they use a train of 180° RF pulses.

Radio frequency irradiation

As the energy level of frequencies used in clinical MR imaging is relatively low and non-ionizing compared with X-rays, visible light and microwaves, the predominant biological effect of RF irradiation absorption is the potential heating of tissue. Although non-thermal effects have been reported, they have not yet been confirmed. As an excitation pulse is applied, some nuclei absorb the RF energy and enter the high-energy state. As they relax, nuclei give off this absorbed energy to the surrounding lattice. In frequencies below 100 MHz, 90% of absorbed energy results from tissue currents (eddy currents in tissues) induced by the magnetic component of the radio frequency field. As frequency is increased, absorbed energy is also increased, so heating of tissue is largely frequency dependent. For this reason, RF heating is less of a concern in MR systems operating below 1 T.

Table 10.1 SAR limits in the USA.

Area	Dose	Time (minutes)	SAR (Watts/kg)
Whole body	averaged over	15	4
Head	averaged over	10	3
Head or torso	per gram of tissue	5	8
Extremities	per gram of tissue	5	12

Specific absorption rate (SAR)

The FDA limit for RF exposure is measured as either an increase in body temperature or as the **specific absorption rate** (SAR). The FDA limit for temperature is an increase of 18°C in the core of the body. In the periphery, higher increases to 38°C in the head, 39°C in the trunk and 40°C in the extremities are permitted. It is therefore necessary to measure RF absorption. This is manifested as tissue heating and the patient's ability to dissipate excess heat. RF absorption can be expressed in terms of SAR, which in turn is expressed in watts per kilogram (W/kg) a quantity that depends on induced electric field, pulse duty cycle, tissue density, conductivity and the patient's size. The patient's weight and the pulse sequence parameters selected are important factors when monitoring SAR.

Care must therefore be taken in recording the patient's proper weight to ensure the SAR does not exceed the permitted levels. SAR can be used to calculate an expected increase in body temperature during an average examination. In the USA the recommended SAR level for imaging used to be 0.4 W/kg (whole body), 3.2 W/kg (head) and 8 W/kg (small volume). As of July 2004 these limits have been increased. Today SAR limits have been increased and are shown in Table 10.1.

In Canada, the recommended SAR level is 2 W/kg. The FDA has reclassified MRI facilities. Sites that are studying the safety of scanning at SAR values above 4 W/kg whole body average are no longer required to limit their capabilities for proton imaging. Sites using research software may still require approval. The FDA also permits an attenuate criterion relying on temperature of the tissues. This is what most sites adhere to. For non-investigational MR sites, new modifications have been established to allow more slices per scan on body imaging. The FDA has acknowledged MR as an established diagnostic tool with recognized risks that are well controlled by the design and use of the equipment.

Studies show that patient exposure up to ten times the recommended levels produces no serious adverse effects, despite elevations in skin and body temperatures. As body temperature increases, blood pressure and heart rate also increase slightly. Even though these effects seem insignificant, patients with compromised thermoregulatory systems may not be candidates for MR. In addition, those areas of the body with an inability to dissipate heat (the orbits and the testicles) have been evaluated independently, and in standard pulse sequences have shown no significant increase

10

in temperature. Corneal temperatures were shown to increase from 0° to 1.8°C. However, as some faster imaging sequences are developed which increase RF deposition to the patient, these areas may need to be re-evaluated.

RF antennae effects

Radio frequency fields can be responsible for significant burn hazards due to electrical currents that are produced in conductive loops. Equipment used in MRI, such as ECG leads and surface coils, should therefore be used with extreme caution. When using a surface coil, the operator must be careful to prevent any electrically conductive material (i.e. cable of surface coil) from forming a 'conductive loop' with itself or with the patient. Tissue or clothing could be potentially ignited by uninsulated cables. Coupling of a transmitting coil to a receive coil may also cause severe thermal injury. The site's engineer should perform routine checks of surface coils to ensure proper function.

At a conference in which they presented *Biological Effects and Safety Aspects of NMR*, the New York Academy of Science recommended that wires used in MR imaging systems should be electrically and thermally insulated.

Claustrophobia

Although claustrophobia does not seem to be a safety issue, it is a condition that commonly affects patients and which MR operators should appreciate. RF heating, gradient noise and the confines of the magnet add to the possibility of claustrophobic reactions.

Although most of these effects are transient, there have been two reported cases of patients who did not suffer from claustrophobia before the MR examination, but who had great difficulty in completing the examination, and developed persistent claustrophobia. These patients required long-term psychiatric treatment. Therefore, it is important to try to reduce the incidence of claustrophobia. Controllable air movement within the bore of the magnet – along with good patient contact and education – should help reduce claustrophobic reactions.

Quenching

Quenching is a sudden loss of absolute zero of temperature in the magnet coils, so that they cease to be superconducting and become resistive. This results in helium escaping from the cryogen bath extremely rapidly. It may happen accidentally or can be manually instigated in the case of an emergency. Quenching may cause severe and irreparable damage to the superconducting coils, so a manual quench should only be performed in extreme cases when the physician and service engineer are involved in the decision to quench.

A fire in the scan room may also be a cause to quench the magnet, so that firefighting personnel can safely enter the room. All systems should have helium-venting equipment, which removes the helium to the outside environment in the event of a quench. If this fails, helium will vent into the room and replace the oxygen. For this reason, all scan rooms should contain an oxygen monitor that sounds an alarm if the oxygen falls below a certain level. Under these circumstances immediate evacuation of the patient and personnel is necessary.

If the scan room door is closed when a quench occurs and helium escapes into the scan room, the depletion of oxygen causes a critical increase in pressure in the room compared with the control area. This produces high pressure in the scan room, which may prevent opening of the door. This should only occur several minutes after a quench but if it does happen, the glass partition between the scan and control rooms should be broken to release the pressure. To expedite this process, many systems have been equipped with 'pop-out' windows that are designed to 'pop out' in the event of an increase in pressure in the MR scan room. The scan room door can then be opened as usual and the patient evacuated. In such a case the patient should be immediately evacuated and evaluated for asphyxia, hypothermia and ruptured eardrums.

Safety education

10

Patient and personnel screening is the most effective way to avoid potential safety hazards to patients. Patients and MR employees with questionable ferromagnetic foreign objects either in or on their bodies should be rigorously examined to avoid any serious health risks and accidents. This controlled environment can be maintained by carefully questioning and educating all patients and personnel. This is usually achieved via a screening questionnaire completed by all persons entering the magnetic field. The ISMRM has published a questionnaire that should be used as a guideline for screening forms. This must include patients, those accompanying patients for their examinations, staff and visitors.

Patient monitoring

The ISMRM Safety Committee recommends that all patients are monitored *'verbally and visually'*. Patients who cannot be contacted verbally

Safety tips – environment

Here are some tips for maintaining a safe environment for patients and their relatives.

- Before sending the patient an appointment, check with them – or the referring clinician – that they do not have a pacemaker or other contraindicated implants.
- Try to ascertain whether they are likely to suffer from claustrophobia – forewarned is forearmed. But be careful how you question the patient – the mere suggestion of claustrophobia may create the problem itself.
- When sending out the appointment, include any relevant safety information and details of the examination – most of a patient's anxiety is fear of the unknown.
- Try to ensure that the waiting area is calming and pleasant.
- Carefully screen the patient and anyone else accompanying the patient into the scan room. This should include questions about surgical procedures, metal injury to the eye and pacemakers.
- Ensure that the patient and relatives/friends remove all credit cards, loose metal items, keys, jewelry, etc.
- Check for body piercing (any body part can be pierced!).
- Tattoos can heat up during image acquisition. A cool wet cloth placed over the tattoo acts as a good heat dissipater. Tattooed eyeliner may be contraindicated as heat can cause ocular damage.
- Bras and belts should also be removed even if they are non-ferrous and are not in the imaging field. They may still heat up and reduce image quality by locally altering the magnetic field.
- Ask the patient to change into a gown for all examinations, as this is really the only way of ensuring that the patient has removed all dangerous objects.
- Always re-check the patient before they are taken into the magnetic field, regardless of how many times they have been checked before. It is the radiographer's responsibility to keep the MR environment safe.
- Remember that patients may know nothing about magnetism and the potential hazards.
- Anxious and sick patients especially cannot be trusted to give you correct information. Be extra vigilant with these types of patients. If you are in any doubt about their safety DO NOT TAKE THEM INTO THE MAGNETIC FIELD.

10

Safety tips for dealing with claustrophobic patients

This is a real art and every radiographer, nurse and radiologist has their own way of coaxing a patient into the magnet. Here are a few suggestions:

- Use a mirror so that the patient can see out of the magnet.
- Examine the patient prone when using the body coil.
- Remove the pillow so that the patient's face is further away from the roof of the bore.
- Ask the patient to close their eyes or place a piece of paper towel over their face.
- Tell the patient that they do not have to have the examination and that although MR may be the best way of sorting out their problem, it is by no means the only way. This gives the patient a feeling of control over their own destiny. It is astonishing how many times these few words have worked!
- Bring the patient out of the magnet in between each sequence, especially in long procedures.
- Reassure them that the magnet is open at both ends and that they are not shut in.
- Use the bore light, the air circulation fan and the patient alarm system wherever possible.
- Encourage a relative or friend to accompany them and to maintain physical contact with them throughout the examination.
- Always communicate with the patient during the examination to check that they are OK, and tell them how long the pulse sequences are. Also remember to tell them what is happening in between sequences. There is nothing worse than lying in the magnet and thinking that everyone has gone home and left you.

10

and visually require more rigorous monitoring by pulse dosimetry. These patients include those who are not responsive, those who are comatose, unconscious, sedated or hearing impaired, those who have weak voices or speak another language and pediatric patients. The ECG used for cardiac gating is not acceptable for monitoring the patient as it has been modified to compensate for the magneto-hemodynamic effect.

Monitors and devices in MRI

There are specific criteria by which ancillary devices are deemed MR compatible. Such criteria recommended by the ISMRM include:

- FDA approval
- manufacturer declaration
- prior testing.

It is probably prudent to trust no-one and test each device yourself before risking patient safety.

Site planning

There are many difficult decisions to be made when installing a magnet system. Careful consideration of these before a magnet is purchased prevents unnecessary expenditure and wastage. Architectural requirements include:

- structural reinforcement
- spatial dimensions
- mechanical and electrical components.

The decision to house the system in an existing building or whether a new building has to be constructed is the primary consideration as the cost implications are considerable. Very often the field strength of the magnet is a limiting factor. At present, there are no real guidelines for determining the optimal field strength. Each facility has to evaluate the purpose of the system and, along with the local site considerations, decide on the field strength required. For example, 0.5 T is probably adequate for imaging purposes, while at least 1.5 T is necessary if spectroscopy is to be carried out. The field strength is important because the size of the fringe field increases at higher field strengths. Shielding can control this, but it also adds significantly to the cost of the unit.

The magnetic safety of personnel, equipment and structures and monitors outside the unit must be considered. The static field is three-dimensional and extends above and below the magnet and to the sides. The magnetic field strength decreases with the cube of the distance from the magnet, and any monitoring and computer devices should be located beyond the 5 G line. In addition, the entrance to the unit and the area surrounding the building must be free from magnetic field effects, to avoid people with pacemakers inadvertently walking into the field. Walls built around the building usually suffice.

Mobile MR units located in trucks have additional hazards. They must comply with road traffic regulations such as weight and wheel base area, and have a very restricted fringe field. For this reason most mobile units are 0.5 T or below. Some high-field mobile systems can be ramped down for relocation. In addition, the site where the truck is parked must be level, and strong enough to take the standing weight of the truck and its contents.

At any site, cooling and air conditioning requirements for the computer and its components should be assessed. Helium venting in the event of a quench, power supply and adequate door and room dimensions need to be taken into account. Adequate RF shielding should be installed and checks made to ensure that monitors and computers located in the vicinity do not interfere with the image. The floor plan of the scan room and the control room should be designed so that there can be rapid straight-line evacuation to an area where emergency equipment can function properly.

In short, the entire facility should be designed with the safety of the patients and personnel in mind. Magnetically controlled security doors located at all entrances to the magnetic field are often the best way of achieving this. Routine preventive maintenance checks by the service engineer and continuing education are also important. Careful planning and diligent upkeep of an MR facility can provide a safe environment for patients and employees.

Questions

1 What is the name of the effect that causes elevation of the T wave in cardiac gating?

2 What velocity does a paper clip have at 1.5 T?

3 What is the SAR limit for the head in the USA?

4 What effects do gradients have on patients using EPI?

5 What is the name of the most up-to-date MRI safety web site?

10

11

Contrast agents in MRI

Introduction

In previous chapters it has been discussed that multiple imaging acquisitions are required to adequately evaluate the patient. Clinical MRI typically uses T1 weighted images with high intrinsic SNR to evaluate anatomy, and T2 weighted images with low SNR and high intrinsic contrast to evaluate pathology. On T1 weighted images, tissues with short T1 relaxation times (fat) appear bright and tissues with long T1 relaxation times (water) appear dark. On T2 weighted images, tissues with short T2 decay times (fat) appear dark and tissues with long T2 decay times (water) appear bright.

Since water demonstrates high signal intensity on T2 weighted images and tumors have a high content of free water, T2 weighted images are used to evaluate such lesions. However, there are pathological conditions in which the high intrinsic contrast provided by T2 weighted images may be insufficient to detect lesions accurately. Although SNR is increased in T1 weighted images, most lesions are inconspicuous because both water and tumors demonstrate low signal intensities. To increase contrast between pathology and normal tissue, enhancement agents may be introduced that selectively affect the T1 and T2 relaxation times in these tissues. This chapter discusses the clinical applications, methodology, administration and precautions of several different enhancement agents used in MRI.

It has been clearly shown that enhancement agents are valuable in detecting tumors, infection, infarction, inflammation, and post-traumatic lesions in the central nervous system (CNS) and in the body. There are MR enhancement agents that affect the T1 and/or T2 relaxation times of different tissues, introducing a contrast difference. The way in which this occurs is best understood by reviewing the basic principles of weighting in MRI.

Review of weighting

Parameters

Several parameters influence inherent image contrast. These include those over which there is no control, and those which can be controlled (*see* Chapter 2). The extrinsic parameters that can be controlled to acquire the MR image include:

> pulse sequence type (spin echo, inversion recovery and gradient echo)
> TR
> TE
> TI
> flip angle

Parameters that previously could not be controlled are:

> T1 recovery time
> T2 decay time
> relative proton density within the tissue

11

Proton density

The proton density is the relative amount of mobile water and fat protons available within the sample of tissue that is being imaged. Proton density is responsible for the initial amplitude of the signal or the height of the FID. In MRI since TR controls T1 weighting and TE controls T2 weighting, the effects of proton density on the images is manipulated by selecting a TR longer than the T1 recovery time of most tissues (more than 2000 ms), and a TE shorter than the T2 decay time of most tissues (less than 20 ms). This results in proton density weighted images, where tissues with high proton densities such as CSF, tumors and fat appear bright.

T2 decay

T2 relaxation occurs as a loss of phase coherence among proton spins. After the RF pulse is withdrawn, nuclei are in phase with each other (coherent). Since the magnetic field strength experienced by the nuclei determines their precessional frequency, changes in B_0 and local inhomogeneities alter the individual precessional frequencies of the nuclei, causing them to dephase. This reduces their T2 decay times and, as dephasing increases, the signal intensity decreases as there is less coherent magnetization present in the transverse plane. To exploit this effect, a short TE is selected to minimize T2 weighting and a long TE is selected to maximize it.

In MRI since TE controls T2 weighting, the effect of T2 decay in the images is manipulated by selecting a TR longer than the T1 recovery time of most tissues (more than 2000 ms), and a TE during the time in which T2 decay is occurring in most tissues (more than 80 ms). This results in a T2 weighted image where tissues with long T2 relaxation times (water and tumor) appear bright, and tissues with short T2 times (fat) appear dark.

T1 recovery

T1 recovery is the longitudinal recovery of the NMV. Before the RF excitation pulse is applied, some magnetic moments are said to be in thermal equilibrium as more nuclei align parallel with the field (low-energy state), than oppose the field (high-energy state). The NMV that represents the sum of the magnetic moments is therefore parallel to B_0. During RF pulse excitation, some nuclei absorb transmitted RF energy and enter the high-energy state. The resultant sum of the magnetic moments causes the NMV to lie in the transverse plane.

After the withdrawal of the RF pulse some high-energy nuclei transfer their absorbed energy and return to the low-energy state. As this occurs, the NMV returns to its original orientation parallel to B_0 and so recovers longitudinally. To exploit this effect, the TR is selected to control the amount of longitudinal recovery permitted between excitation pulses. Short TRs maximize T1 weighting, longer TRs minimize it.

In MRI, since TR controls T1 weighting the effect of T1 recovery in the images is manipulated by selecting a TR during the time in which T1 recovery time is occurring in most tissues (less than 1000 ms), and TE shorter than the T2 decay time of most tissues (less than 20 ms). The result is a T1 weighted image where tissues with short T1 times appear bright (fat), and tissues with long T1 relaxation times (water and tumors) appear dark.

Mechanism of action

Both T1 recovery and T2 decay are influenced by the magnetic field experienced locally within the nucleus. The local magnetic field responsible for these processes is caused by:

- the main magnetic field
- the fluctuations caused by the magnetic moments of nuclear spins in neighboring molecules.

These molecules rotate or tumble, and the rate of rotation of the molecules is a characteristic property of the solution. It depends on:

- the viscosity of the solution
- the temperature of the solution.

Both T1 and T2 recovery times can be changed by the introduction of contrast agents. Some agents *primarily* shorten T1 and some shorten T2. When the predominant effect is T1 shortening, structures with a reduced T1 relaxation time appear bright on T1 weighted images. When the predominant effect is T2 shortening, structures with a reduced T2 relaxation time appear dark on T2 weighted images. The former are known as T1 agents and the latter as T2 agents. These effects are now described in more detail. However, agents that affect T1 also affect T2 as these effects occur simultaneously. An agent that shortens T1 also shortens T2, but can have a greater effect on one or the other depending upon dose (concentration), imaging parameters (scan type, TR, TE, flip) or magnetic field strength.

At magnetic field strengths commonly used in MRI, the speed of the molecular rotation is closely matched to the precessional frequency of the nuclei. As molecules tumble, magnetic moments within the molecules have varying effects on the externally applied magnetic field, and ultimately the field experienced by the nucleus. In Figure 11.1, the tumbling or rotation of the magnetic moments of hydrogen in water molecules is illustrated.

During time 1, the magnetic moments of the hydrogen nuclei add to B_0, during times 2 and 3 there is no net effect as the magnetic moments lie perpendicular to B_0, and at time 4 they impose a negative effect on the applied field B_0. This tumbling therefore results in local fluctuations in the magnetic field. Molecules that tumble with a frequency at or near the Larmor frequency have more efficient T1 recovery times than other molecules. Therefore, when local magnetic field fluctuations occur at or near the Larmor frequency of hydrogen, the T1 relaxation time of hydrogen is reduced.

11

Dipole–dipole interactions

The phenomenon by which excited protons are affected by nearby excited protons and electrons is called dipole–dipole interaction. Water within the body tumbles much faster than the Larmor frequency, resulting in inefficient relaxation and a long T1 relaxation time. If a tumbling molecule with a large magnetic moment is placed in the presence of water protons, local magnetic field fluctuations occur.

Molecular tumbling creates fluctuations in a magnetic field near the Larmor frequency, and so T1 relaxation times of nearby protons can be

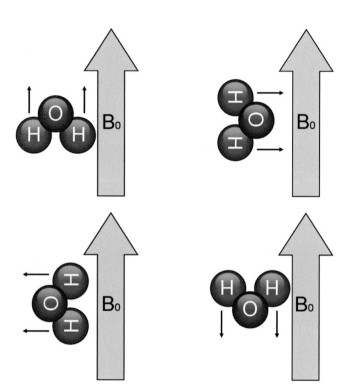

Figure 11.1 Tumbling of water molecules. Top left (time 1), top right (time 2), bottom left (time 3) bottom right (time 4).

11

reduced. This is the effect that occurs when enhancement agents that have large magnetic moments come into contact with water protons – the T1 relaxation times of the protons is reduced so they appear bright (not dark) on a T1 weighted image. In addition, when a substance that demonstrates high positive magnetic susceptibility comes into contact with tissues with long T2 decay times, they too can be reduced so they appear dark (not bright) on T2 weighted images.

Magnetic susceptibility

When evaluating suitable enhancement agents, their magnetic susceptibility must be considered. Magnetic susceptibility is a fundamental property of matter and is defined as the ability of the external magnetic field to affect the nucleus of an atom and magnetize it. Magnetic susceptibility effects include diamagnetism, paramagnetism and ferromagnetism. As discussed in Chapter 9:

- diamagnetic substances such as gold and silver show mild negative effects on the local magnetic field within the nucleus
- paramagnetic substances such as gadolinium chelates have a positive effect on the local magnetic field

- superparamagnetic substances have large magnetic moments and create large disruptive changes in local magnetic fields
- ferromagnetic substances such as iron acquire large magnetic moments when placed in a magnetic field and retain this magnetization even when the external field is removed.

T1 agents

As paramagnetic substances have positive magnetic susceptibilities, they provide a suitable choice for an enhancement agent in MRI. Gadolinium (Gd), a trivalent lanthanide element, is ideal because it has seven unpaired electrons and an ability to allow rapid exchange of bulk water. Water within the body (such as that found in tumors) tumbles much faster than the Larmor frequency, resulting in inefficient relaxation that is demonstrated by long T1 and T2 relaxation times. If a substance with a large magnetic moment (such as gadolinium) is placed in the presence of tumbling water protons, fluctuations in the local magnetic field are created.

When molecular tumbling creates fluctuations in a magnetic field near the Larmor frequency, the T1 relaxation times of nearby water protons can be reduced. This results in an increased signal intensity of these protons on T1 weighted images. For this reason, gadolinium is known as a **T1 enhancement agent**. Other T1 enhancement agents include manganese, an intravenous agent used in liver imaging, and hyperpolarized helium – a T1 ventilation agent used for the evaluation of the lungs (Figure 11.2).

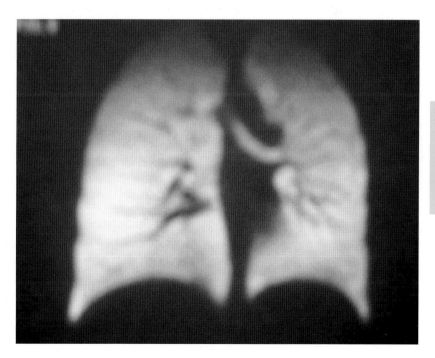

Figure 11.2   Image of the lungs after inhalation of hyper-polarized helium.

11

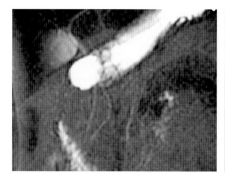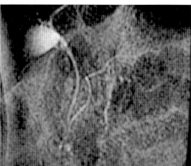

Figure 11.3 These images were acquired for the biliary system. The image on the left is a coronal, T1 weighted before contrast and on the right after the iron oxide oral agent (Gastromark™).

T2 agents

Paramagnetic agents have been used effectively for several years. However, there are superparamagnetic agents that can be used as **T2 enhancement agents**. To increase contrast in a specific tissue, an area must be either brighter or darker than the surrounding structures. Substances such as iron oxides can be used to shorten the T2 decay times and thus decrease signal intensity on T2 weighted images. Iron oxides shorten relaxation times of nearby hydrogen atoms and therefore reduce the signal intensity in normal tissues. This results in a signal loss on proton density weighted or heavily T2 weighted images. For this reason, superparamagnetic iron oxides are known as T2 enhancement agents. One such agent is an intravenous agent for the liver made from iron oxide particles known as Feridex™. Other T2 agents include oral agents for MRCP (MR cholangiopancreatography) known as Gastromark™ and a more natural agent, blueberry juice. Both of these agents make bowel appear dark on T2 weighted images (Figure 11.3).

Relaxivity

When contrast agents are used in computed tomography (CT), the enhancement is due to concentrations of the agent. When contrast agents are used in MRI it is not the agent itself but the effects of the agent that are measured.

The effect of a substance on relaxation rate is known as its **relaxivity**. As previously discussed, water tumbles much faster than the Larmor frequency resulting in inefficient relaxation and persistence of phase coherence. T1 and T2 times are directly affected by local magnetic fields and any substance that affects T1 also affects T2 as they do not occur independently of one another. Since short T1 and long T2 relaxation times both increase signal intensity, it would seem difficult to find a substance that both shortens the T1 time and lengthens the T2 time.

Relaxivity is expressed in the following equation where:

$(1/T1)$observed $= (P)(1/T1)$enhanced $+ (1 - P)(1/T1)$bulk water, and,

$(1/T2)$observed $= (P)(1/T2)$enhanced $+ (1 - P)(1/T2)$bulk water

The relaxivity equation shows that the inverse of T1 in bulk water combined with an enhancement agent results in a new relaxivity, $(1/T)$-enhanced. P is the fraction or concentration of the substance, and therefore as the concentration is increased the effect of the agent is also increased. The equation also demonstrates that T1 and T2 are equally affected by enhancement agents. However, since the T2 relaxation time of biological fluids (approximately 100 ms) is much shorter then the T1 relaxation time (approximately 2000 ms), a higher effective concentration of the enhancement agent is needed to produce significant shortening of T2.

As the static magnetic field B_0 is responsible for altering the precessional frequency of protons bound to different sites on the molecule, it produces an effect (previously described) known as chemical shift. Chemical shift increases as the magnitude of B_0 increases. Substances such as gadolinium do not affect the static magnetic field and subsequently have little effect on chemical shift. Therefore at recommended doses gadolinium has the greatest effect on altering T1 relaxation times. However, substances such as iron oxides do affect the static magnetic field and thus the precessional frequencies of individual nuclei. This results in an increase in dephasing and a shortening of T2 decay times. These agents are known as selective T2 agents. The relaxivity equation assumes no chemical shift and so a chemical exchange broadening term must be added to evaluate iron oxides accurately.

Gadolinium safety

Gadolinium is a rare earth metal (lanthanide) more commonly known as a 'heavy metal'. Metal ions with free electrons tend to accumulate in tissues with a natural affinity for metals (binding sites). Sites within the body that bind Gd + 3 include membranes, transport proteins, enzymes and the osseous matrix (lungs, liver, spleen and bone). As the body is unable to excrete these metals, they can remain for a long period of time.

Fortunately there are substances with a high affinity for metal ions. These substances are known as chelates. The chelate (from the Greek word *khele*, meaning 'claw') binds some of the available sites of the metal ion. A commonly used chelate is diethylene triaminepentaacetic acid (DTPA). DTPA binds eight of the nine binding sites of the gadolinium ion leaving the ninth free for close approach of water molecules to the paramagnetic center. By binding the rare earth metal ion gadolinium, with the chelate DTPA (a ligand), Gd-DTPA (gadopentetate) is formed. It is a relatively safe, water-soluble contrast enhancement agent for MRI.

11

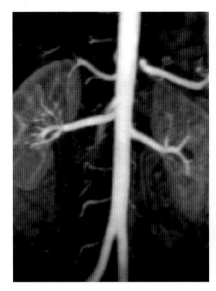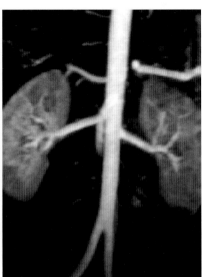

Figure 11.4 These images were acquired for the renal arteries. The image on the left was acquired with the new (higher relaxivity) agent with 20 cc. The image on the right with standard gadolinium with a standard MRA (40 cc) dose.

11

The gadopentetate molecule has two negative charges that must be balanced in solution by two positively charged meglumine ions, and it is therefore ionic. Another agent that received FDA approval is Gd-HP-DO3A (gadoteridol) in which the charges have been balanced to produce a non-ionic contrast agent. The structure of the HP-DO3A ligand differs from that of DTPA as it is macrocyclic, affording greater stability and a reduced tendency for release of the toxic gadolinium atom. Other chelates soon to be available include Gd-DTPA-BMA (gadodiamide), a non-ionic derivative of Gd-DTPA, and Gd-DOTA, an ionic macrocyclic molecule.

There is yet another gadolinium chelate that has been in use in Europe for several years and is about to become available in the United States known as Gd-BOPTA. This gadolinium contrast agent has shown promise for use in the liver as it is excreted by the renal and hepato-biliary systems. In addition, this agent has a higher relaxivity than the more mainstream gadolinium agents. Due to this higher relaxivity, Gd-BOPTA can either demonstrate more enhancing structures at the standard doses, or similar structures at lower doses (Figure 11.4).

Gadolinium side effects and contraindications

At standard doses the side effects of gadolinium chelates are minimal when compared with those of iodinated contrast agents that can cause anaphylaxis and even death. Studies show that the side effects associated with gadolinium contrast agents include:

- a slight transitory increase in bilirubin and blood iron
- 9.8% mild transitory headaches
- 4.1% nausea

- 2% vomiting
- less than 1% hypotension, gastrointestinal upset or rash.

At present, there have been two reported cases (out of 500 000 injections) of death attributed to the introduction of gadolinium into the body. Approximately 80% of gadolinium is excreted by the kidneys in three hours and 98% is recovered by feces and urine in one week. Although there are no known contraindications for the use of gadolinium at this time, there are several situations where caution should be used before administering gadolinium. These include pregnancy and lactation, respiratory disorders, asthma, previous allergic history and hematological disorders such as hemolytic and sickle cell anemias.

Gadolinium administration

The effective dosage of Gd and Gd is 0.1 millimoles per kilogram (mmol/kg) of body weight (0.2 ml/kg or approximately 0.1 ml/lb) with a maximum dose of 20 ml. Gd-HP-DO3A has been approved for up to 0.3 mmol/kg or three times the dose of Gd-DTPA. The lethal dose, determined in rat studies, is never approached in the clinical situation and is 10 mmol/kg. This is a similar safety factor to the 400 mg/kg effective and the 6000 mg/kg lethal dose of iodine.

Iron oxide safety

Feridex™ (a typical iron oxide used in clinical MRI) is a superparamagnetic iron oxide with dextran for intravenous administration. Chemically, ferrous oxide is a non-stoichiometric magnetic. The iron in Feridex™ enters the normal body iron metabolism demonstrated by a transient increase in serum iron values one day after injection and increased serum ferritin values seven days after administration.

Iron oxide side effects and contraindications

Adverse side effects occur in less than 5% of the population who receive the agent. These include mild to severe back, leg and groin pain and, in a few cases, head and neck pain. In clinical trials, 2.5% of subjects experienced pain severe enough to cause interruption or discontinuation of the drug. A few patients experience digestive side effects including nausea, vomiting and diarrhea. Anaphylactic-like reactions and hypotension have been reported in a few patients receiving Feridex™. Feridex™ is contraindicated in patients with known allergies or hypersensitivity to iron, parenteral dextran, parenteral iron-dextran or parenteral iron-polysaccharide preparations. After administration of the contrast agent,

11

full resuscitation facilities should be available. In addition, since the infusion is dark in color, skin surrounding the infusion site might discolor if there is extravasation.

Iron oxide administration

The recommended dose of Feridex™ iron oxide is 0.56 mg of iron (0.05 ml Feridex™ I.V.) per kg of body weight. This should be diluted in 100 ml of 50% dextrose and given intravenously over 30 min. The diluted drug is administered through a 5 micron filter at a rate of 2–4 mm per min. This agent should be used within 8 hours following dilution.

Current applications of contrast agents

Gadolinium has proven invaluable in imaging the central nervous system because of its ability to pass through breakdowns in the blood–brain barrier (BBB). Clinical indications for the head, spine and body for gadolinium include:

- tumors pre- and post-operation
- pre- and post-radiotherapy
- infection
- infarction
- inflammation
- post-traumatic lesions
- post-operation lumbar disc.

Head and spine (Figures 11.5 to 11.8)

Extra-axial areas or areas outside the BBB demonstrate normal enhancement. These areas include the falx, petrous matrix, choroid plexus, pineal gland, pituitary gland, and the infundibulum. The diagnosis of other extra-axial lesions such as acoustic neuromas and meningiomas has been facilitated by the use of gadolinium (Figure 11.6). Areas with slow-flowing blood such as the cavernous sinus and the venous drainage system may also demonstrate enhancement. Therefore, fat and slow-flowing blood can often be mistaken for blood products. In the pituitary gland a macro adenoma enhances rapidly but a micro adenoma, because of its densely-packed cells, does not enhance and therefore appears dense compared with the normal enhancement of the sella tursica.

Intra-axial lesions such as infarcts and tumors enhance due to the breakdown in their BBB, but peri-infarctal edema does not enhance (Figure 11.5). Although recent infarctions do not enhance until the BBB

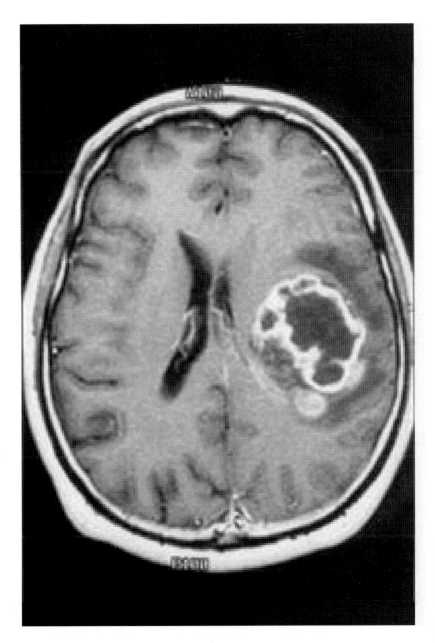

Figure 11.5 Axial T1 weighted image of a cerebral tumor after administration of gadolinium.

11

has been disrupted, some evidence suggests that arterial vessels in the brain enhance and therefore any occlusion or slow flow in these vessels can be demonstrated.

Metastatic disease can be demonstrated with the use of gadolinium. Studies have shown that at higher doses metastatic lesions are more conspicuous. As patient management often changes according to the number of intracranial metastases demonstrated, the ability to demonstrate these lesions can be important.

11

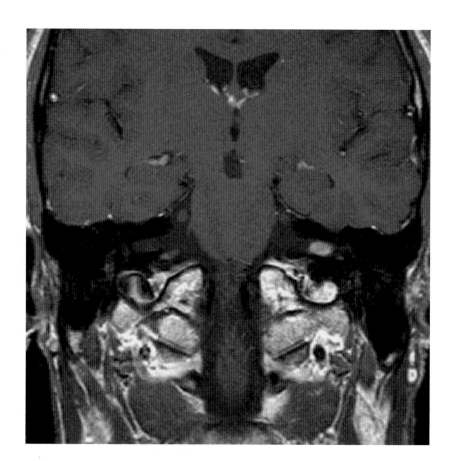

Figure 11.6 Coronal T1 weighted image of a small acoustic neuroma after administration of gadolinium.

Spinal cord lesions may also be well visualized with the use of gadolinium. Although lesions can sometimes be detected without the use of gadolinium, in some cases circumscribing the lesion with enhancement agents can demonstrate the presence of other anomalies such as a syrinx. Lesions such as in MS and other infectious disorders, including AIDS and abscesses, also enhance with the use of gadolinium. Enhancing MS plaques may indicate activity within the plaque.

Perfusion is micro-circulation or the delivery of blood to tissues. Perfusion imaging is the measurement of blood volume in these areas. This measurement, however, is complicated because less than 5% of tissue protons are intravascular. To measure perfusion the signal intensity in perfusing spins may be suppressed or increased. This can be achieved by either employing motion sensitive gradients (as in diffusion imaging), or by introducing enhancement agents (*see* Chapter 12). Agents like gadolinium and iron oxide may be localized in the capillary bed and produce large magnetic moments in the capillary network, creating magnetic fields that extend into the adjacent tissues. This results in perfusion information in patients with ischemia in brain parenchyma, liver parenchyma and in myocardial infarction.

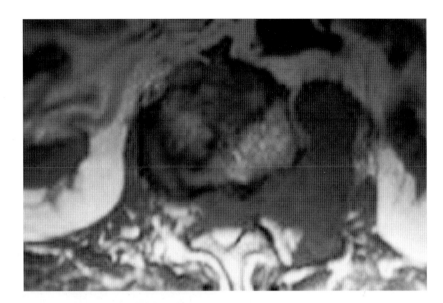

Figure 11.7 Axial T1 weighted image of a lumbar vertebra without gadolinium. Bony metastases are seen.

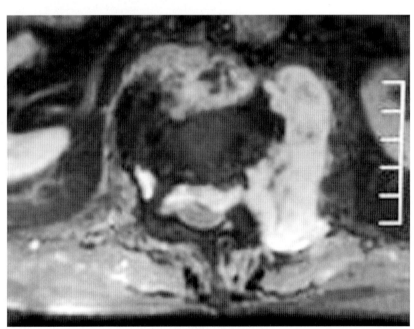

Figure 11.8 Same patient as in Figure 11.7 after gadolinium. Enhancement is clearly seen.

Subtle enhancement can be shown in the scar in post-operative discectomy patients when differentiating between scar tissue and recurrent herniated disc – scar enhances and disc does not. However, after approximately 30 min, disc matter shows signs of enhancement. For this reason, it is advisable to scan immediately after injection in cases where scar is suspected.

Bone lesions of the spine can be well visualized with the use of gadolinium (Figures 11.7 and 11.8). However, some metastatic lesions of the

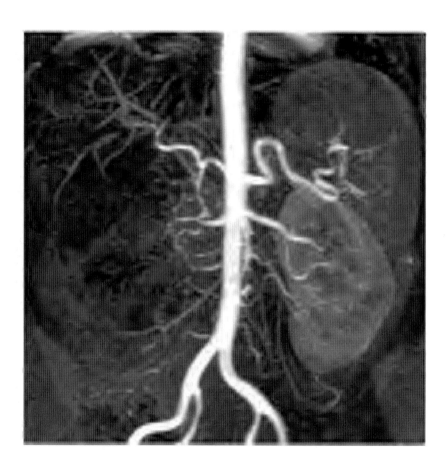

Figure 11.9 Abdominal vessels after gadolinium administration – arterial phase.

spine appear as low signal intensities on T1 weighted images relative to the high signal intensities caused by fat in the bone marrow. Enhancement can raise the signal intensity of the bone lesion to that of normal marrow making the lesion iso-intense with normal bone. Fat selective saturation pulses (fat sat) can be used to suppress fat marrow and so visualize enhancing lesions.

Body (Figures 11.9 to 11.13)

Many lesions in the abdomen have been demonstrated on T2 weighted sequences without the use of relaxation enhancing agents. However, it is the enhanced images of the visceral structures of the abdomen, acquired dynamically, that typically help to finalize the diagnosis. The use of gadolinium in body imaging is increasing. Even though contrast does not enhance all lesions within the body, gadolinium has shown some promising effects.

Gadolinium has been used for perfusion studies of the kidneys, liver, spleen, pancreas, adrenals, vascular structures and pelvis structures. Since the liver, spleen and kidneys are vascular organs contrast enhances these

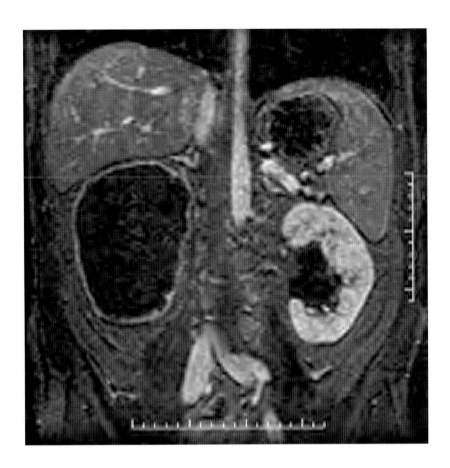

Figure 11.10 Abdominal vessels after gadolinium administration – middle phase.

structures almost immediately after injection. For this reason, rapid imaging is recommended. Dynamic enhancement and rapid imaging can be used to evaluate arterial flow in abdominal vessels by using 3D T1 gradient echo breath-hold acquisitions after gadolinium (Figures 11.9 to 11.11). Peak enhancement differences occur shortly after injection, and by two minutes after injection lesions begin to enhance so that they are iso-intense with normal organ parenchyma. For this reason, rapid imaging acquisitions should be used when imaging the abdomen to maximize the enhancement effect.

Metastatic lesions of the bone have been more clearly delineated by the use of gadolinium. If bony lesions are to be evaluated with gadolinium on T1WI, fat saturation techniques should be used. Since the gadolinium will make the signal from the lesion bright and the fat in the marrow is also bright, the lesion will be difficult to visualize. Therefore the use of fat sat will suppress the signal from fat in the marrow allowing for the visualization within the bone. Superparamagnetic iron oxides are commonly used for liver imaging by reducing the signal intensity in normal liver parenchyma, hence increasing the CNR between lesions and normal liver on T2 weighted images (Figure 11.12). These agents are also useful in imaging bony metastases by suppressing normal fatty marrow.

11

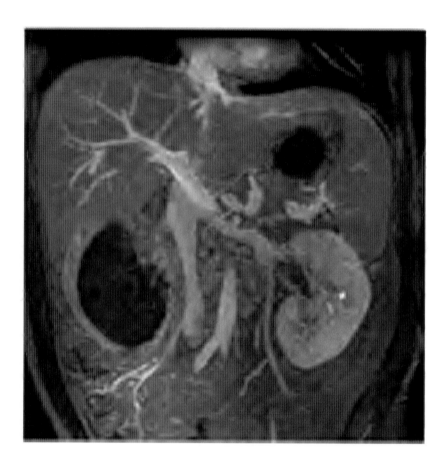

Figure 11.11 Abdominal vessels after gadolinium administration – venous phase.

In cardiac imaging, myocardial infarctions (MI) have been shown to be enhanced. This can be best visualized by cardiac perfusion sequences. These sequences are acquired dynamically with gadolinium enhancement for the evaluation of MIs during rest and during physical or pharmacologic induced stress (*see* Chapter 8).

In breast imaging, the use of gadolinium followed by repeated rapid acquisition, acquired with fat saturation and/or followed by subtraction techniques, is proving to help determine the nature of suspicious lesions within the breast tissue (Figure 11.13). In general many rapidly enhancing and/or spiculated enhanced lesions are thought to be malignant. In addition, this technique seems to demonstrate multi-focal lesions that are not always apparent on plain mammography.

Oral and rectal enhancement agents

Gastrointestinal contrast agents are not as widely used as intravascular agents at present but may increase in use in the future. Oral contrast agents

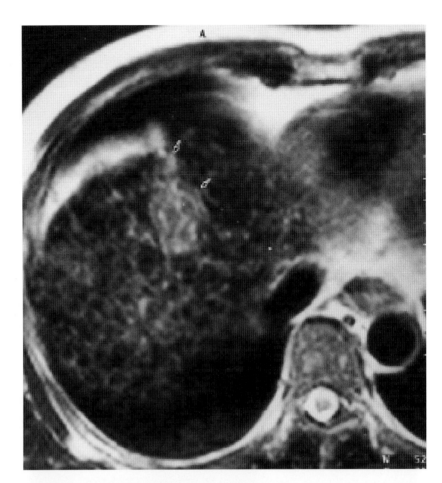

Figure 11.12 Axial T2 weighted image after administration of superparamagnetic iron oxide. A lesion within the liver is shown.

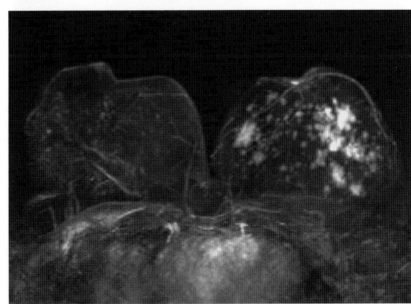

Figure 11.13 Axial T1 weighted subtracted image of the breast. Lesions are clearly seen after enhancement with gadolinium.

Image reproduced with kind permission of Dr Christiane Kuhl, University of Bonn.

11

11

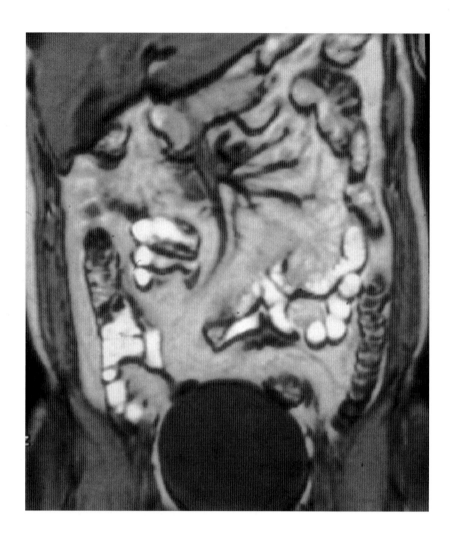

Figure 11.14 Coronal image of the abdomen with bowel contrast enhancement.

have been researched for bowel enhancement. Iron oxides and fatty substances have been used orally to try to enhance effectively the gastrointestinal tract (Figure 11.14). However, due to constant peristalsis, these agents enhance bowel motion artefacts more often than enhancing pathologic lesions. The use of antispasmodic agents helps to retard peristalsis and/or ultra-fast imaging techniques to decrease these artefacts.

Some facilities have used blueberry juice (makes bowel dark on T2 weighted images) and dilute gadolinium (makes bowel bright on T1 weighted images) to enhance bowel. In addition, agents such as dilute barium solutions can be used to make bowel contents appear dark. Air has also been used as an effective contrast agent in the rectum. By showing a signal intensity void in the distended rectum, the prostate in males and the uterus in females can be more clearly demonstrated when imaging the pelvis.

Musculo-skeletal

Contrast agents are rarely used in the musculo-skeletal system. Gadolinium is occasionally used in soft tissue tumors. However, its primary role is in MR arthrography where it is mixed with saline and injected directly into a joint to improve visualisation of intra-capsular structures.

Conclusion

Overall examination time may lengthen with the use of intravenous contrast in MRI as additional sequences are performed. In most cases T1 and T2 weighted sequences should be performed before the use of gadolinium followed by contrast and another T1 weighted series. Gadolinium has improved the visualization of lesions in many cases and it has enabled a more precise delineation of lesions in T1 weighted images. It is also a safer form of enhancing agent than iodine and currently the most effective contrast agent in MRI.

The greatest effect of the increased use of enhancement agents has been on the system operator. The operator should be aware that contrast enhances lesions and slow-flowing vessels. Flow motion artefacts increase with the use of gadolinium and should therefore be anticipated and compensated for by the operator especially when imaging vascular areas of the body. In addition, gadolinium should be used in conjunction with fat suppression techniques in areas where it is suspected that the increased signal from enhancement will become iso-intense with fatty tissues.

Lastly, different concentrations of gadolinium will affect image contrast and produce a layering effect in the bladder.

Questions

11

1   Gadolinium chelates are ferromagnetic. True or false?

2   What are the contraindications for gadolinium?

3   What is the recommended dose for gadolinium?

4   What structures normally enhance with gadolinium?

5   What intrinsic contrast parameter does iron oxide affect?

Functional imaging techniques

Introduction

The previous chapters introduce the basis for MRI by describing fundamental pulse sequences and image formation. Technical developments in system hardware and software have allowed for ultra-fast imaging sequences in the order of milliseconds. Ultra-fast imaging sequences permit an almost unlimited range of applications that were never possible with conventional MR imaging sequences. Most of these are now collectively called **functional imaging techniques** because they allow MRI to be used to assess function and physiology as opposed to merely conventional structural imaging.

Such applications include:

- diffusion weighted imaging (DWI)
- perfusion imaging
- functional brain imaging (fMRI)
- real-time imaging of cardiac motion and perfusion (described in Chapter 8)
- spectroscopy (MRS)
- whole body imaging
- MR microscopy (MRM).

This chapter describes these functional imaging techniques and their potential applications.

12

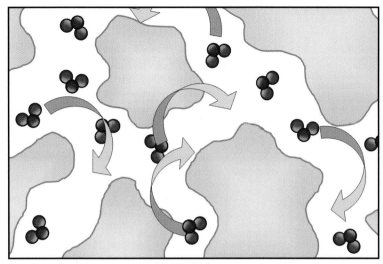

freely diffusing water

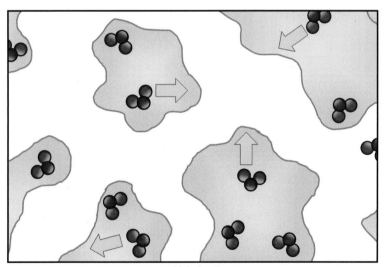

Figure 12.1 Free and restricted diffusion in water.

restricted water

Diffusion weighted imaging (DWI)

Diffusion is a term used to describe the movement of molecules due to random thermal motion. This motion is restricted by boundaries such as ligaments, membranes and macromolecules (Figure 12.1). Sometimes restrictions in diffusion are directional, depending on the structure of the tissues. Diffusion of molecules also occurs across tissues, especially from areas of restricted diffusion to areas with free diffusion. The net displacement of molecules is called the **apparent diffusion coefficient** (**ADC**) and a

12

sequence can be sensitized to this motion by applying two gradients on either side of the 180° RF pulse. This works in a similar way to phase contrast MRA (*see* Chapter 8) in that stationary spins will acquire no net phase change after the gradients have been applied. Moving spins, however, will acquire this phase change and result in a signal loss. In diffusion imaging, normal tissue has a lower signal intensity than abnormal tissue as the molecules within it are free to move, while diffusion becomes restricted when pathology is present.

Learning point: diffusion is another type of weighting

The signal change depends on the ADC of the tissue and the strength of the gradients. The amplitude of these are controlled by the **b factor/value** (which is similar to the VENC in phase contrast MRA, *see* Chapter 8). This is another type of weighting. In Chapter 2 we discussed how extrinsic contrast parameters such as the TR and TE control how much an intrinsic contrast parameter such as T1, T2 and PD contribute to the overall image contrast. For example, TE controls how much T2 contrast is displayed in the image. In diffusion imaging an extrinsic contrast parameter (b factor) controls how much a tissue's ADC contributes towards image weighting. If the TE and TR are long and b = 0 then the image is T2 weighted.

If we then increase the b factor then the image weighting changes from T2 to diffusion weighting. By this we mean that areas will have a high signal not because they have a long T2 time but because they have a low ADC. This is why this technique is called **diffusion weighted imaging (DWI)**. It is, in fact, another type of weighting. 'b' is expressed in units of s/mm^2. Typical 'b' values range from 500 s/mm^2 to 1000 s/mm^2.

DWI and directional effects

The diffusion gradient discussed above can be applied along all three axes, either individually or together. Individual acquisitions with different gradients sensitize the sequence to restricted diffusion along a particular axis. This is useful when imaging areas that have a directional difference in diffusion. The best example of this is in white matter, where white matter tracts take specific courses through the brain and spinal cord. Using DWI with a particular gradient applied allows us to see these white matter tracts in separate images. Tissues that display this characteristic are called **anisotropic**; tissues where this does not occur (such as gray matter) are called **isotropic**.

12

DWI and sequences

In DWI we need to use spin echo sequences as gradients must be applied on either side of a 180° RF to sensitize the sequence to changes in diffusion. Usually very fast types of spin are used, such as SS-SE-EPI (*see* Chapter 5). This is not because diffusion happens particularly quickly but because we need to reduce other types of motion such as flow, so that only motion from diffusion is measured. Typically single or multi-shot SE-EPI is used to acquire images in a few seconds. However, conventional spin echo can be used in areas with few motion artefacts.

There are two types of DW images:

- Diffusion or **trace images** are those where damaged tissue that has restricted diffusion (low ADC) is brighter than normal tissues where diffusion is free (high ADC). This is because spins in restricted tissue are refocused as they stay in the same place during excitation and refocusing. However, in normal tissue where diffusion is random, refocusing is not complete and signals cancel. If motion varies rapidly, diffusion attenuation occurs and signal is lost in that area. Hence abnormal tissue is brighter than normal tissue.
- **ADC maps** are acquired via post-processing by calculating the ADC for each voxel of tissue and allocating a signal intensity according to its value. Therefore restricted tissue, which has a low ADC, is darker than free diffusing areas that have a high ADC. The contrast is therefore the mirror of the trace images. This is useful when **T2 shine through** is a problem.

T2 shine through occurs when lesions or areas with a very long T2 decay time remain bright on the DW or trace image. It is therefore difficult to know whether they represent an area of restricted diffusion or not. By producing ADC maps it is possible to differentiate between areas with a low ADC and those with a long T2 decay time. Look at Figures 12.2 and 12.3. On the trace image the infarcted tissue is bright while on the ADC map it is dark. The ADC map enables differentiation of this area from the other high signal intensities seen on the ADC map. These areas represent tissues with a long T2 decay time, not those with a low ADC.

DWI uses

The most common use of DWI is in the brain after infarction. In early stroke, soon after the onset of ischemia but before infarct or permanent tissue damage, cells swell and absorb water from the extra-cellular space. Since cells are full of large molecules and membranes, diffusion is restricted and the ADC of the tissue is reduced. These areas appear bright on trace images and these changes can be seen within minutes of infarction as opposed to hours or days using conventional MRI techniques. Diffusion MRI can show irreversible and reversible ischemia lesions, so has a potential to discriminate salvageable tissues from irreversibly damaged

12

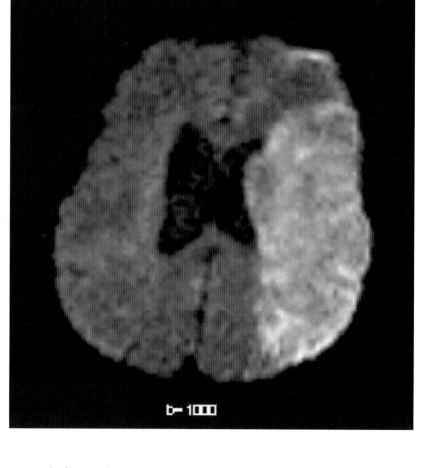

Figure 12.2 Axial trace image. Abnormality returns a higher signal than normal brain.

tissues before a therapeutic intervention. However, timing of diffusion MRI is important – it can only visualize fresh lesions as water diffusion is decreased several days after stroke onset.

DWI can also be used to differentiate malignant from benign lesions and tumor from edema and infarction. This is because these disease processes have different ADC values. In addition DWI is proving a useful tool to image neonatal brains where it is sometimes difficult to discriminate between infarction and myelinating brain. DWI has also been used to map out myelination patterns in pre-term infants to assist in our understanding of this process and how hypoxic events cause certain types of brain damage. The anatomy of white matter tracts can be mapped using different gradients in DWI (diffusion tensor imaging) (Figure 12.4). This has enabled very detailed imaging of white matter *in vivo* and may enable the use of DWI to image certain white matter diseases.

Several studies are exploring the use of DWI in other areas and pathologies. So far these include:

- characterizing liver lesions such as hepato-cellular carcinoma, metastases and hemangiomas

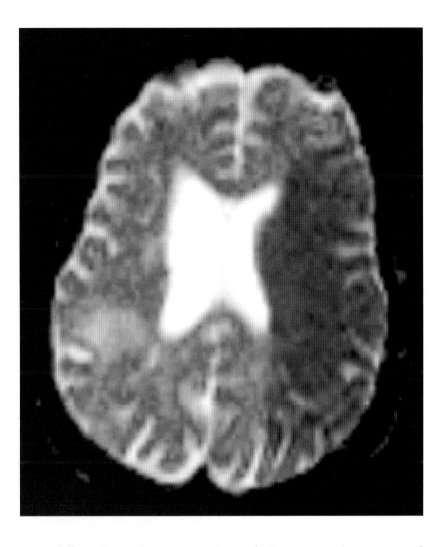

Figure 12.3 ADC map. Area of abnormality now has a low signal as it has a low ADC.

- differentiating between mucin-producing pancreatic tumors and other tumors
- discriminating between pathological and traumatic fractures
- assessing bone bruising.

It is clear that DWI has applications in many areas of the body and that its use will increase in the future.

Perfusion imaging

Clinical perfusion measurements can be made with radio tracers, but as MRI is a non-ionizing technique with high spatial and temporal resolution that can be co-registered with anatomic information, there is much

12

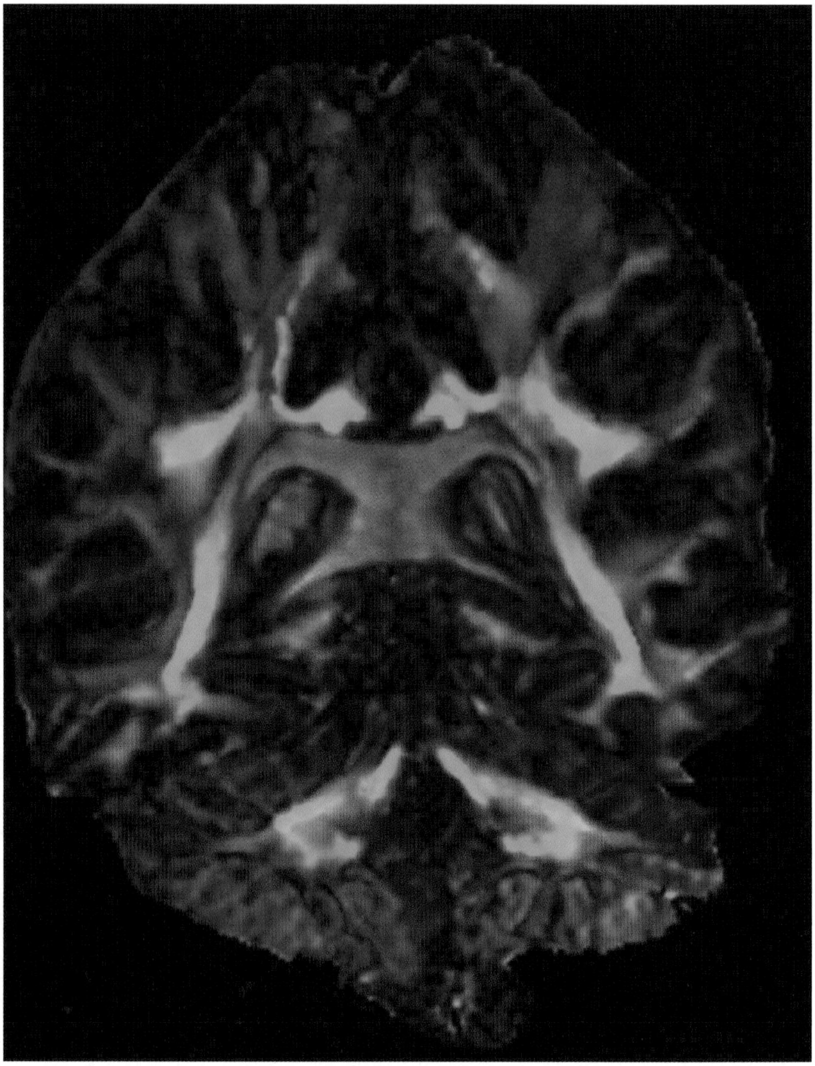

Figure 12.4 Diffusion tensor image showing white matter tracts.

interest in perfusion MRI studies. Perfusion is the regional blood flow in tissues and is defined as the volume of blood that flows into one gram of tissue. Perfusion is a measure of the quality of vascular supply to a tissue and, since vascular supply and metabolism are usually related, perfusion can also be used to measure tissue activity.

Perfusion is measured using MRI by tagging the water in arterial blood during image acquisition. Tagging can be achieved by either a bolus injection of exogenous contrast agent like gadolinium, or by saturating the protons in arterial blood with RF inversion or saturation pulses. As the difference between tagged and untagged images is so small, ultra-fast imaging methods are desirable for reducing artefact. In their simplest form, perfusion images can be acquired with fast scanning acquisitions before, during and after a bolus injection of intravenous contrast. In this

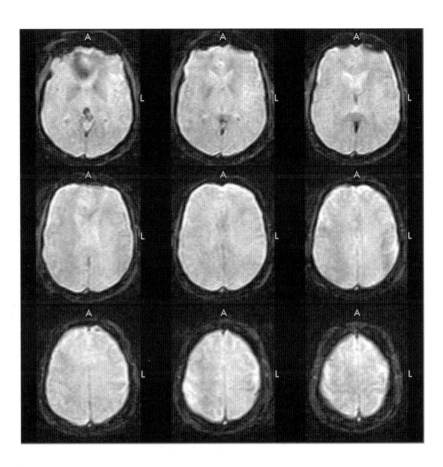

Figure 12.5 Perfusion imaging.

case several ultra-fast incoherent gradient echoes are acquired during breath hold at the same slice location. Since gadolinium shortens T1 recovery, visceral structures with high perfusion appear bright on T1 weighted fast gradient echoes. This technique is useful for the evaluation of visceral structures such as the kidneys, liver and spleen.

Another technique to evaluate perfusion uses a bolus injection of gadolinium administered intravenously during ultra-fast T2 or T2* acquisitions. In this case, the contrast agent causes transient decreases in T2 and T2* decay in and around the microvasculature perfused with contrast. SS-GE-EPI sequences are usually used as they produce the required temporal resolution to measure such transient changes (Figure 12.5). Gradient echo EPI, especially when used with echo shifting (where the TE is longer than the TR) maximizes the susceptibility effects. After data acquisition, a signal decay curve is used to ascertain blood volume, transient time and measurement of perfusion. This curve is known as a **time intensity curve**. Time intensity curves for multiple images acquired during and after injection are combined to generate a cerebral blood volume (CBV) map.

Perfusion imaging with arterial spin tagging is another perfusion technique. With continuous arterial spin labeling (CASL), arterial spins are attenuated by inversion or saturation pulses outside the FOV. An

12

untagged image is also acquired as a reference image. In this technique the reference image is subtracted from the tagged image. Spin tagging is a non-invasive alternative to the introduction of exogenous contrast agents that is potentially quantitative.

Perfusion imaging uses

These techniques can be used to evaluate ischemia disease or metabolism at rest or during exercise. In addition, the malignancy of neoplasms can be reflected in increased tissue metabolism or perfusion. On the CBV map, areas of low perfusion appear dark (stroke) while areas of higher perfusion appear bright (malignancies). Such techniques show great potential in the evaluation of tissue viability and metabolism of vascular organs such as the heart, visceral structures and the brain. In particular, characteristic perfusion patterns are seen in hepato-cellular carcinoma, metastases and hemangiomas. In renal imaging acute focal changes can be seen in renal artery stenosis using perfusion techniques.

Functional imaging (fMRI)

Functional MR imaging (fMRI) is a rapid MR imaging technique that acquires images of the brain during activity or stimulus and at rest. The two sets of images are then subtracted, demonstrating functional brain activity as the result of increased blood flow to the activated cortex. In the early days of this technique, visualization of blood flow was achieved using contrast agents. More recently, blood has been used as an internal contrast.

The magnetic properties of blood are important in the understanding of this technique. Hemoglobin is a molecule that contains iron and transports oxygen in the vascular system as oxygen binds directly to iron. When oxygen is bound (oxyhemoglobin), the magnetic properties of iron are largely suppressed but when oxygen is not bound (deoxyhemoglobin) the molecule becomes more magnetic. Therefore oxyhemoglobin is diamagnetic and deoxyhemoglobin is paramagnetic. Paramagnetic deoxyhemoglobin creates an inhomogeneous magnetic field in its immediate vicinity. This inhomogeneous magnetic field increases $T2^*$ decay and attenuates signal from regions containing deoxyhemoglobin.

At rest, tissue uses a substantial fraction of the blood flowing through the capillaries, so venous blood contains an almost equal mix of oxyhemoglobin and deoxyhemoglobin. During exercise, however, when metabolism is increased, more oxygen is needed and hence more is extracted from the capillaries. In muscle tissue the concentration of oxyhemoglobin in the venous system can become very low. The brain, however, is very sensitive to low concentrations of oxyhemoglobin and therefore the cerebral vascular system increases blood flow to the activated area. Blood oxygenation increases during brain activity and specific locations of the cerebral cortex are activated during specific tasks. For example, seeing activates the visual cortex, hearing the auditory cortex, finger tapping the motor cortex, etc. More sophisticated tasks, including maze paradigms and other thought-provoking tasks, stimulate other brain cortices.

The most important physiological effect that produces MR signal intensity changes between stimulus and rest is called the **blood oxygenation level dependent (BOLD)** effect. BOLD imaging exploits differences in the magnetic susceptibility of oxyhemoglobin and deoxyhemoglobin as a result of increased cerebral blood flow and little or no increase in local oxygen consumption that occurs during stimulation. Because deoxyhemoglobin is paramagnetic, vessels containing a significant amount of this molecule create local field inhomogeneities causing dephasing and therefore signal loss. During activity, blood flow to the cortex increases causing a drop in deoxyhemoglobin, which results in a decrease in dephasing and a corresponding increase in signal intensity. These effects are very short lived and therefore require extremely rapid sequences such as EPI or fast gradient echo. To exploit T2* effects, BOLD images are usually acquired with long TEs (40–70 ms) while the task is modulated on and off. The 'off' images are then subtracted from the 'on' images and a more sophisticated statistical analysis is performed. Regions that were activated above some threshold level are overlaid on anatomical images (Figure 12.6). It is these regions that reflect brain activity. With EPI, images can be collected in a very short time and therefore, in principle, high temporal resolution is possible. However, the temporal resolution is limited by a blurred intrinsic hemodynamic response and a finite SNR.

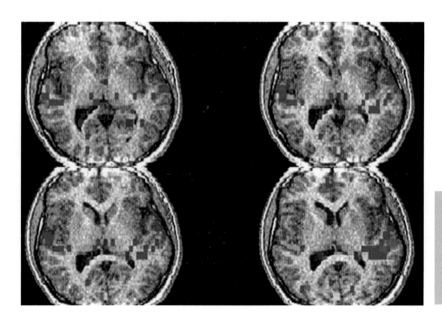

Figure 12.6   BOLD images of the brain. Functional areas shown in red.

12

Despite these limitations there is no doubt that this sophisticated technique will develop our understanding of brain function and will have several clinical applications including the evaluation of stroke, epilepsy, pain and behavioral problems. There is also some potential in abdominal imaging. In particular BOLD imaging has been used to predict tubular necrosis in the kidneys, and mesenteric ischemia.

Interventional MRI

MRI is now used for operative interventional procedures in some centers. The inherent safety and multi-planar facility of MRI makes it an ideal modality for some operative procedures. However, the development of this technique has required several modifications to existing hardware and software options.

Due to the restricted nature of conventional semi-conducting systems, a more open magnet design is required to permit easy access to the patient during the procedure. Low field permanent magnets are well suited from an access point of view, but image quality and acquisition times restrict their use to simple interventions. An interventional system uses a semi-conducting 0.5 T system shaped liked two doughnuts which readily permits access to the patient and allows real-time image acquisition (Figure 12.7). This system permits:

- intra-operative acquisition of MR images without moving the patient
- online image-guided stereotaxy without pre-operative imaging
- 'real-time' tracking of instruments in the operative field registered to the MR images
- precise location of the area under examination (achieved via triangulation)

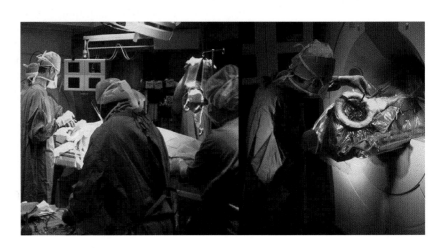

Figure 12.7 Interventional magnet system.

12

- continual monitoring of the procedure in three dimensions (using in-bore monitors).

This is an expensive technique, however. Flexible transmit and receive coils have been especially designed to fit around the operative area while allowing access for intervention. Endovascular coils have been developed to allow real-time tracking within vessels. In addition, all surgical instruments must be non-ferromagnetic and produce minimum susceptibility artefact so that they do not obscure the operating field. Anesthetic and monitoring equipment must also be MR safe.

Interventional MRI uses

Despite these design and safety implications, interventional MR has been used in many operative techniques including:

- liver imaging and tumor ablation
- breast imaging and benign lump excision
- orthopedic and kinematic studies
- congenital hip dislocation manipulation and correction
- biopsies
- functional endoscopic sinus surgery.

One important application is tumor ablation using either laser therapy (in which heat is used to ablate the tumor) or cryotherapy (when extreme cold is used for ablation). MRI is the only imaging technique that can discriminate tissue of different temperatures. Since T1 recovery and T2 decay are temperature dependent, temperature changes alter image contrast. For this reason, techniques such as laser and cryotherapy can be monitored using MRI.

Interstitial laser therapy (ILT) is a promising therapeutic technique in which laser energy is delivered percutaneously to various depths in tissue. Previously the extent of heat distribution from the laser was difficult to assess. The use of EPI sequences has enabled real-time monitoring of laser-induced therapy providing a non-invasive method for intra-operative assessment of heat distribution during ILT. Similarly, interventional MR has enormous potential in the evaluation of cryotherapy. This exciting technique may have profound influences on interventional radiology. It is likely that in the future interventional vascular suites will be replaced by interventional MR systems and many surgical and interventional procedures will be carried out using MR technology.

MR spectroscopy (MRS)

12

MR spectroscopy produces a spectrum as opposed to an MR image. A spectrum is a plot of signal intensity vs frequency that shows the chemical

Table 12.1 Typical hydrogen or proton spectra available in human tissue.

Spectrum	Abbreviation	Effect	Resonance
NAA-N-acetyl aspartate	NAA	neuronal marker	2.0 ppm
Lactate	Lac	product of anaerobic glycosis	1.3 ppm
Choline	Cho	present in cell membrane	3.2 ppm
Creatine	Cr-PCr		3.0 ppm
Lipids	Lip	result of cellular decay	0.9, 1.3 ppm
Myo-inositol	Ins	glial cell marker	3.5, 3.6 ppm
Glutamine/Glutamate	Glx	neurotransmitter	2.1, 3.8 ppm

shift or frequency difference between different elements. This chemical shift is caused by the electron shielding of a specific atom to create a difference in field strength and therefore frequency. Chemical shift is measured in parts per million in frequency (ppm). Chemical dispersion increases with field strength. Fluorine, carbon and sodium can be measured using MR spectroscopy but hydrogen is the most widely used in clinical imaging. Table 12.1 shows the typical hydrogen or proton spectra available in human tissue.

A spectrum is located in one of two ways. Both use an image for guidance:

- **Single voxel** techniques use three intersecting slices to locate a single voxel from which to measure the spectrum. Currently there are two types of single voxel technique:
  - **stimulated echo acquisition mode (STEAM)**
  - **point resolved spectroscopy spin echo (PRESS)**.

  Both localize in a single acquisition but suffer from SNR and chemical shift artefacts. Motion is sometimes a problem if multiple TR periods are used.
- **Multi-voxel** techniques are more time efficient as they acquire multiple voxels by encoding in K space as in conventional imaging.

By viewing spectra from either single or multi voxels it is possible to compare the relative amounts of each to determine a disease process (Figures 12.8 and Figure 12.9). For example, elevations in the following are indicators for tumors:

- NAA drop indicates tumor cell invasion
- choline elevation indicates tumor growth
- lactate changes indicate anaerobic status
- lipid elevation indicates tumor necrosis.

12

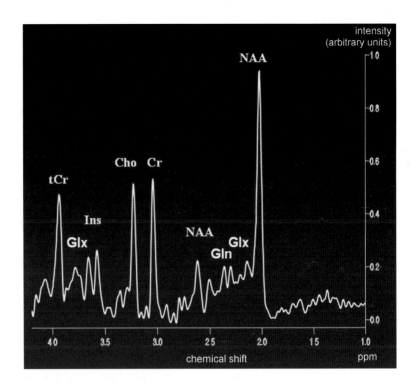

Figure 12.8 MR spectra of the brain.

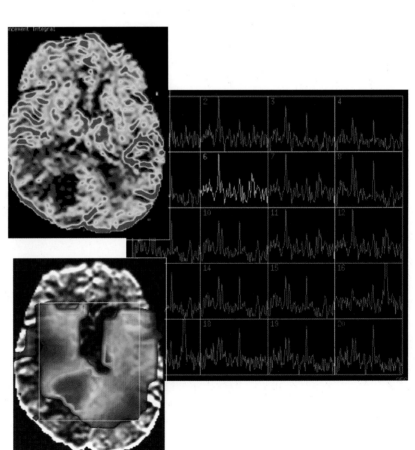

Figure 12.9 Multi-voxel MRS technique.

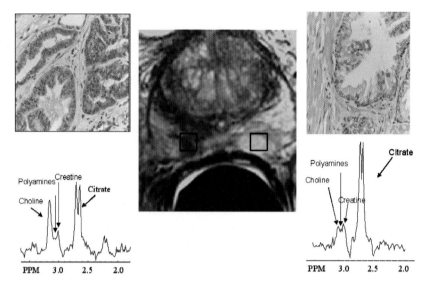

Figure 12.10 MRS for prostate imaging.

MR spectroscopy uses

MRS is used in the following ways:

- to diagnose in conjunction with MRI
- to plan therapy (Figure 12.10)
- biopsy guidance
- to aid in prognosis
- therapy monitoring.

In particular MRS is useful in stroke and tumor staging especially in the brain, breast and prostate. It may also have some use in the diagnosis and understanding of depression, epilepsy and schizophrenia.

Whole body imaging

Researchers have been investigating the use of MRI to image the whole body in a single examination. This may prove useful for screening patients for common diseases such as cancer and cardiovascular disease and for skeletal surveys in patients with widespread bone disease. Most centers have devised protocols that image areas independently using fast imaging sequences such as EPI and turbo gradient echo.

Extra studies are performed in patients with a particular risk of disease. For example, breast imaging is added onto the standard protocol in patients with specific concerns over breast pathology. Manufacturers are developing hardware and software tools to enable fast imaging of the whole body in a single examination (not unlike CT scanning). This includes having multiple coil elements and independent receiver channels enabling a FOV of over 200 cm.

MR microscopy (MRM)

Magnetic resonance microscopy (MRM) uses extremely fine resolution data to image structures with the same resolution as pathology sections. It is therefore an ideal research tool as it allows study in detail of very small areas of tissue. Pathologists can use MRM to examine tissue samples without conventional sectioning. With MRM, investigators can study models of disease, toxicology, and the effects of drug therapies. Because of the SNR problems associated with very small voxels (*see* Chapter 4), very high fields and dedicated ultra-small coils are necessary to image in this manner. MRM is being used in many areas but in clinical use the main application appears to be in bone and joint imaging, especially of hyaline cartilage (Figure 12.11).

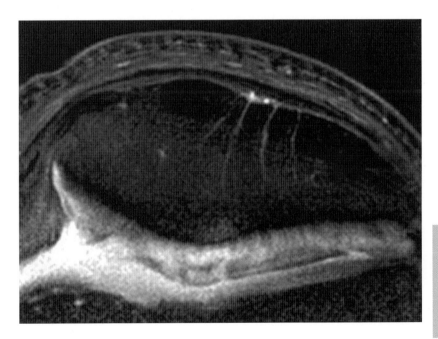

Figure 12.11 MR microscopy of the patellar cartilage. Voxels many, many times smaller than in conventional imaging are used.

12

Questions

1   Name the term used to describe the net displacement of diffusion spins across a tissue.

2   What is the extrinsic parameter that controls the amount of diffusion seen on an image?

3   What signal intensity is an area of abnormality likely to have on an ADC map?

4   What sequence should be used in perfusion imaging when the transient change in T2* is measured and why?

5   What does BOLD stand for?

6   What is chemical shift?

Answers to questions

Chapter 1

1   The Classical and Quantum Theories.

2   Atoms are tiny structures that are the basis for all things.
Molecules are two or more atoms arranged together.
Nucleons are particles within the nucleus of an atom.
Protons are the positively charged elements within an atomic nucleus.
Neutrons are the neutrally charge elements within an atomic nucleus.
Electrons are particles that spin around the nucleus.
Isotopes are atoms with an odd mass number.
Ions are atoms that are electrically unstable because electrons have been knocked out of their shells.

3   The mass number is the total number of nucleons in a nucleus, and it is important in MRI because it determines whether a nucleus has a net magnetic moment.

4   Energy must be applied at the precessional frequency of the nucleus being imaged and at right angles to the main field.

5   Frequency is the number of revolutions per second or the speed of precession. Phase is the position of a magnetic moment at any moment in time.

Chapter 2

1   Inherent energy of the tissue.
How well the molecular tumbling rate matches the Larmor frequency.
How closely spaced the molecules are.

2   Because fat has a low inherent energy, a slow molecular tumbling rate and its molecules are packed together. This means energy exchange is efficient and therefore relaxation occurs quickly.

3   Weighting means that parameters are selected to make one contrast mechanism dominate over the others.

4   The TR must be long so that neither fat nor water has had time to fully recover their longitudinal magnetization. The TE must also be short to minimize the T2 differences between the tissues.

5   Variable flip angles, gradient rephasing, shorter TRs and scan times.

6   The TE controls T2 decay as it determines how much is allowed to occur before the signal is read.

7   (a)   T1 weighting.
              (b)   T2* weighting.

Chapter 3

1	The direction of the current through the gradient coil.
2	The FOV.
3	The frequency matrix.
4	Radians per cm.
5	Aliasing.
6	Outer areas.
7	Left to right.

Chapter 4

1   (a) 512×256, 4 mm slices, 8 cm FOV, 2 NEX.
           (b) 256×128, 8 mm slice thickness, 40 cm FOV, 4 NEX.

2   Field strength
Proton density
Coil type
TR
TE
Flip angle
Slice thickness
Matrix
FOV
Receive bandwidth
NEX.

3   Slice thickness, FOV and coil.

4   MTC, T2 weighted images, contrast enhancement.

5   The incremental step between each phase encode is doubled, which halves the FOV in the phase direction and halves the number of phase encodes performed. The resolution is maintained but the scan time is halved.

6   Voxel must be isotropic, i.e. equal dimensions in all planes. Keep matrix square. Calculate pixel dimension by dividing FOV by number of pixels. Select slice thickness that equals this dimension.

7   The ability to resolve. The minimum distance between two points at which they can be seen as distinct and separate.

Chapter 5

1   RF spoiling eliminates residual transverse magnetization that causes increased T2* weighting.

2   Balanced gradients on all three axes, large flip angle with alternating phase.

3   Long TI to suppress CSF, long TE to enhance T2 weighting, long TR to allow full recovery of spins from saturation.

4	Shorter scan times, more T2 weighting, less slices per TR.
5	In SSFP the stimulated echo only is sampled.
6	Two coils.

Chapter 6

1	TE, slice thickness, velocity of flow.
2	TR, slice thickness velocity of flow, direction of flow.
3	Counter-current.
4	Reduced ghosting, high signal in vessel, increased TE, fewer slices for a given TR.
5	Volumes should be placed inferioraly and on the right to null signal coming up the arm and from the chest.
6	SPIR has fewer inhomogeneity problems than fat saturation. SPIR can used after gadolinium administration whereas STIR cannot.

Chapter 7

1	Magnetic susceptibility artefact is the ability of an object to become magnetized. Metal objects cause an artefact because they magnetize to a different degree than tissue.
2	Magnetic susceptibility: always scan using spin echo pulse sequences.
3	Chemical shift occurs in frequency axis. Increased at high field strengths and when using reduced receive bandwidths. Chemical mis-registration occurs along the phase axis and is increased when using gradient echo sequences and a TE that regenerates an echo when fat and water are out of phase.
4	When anatomy that is producing signal occurs outside the FOV in the phase direction.
5	Cross talk occurs when energy is given up to nuclei in adjacent slices during relaxation. Cross excitation is caused by RF pulses exciting nuclei in adjacent slices. Only this can be compensated for by having a gap between slices, squaring the RF pulses off so that they fit the slices or by interleaving the slice acquisition.
6	Respiratory compensation, increasing NEX, gating, gradient moment rephasing, pre-saturation, breath-holding techniques, compression.

Chapter 8

1	Using coherent and balanced gradient echo sequences and gradient moment rephasing.
2	Using an out of phase TE and MTC.
3	To give the system time to wait for the next R wave.
4	716 ms.

5   Peripheral.
                None.
                Peripheral.
                ECG.

Chapter 9

1   Diamagnetism, paramagnetism and ferromagnetism.

2   Vertical.

3   Right-hand thumb rule.

4   8 T.

5   To correct for field inhomogeneity.

6   To reduce the fringe field.

7   Good SNR from small coils, combined with coverage.

Chapter 10

1   Magneto-hemodynamic effect.

2   40 mph.

3   3.

4   Mild cutaneous sensations and involuntary muscle contractions.

5   www.mrisafety.com.

Chapter 11

1   False. They are paramagnetic.

2   None known although should use with caution in pregnancy.

3   Recommended dose is 0.1 mm/kg.

4   Pituitary and the falx.

5   T2 relaxation times.

Chapter 12

1   ADC.

2   b factor or value.

3   Dark.

4   GE-EPI for speed and to accentuate T* effects with a gradient echo.

5   Blood oxygenation level dependent.

6   Difference in frequency as a result of a magnetic field.

Glossary

A

Actual TE   the time between the echo and the next RF pulse in SSFP.

Acquisition window   *see* **sampling time**.

Active shielding   uses additional superconducting coils located at each end of the main magnet inside the cryostat to shield the system.

Active shimming   additional solenoid magnets to adjust field homogeneity.

ADC map   post-processing in DWI that produces images where abnormal tissue is darker than normal tissue.

Aliasing   artefact produced when anatomy outside the FOV is mismapped inside the FOV.

Alnico   alloy used to make permanent magnets.

Angular momentum   the spin of MR active nuclei which depends on the balance between the number of protons and neutrons in the nucleus.

Anisotropic   voxels that are not the same dimension in all three planes.

Anti-foldover   also called **no phase wrap** oversamples along the phase encoding axis by increasing the number of phase encodings performed.

Apparent diffusion coefficient (ADC)   the net displacement of molecules.

Atom   a tiny element that is the basis for all things.

Atomic number   sum of protons in the nucleus – this number gives an atom its chemical identity.

B

B_0   the main magnetic field measured in tesla.

b factor   strength and duration of the gradients in DWI.

Bandwidth   a range of frequencies.

Black blood imaging   acquisitions in which blood vessels are black.

Blipping   used in EPI to step down through phase encoding steps.

Blood oxygen level dependent (BOLD) imaging   a functional MRI technique that uses the differences in magnetic susceptibility between oxyhemoglobin and deoxyhemoglobin to image areas of activated cerebral cortex.

Blurring   the result of T2* decay during the course of the EPI acquisition.

Bright blood imaging   acquisitions in which blood vessels are bright.

C

CASL   continuous arterial spin labelling – attenuates arterial spins by inversion or saturation pulses outside the FOV.

CBV   cerebral blood volume.

Central lines   area of K space filled with the shallowest phase encoding slopes.

Chemical misregistration   artefact along the phase axis caused by the phase difference between fat and water.

Chemical shift artefact	artefact along the frequency axis caused by the frequency difference between fat and water.
Coarse matrix	a matrix with a low number of frequency encodings and/or phase encodings and results in a low number of pixels in the FOV.
Co-current flow	flow in the same direction as slice excitation.
Coherent	*see* in phase.
Conjugate symmetry	the symmetry of data in K space.
Contrast to noise ratio (CNR)	difference in SNR between two points.
Counter current flow	flow in the opposite direction to slice excitation.
Cross excitation	energy given to nuclei in adjacent slices by the RF pulse.
Cross talk	energy given to nuclei in adjacent slices due to spin lattice relaxation.
Cryogens	substances used to supercool the coils of wire in a superconducting magnet.
Cryogen bath	area around the coils of wire in which cryogens are placed.

D

Data point	point in K space that contains digitized information from encoding.
Decay	loss of transverse magnetization.
Diffusion	the movement of molecules due to random thermal motion.
Diffusion weighted imaging (DWI)	technique that produces images whose contrast is due to the differences in ADC between tissues.
Double IR prep	sequence in which two 180° pulses are used to saturate blood in black blood imaging.
DRIVE	driven equilibrium – a pulse sequence that achieves a very high signal intensity from water even when using short TRs.
DS-MRA	digital subtraction MR angiography – contrast is selectively produced for moving spins during two acquisitions. These are then subtracted to remove the signal from the stationary spins, leaving behind an image of only the moving spins.
DTPA	diethylene triaminepentaacetic acid, a gadolinium chelate.

E

Echo time (TE)	time in milliseconds from the application of the RF pulse to the peak of the signal induced in the coil – TE determines how much decay of transverse magnetization is allowed to occur.
Echo train	series of 180° rephasing pulse and echoes in a fast spin echo pulse sequence.
Echo train length	the number of 180° rephasing pulse/echoes/phase encodings per TR in fast spin echo.
Effective TE	the time between the echo and the RF pulse that initiated it in SSFP – also the TE used in FSE.
Electrons	particles that spin around the nucleus.
Encoding	once a slice is selected, the signal is located or **encoded** along both axes of the image.
Entry slice phenomena	contrast difference of flowing nuclei relative to the stationary nuclei because they are fresh.
Even echo rephasing	technique that uses two echoes to reduce flow artefact.
Excitation	application of an RF pulse that causes resonance to occur.
Extrinsic contrast parameters	those parameters that can be changed at the operator console.

F

Fat saturation	technique that nulls signal from fat by applying an RF pulse at the frequency of fat to the imaging volume before slice excitation.
Fast Fourier transform (FFT)	mathematical conversion of frequency/time domain to frequency/amplitude.
Field of view (FOV)	area of anatomy covered in an image.
Fine matrix	matrix where there are a high number of frequency encodings and/or phase encodings, and results in a large number of pixels in the FOV.
First order motion compensation	gradient moment nulling.
Flip angle	the angle of the NMV to B_0.
Flow encoding axes	axes along which bipolar gradients act in order to sensitize flow along the axis of the gradient used in phase contrast MRA.
Flow phenomena	artefacts produced by flowing nuclei.
Flow related enhancement	decrease in time of flight due to a decrease in velocity of flow.
Fractional averaging	*see* **partial averaging.**
Fractional echo	*see* **partial echo.**
Free induction decay (FID)	loss of signal due to relaxation.
Frequency encoding	locating a signal according to its frequency.
Frequency wrap	aliasing along the frequency encoding axis.
Fresh spins	nuclei that have not been beaten down by repeated RF pulses.
Fringe field	stray magnetic field outside the bore of the magnet.
Fully saturated	when the NMV is pushed to a full 180°.
Functional imaging techniques	these allow MRI to be used to assess function and physiology.

G

Gd-BOPTA	gadobenate dimeglumine.
Gd-DOTA	gadoterate meglumine.
Gd-DTPA	gadopentetate.
Gd-DTPA-BMA	gadodiamide.
Gd-HP-DO3A	gadoteridol.
Ghosting	motion artefact in the phase axis.
Gibbs artefact	line of low signal in the cervical cord image due to truncation.
Gradient amplifier	supplies power to the gradient coils.
Gradient echo	echo produced as a result of gradient rephasing.
Gradient echo-EPI (GE-EPI)	gradient echo sequence with EPI readout.
Gradient echo pulse sequence	one that uses a gradient to regenerate an echo.
Gradient moment nulling (rephasing)	a system of gradients that compensates for intra-voxel dephasing.
Gradients	coils of wire that alter the magnetic field strength in a linear fashion when a current is passed through them.
Gradient spoiling	the use of gradients to dephase magnetic moments – the opposite of rewinding.
GRASE	gradient echo and spin echo.
Gyro-magnetic ratio	the precessional frequency of an element at 1.0 T.

H

Hahn echoes	echoes formed when any two 90° RF pulses are used in steady state sequences.
Half Fourier	*see* **partial averaging**.
High velocity signal loss	increase in time of flight due to an increase in the velocity of flow.
Homogeneity	evenness of the magnetic field.
Hybrid sequences	combination of fast spin echo and EPI sequences where a series of gradient echoes are interspersed with spin echoes – in this way susceptibility artefacts are reduced.
Hydrogen	the most abundant atom in the body.

I

ISMRM	International Society for Magnetic Resonance in Medicine.
IMRSER	Institute for Magnetic Resonance Safety, Education, and Research.
Incoherent	*see* **out of phase**.
Inflow effect	another term for **entry slice phenomenon**.
Inhomogeneities	areas where the magnetic field strength is not exactly the same as the main field strength – magnetic field unevenness.
In phase	magnetic moments that are in the same place on the precessional path around B_0 at any given time.
Interleaving	a method of acquiring data from alternate slices and dividing the sequence into two acquisitions – no slice gap is required.
Intra-voxel dephasing	phase difference between flow and stationary nuclei in a voxel.
Intrinsic contrast parameters	those parameters that cannot be changed because they are inherent to the body's tissues.
Ions	atoms with an excess or deficit of electrons.
Isotopes	atoms with an odd mass number.
Isotropic	voxels that have the same dimension in all three planes.

J

J coupling	causes an increase in the T2 decay time of fat when multiple RF pulses are applied as in fast spin echo.

K

K space	an area in the array processor where data on spatial frequencies are stored.

L

Larmor frequency	*see* **precessional frequency**.
Longitudinal plane	the axis parallel to B_0.

M

Magnetic field gradient	field created by passing current through a gradient coil.
Magneto-hemodynamic effect	effect that causes elevation of the T wave of the ECG of the patient when placed in a magnetic field – this is due to the conductivity of blood.
Magnetic isocentre	the centre of the bore of the magnet in all planes.
Magnetic moment	denotes the direction of the north/south axis of a magnet and the amplitude of the magnetic field.
Magnetic susceptibility	ability of a substance to become magnetized.

Magnetization transfer contrast/coherence (MTC)	technique used to suppress background tissue and increase CNR.
Magnetism	a property of all matter that depends on the magnetic susceptibility of the atom.
Magnitude image	un-subtracted image combination of flow sensitized data.
Mass number	sum of neutrons and protons in the nucleus.
Maximum intensity projection (MIP)	technique that uses a ray passed through an imaging volume to assign signal intensity according to their proximity to the observer.
Molecules	where two or more atoms are arranged together.
MR active nuclei	nuclei that possess an odd mass number.
MR angiography (MRA)	method of visualizing vessels that contain flowing nuclei by producing a contrast between them and the stationary nuclei.
MR signal	the voltage induced in the receiver coil.
Multiple overlapping thin section angiography (MOTSA)	method combining a number of high resolution 3D acquisitions to produce an image that has good resolution and a large area of coverage.
Multi-shot	where K space is divided into segments and one segment is acquired per TR.
Multi-voxel	technique that acquires multiple voxels by encoding in K space in MR signal.

N

Net magnetization vector (NMV)	the magnetic vector produced as a result of the alignment of excess hydrogen nuclei with B_0.
Neutron	neutrally charged element in an atomic nucleus.
NEX	number of excitations (also known as **number of signal averages** or **acquisitions** depending on manufacturer), the number of times an echo is encoded with the same slope of phase encoding gradient.
Noise	frequencies that exist randomly in time and space.
Nucleons	particles in the nucleus.
Null point	the point at which there is no longitudinal magnetization in a tissue in an inversion recovery sequence.
Nyquist theorem	states that a frequency must be sampled at least twice in order to reproduce it reliably.

O

Ohm's law	basic law of electricity – voltage (V) = current (I) × resistance (R).
Outer lines	area of K space filled with the steepest phase encoding gradient slopes.
Out of phase	when magnetic moments are not in the same place on the precessional path.

P

Parallel imaging	a technique that uses multiple coils to fill segments of K space.
Partial averaging	filling only a proportion of K space with data and putting zeros in the remainder.
Partial echo imaging	sampling only part of the echo and extrapolating the remainder in K space.
Partially saturated	occurs when the NMV is flipped beyond 90° (91° to 179°).
Partial voluming	loss of spatial resolution when large voxels are used.
Passive shielding	shielding accomplished by surrounding the magnet with steel plates.

Passive shimming	uses metal discs/plates at installation to adjust for large changes in field homogeneity.
Pathology weighting	achieved in IR pulse sequence with a long TE–pathology appears bright even though the image is T1 weighted.
Permanent magnets	magnets that retain their magnetism.
Phase	the position of a magnetic moment on its precessional path at any given time.
Phase contrast angiography (PCMRA)	technique that generates vascular contrast using the phase difference between stationary and flowing spins.
Phase encoding	locating a signal according to its phase.
Phase image	subtracted image combination of flow sensitized data.
Phase wrap	aliasing along the phase encoding axis.
Polarity	the direction of a gradient, i.e. which end is greater than B_0 and which is lower than B_0. Depends on the direction of the current through the gradient coil.
Point resolved spectroscopy spin echo (PRESS)	single voxel technique in MRS.
Precession	the secondary spin of magnetic moments around B_0.
Precessional (Larmor) frequency	the speed of precession.
Precessional path	the circular pathway of magnetic moments as they precess around B_0.
Proton	positively charged element of an atomic nucleus.
Proton density	number of protons per unit volume of that tissue.
Proton density (PD) weighting	image that demonstrates the differences in the proton densities of the tissues.
Pseudo-frequency	frequency that is indirectly derived from a change of phase.
Pulse control unit	co-ordinates switching on and off the gradient and RF transmitter coils at appropriate times during the pulse sequence.

Q

Quenching	sudden loss of the superconductivity of the magnet coils so that the magnet becomes resistive.

R

Radioactivity	emission of energy caused by a deficit in the number of electrons compared with protons.
Radio frequency (RF)	low energy, low frequency electromagnetic radiation. Used to excite hydrogen nuclei in MRI.
Ramp sampling	where sampling data points are collected when the gradient rise time is almost complete – sampling occurs while the gradient is still reaching maximum amplitude, while the gradient is at maximum amplitude and as it begins to decline.
Readout gradient	the frequency encoding gradient.
Receive bandwidth	range of frequencies that are sampled during readout.
Recovery	growth of longitudinal magnetisation.
Rectangular FOV	also known as **asymmetric FOV** – uses a FOV in the phase direction that is different to that in the frequency direction of the image.
Reduction factor	the factor by which the scan time is reduced using parallel imaging. Equals the number of coils used.

Relaxation	process by which the NMV loses energy.
Relaxivity	the effect of a substance on relaxation rate.
Repetition time TR	time between each excitation pulses.
Residual transverse magnetization	transverse magnetisation left over from previous RF pulses in steady state conditions.
Resistive magnet	another term for solenoid magnet.
Respiratory compensation	uses mechanical motion of air in bellows to order K space filling and reduce respiratory motion artefact.
Respiratory gating/ triggering	gates the sequences to chest wall movements to reduce respiratory motion artefacts.
Rewinders	gradients that rephase.
RF amplifier	supplies power to the RF transmitter coils.
RF pulse	short burst of RF energy that excites nuclei into a high-energy stage.
RF spoiling	the use of digitized RF to transmit and receive at a certain phase.
RF transmitter coil	coil that transmits RF at the resonant frequency of hydrogen to excite nuclei and move them into a high energy state.
Rise time	the time it takes a gradient to switch on, achieve the required gradient slope, and switch off again.
R to R interval	time between each R wave in gated studies.
S	
Sampling rate or frequency	rate at which samples are taken during readout.
Sampling time	the time that the readout gradient is switched on for.
SAR	standardized absorption rate – a way of measuring the USA Food and Drug Administration limit for RF exposure.
SAT TR	time between each pre-saturation pulse.
Saturation	occurs when the NMV is flipped to a full 180°.
Sequential acquisition	acquisition where all the data from each slice is acquired before going on to the next.
Sensitivity encoding	*see* **parallel imaging**.
Shim coil	extra coils used to make the magnetic field as homogeneous as possible.
Shimming	process whereby the evenness of the magnetic field is optimized.
Signal	voltage induced in the receiver coil.
Signal to noise ratio (SNR)	ratio of signal relative to noise.
Single shot FSE (SS-FSE)	a fast spin echo sequence where all the lines of K space are acquired during a single TR period.
Single voxel	techniques that use three intersecting slices to locate a single voxel in MRS.
Slew rate	the strength of the gradient over distance.
Slice encoding	the separation of individual slice locations by phase in volume acquisitions.
Slice selection	selecting a slice using a gradient.
Solenoid electromagnet	magnet that uses current passed through coils of wire to generate a magnetic field.
Spatial encoding	encoding or locating signal in spatial three dimensions of the imaging volume.
Spatial modulation of magnetisation (SPAMM)	creates a saturation effect which produces a cross hatching of stripes on the image. These can be compared with moving anatomy to determine its function.

Spatial resolution	the ability to distinguish two points as separate.
Spin-down	the population of high energy hydrogen nuclei that align their magnetic moments anti-parallel to B_0.
Spin echo	echo produced as a result of a 180° rephasing pulse.
Spin echo–EPI (SE-EPI)	spin echo sequence with EPI readout.
Spin echo pulse sequence	one that uses a 180° rephasing pulse to generate an echo.
Spin lattice relaxation	process by which energy is given up to the surrounding lattice.
Spin-spin relaxation	process by which interactions between the magnetic fields of adjacent nuclei causes dephasing.
Spin-up	the population of low energy hydrogen nuclei that align their magnetic moments parallel to B_0.
Spoilers	gradients that dephase.
Steady state	condition where the TR is less than T1 and T2 relaxation times of the tissues.
Stimulated echoes	echoes formed when any two RF pulses are used in steady state sequences.
Stimulated Echo Acquisition Mode (STEAM)	single voxel technique in MRS.
Superconducting magnet	solenoid electromagnet that uses super-cooled coils of wire so that there is no inherent resistance in the system through which the current flows, and therefore the magnetism is generated without a driving voltage.

T

T1 enhancement agent	a contrast agent that shortens T1 relaxation in tissues that take up the agent.
T1 recovery	growth of longitudinal magnetization as a result of spin lattice relaxation.
T1 relaxation time	time taken for 63% of the longitudinal magnetization to recover.
T1 weighted image	image that demonstrates the differences in the T1 times of the tissues.
T2*	dephasing due to magnetic field inhomogeneities.
T2 enhancement agents	agents that shorten T2 relaxation times in tissues that take up the agent.
T2 decay	loss of transverse magnetization as a result of spin-spin relaxation.
T2 relaxation time	time taken for 63% of the transverse magnetization to decay.
T2 shine through	when lesions remain bright on a trace image in DWI.
T2 weighted image	image that demonstrates the differences in the T2 times of the tissues.
3D volumetric acquisition	acquisition where the whole imaging volume is excited so that the images can be viewed in any plane.
TAU	the time between the excitation pulse and the 180° rephasing pulse and the time between this and the echo. Sometimes used in STIR sequences as an alternative to the TI.
Thermal equilibrium	assumes patient's temperature is constant and therefore does not influence the thermal energy of hydrogen during the MR experiment.
Time intensity curve	curve produce in perfusion imaging to show perfusion kinetics of a tissue.
Time of flight	rate of flow in a given time – causes some flowing nuclei to receive one RF pulse only and therefore produce a signal void.
Time of flight MR angiography (TOF-MRA)	technique that generates vascular contrast by using the inflow effect.
Time to echo (TE)	*see* echo time.

Time from inversion (TI)	time from 180° inverting pulse to 90° excitation pulse in inversion recovery pulse sequences.
TR	*see* **repetition time.**
Trace image	image in DWI where abnormal tissue is brighter than normal tissue.
Transceiver	coil that both transmits RF and receives the MR signal.
Transmit bandwidth	range of frequencies transmitted in an RF pulse.
Transverse plane	the axis perpendicular to B_0.
Trigger delay	waiting period after each R wave – the time between the R wave and the beginning of data acquisition.
Trigger window	waiting period before each R wave in gated studies.
Truncation artefact	artefact caused by under-sampling so that edges of high and low signal are not properly mapped into the image.
Turbo factor	*see* **echo train length.**
2D volumetric acquisition	acquisition where a small amount of data is acquired from each slice before repeating the TR.
V	
Volume coil	coil that transmits and receives signal over a large volume of the patient.
Voxel volume	volume of tissue in the patient.
W	
Water saturation	technique that nulls signal from water by applying an RF pulse at the frequency of water to the imaging volume before slice excitation.
Window levels and settings	settings that control brightness and contrast in MR images.

Index